# Hairdressing
## the complete guide

# Hairdressing
## the complete guide

FIFTH EDITION

PETER CUTTING
RENIE ROSS

Longman

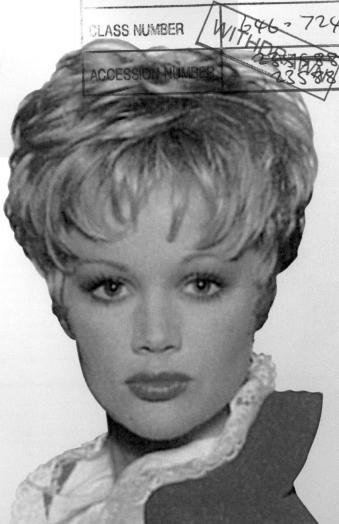

**Pearson Education Limited**
Edinburgh Gate
Harlow
Essex CM20 2JE
England

*and Associated Companies throughout the world*

*Visit us on the World Wide Web at*:
http://www.pearsonededuc.com

First published in Great Britain by Pitman Publishing as *Hairdressing: Theory, Science and Practice* 1988
Second edition 1991
Third edition published as *Hairdressing: The Complete Guide* 1994
Fourth edition 1996
Fifth edition 2000

**British Library Cataloguing in Publication Data**
A catalogue entry for this title is available from the British Library

ISBN 0-582-35798-5

10  9  8  7  6  5  4  3  2
06  05  04  03  02

Set by 30 in Stone Serif and Stone Sans
Printed in Singapore (MPM)

# Contents

# Level 3

# Acknowledgements

We would like to offer our personal thanks to the following:

- The Managing Director at Sabre Europe Ltd for his time an help in providing photographs
- Nicky Keane at Sabre Europe Ltd for her prompt response to photographic requests
- Thea Brunton at L'Oreal for her time and help in providing photographs
- Mr Mayhew at Goldwell for his prompt help and support in providing photographs
- Julie Greatorex at Clynol for providing photographs
- Peter West and his team for providing photographs
- Julian and all the hairdressing staff at the Plassey, Wrexham for their patience and help with additional photographs
- Trevor Sorbie for supplying the front cover photograph
- Mrs E Middleton and Barbara Eden for their help with proofreading
- Lisa Duncalf for her support and help with the basic skills element of level 1
- Nick Stephenson, Barabara Crowther and Jason Thomas for modelling
- The MCI for allowing us to quote freely from their standards and summaries
- The Hairdressing and Beauty Industry Authority for allowing us to use their standards
- Brett Gilbert at Pearson Education
  *and*
- Our families, who suffered long – again, again, and then again.

# Level 1

# 1

In this unit you will learn about:

- Shampooing and conditioning hair.
- Drying one-length, long hair.
- Working safely without wasting any products.
- Working efficiently, without wasting time.
- Caring for your client.

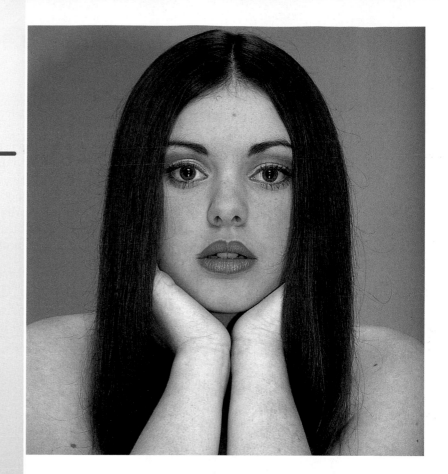

# Introduction to shampooing, conditioning and drying hair

## Shampooing and conditioning hair

### Shampooing hair

Shampooing is one of the most common treatments to be carried out in the salon. We shampoo the hair to clean it before other processes such as conditioning, blow-drying, setting, cutting or perming.

All trainees learn to shampoo hair very soon after starting work and it is always important to listen to the stylist's instructions *carefully* to prevent anything going wrong!

The shampoo and conditioner that the stylist chooses will depend on the type of hair the client has. This can be **greasy**, **normal** or **dry**. The stylist also has to decide whether the hair has been permed, coloured or bleached, and whether it has any dandruff. To choose the right product for the hair, both you and the stylist must:

- **Look** at the hair and scalp very carefully
- **Listen** to what the client tells you
- **Feel** both the hair and the scalp

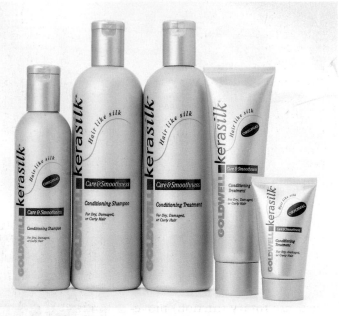

Goldwell/Michael Balfre Photography

### Massage

Massage has been used on the body for thousands of years. It is very relaxing and relieves tension through touch. It also helps the blood flow, which makes the skin and hair healthier.

Massage can be done manually with the hands or mechanically with a vibro machine. Shampoo massage is almost always a hand massage using the pads of the fingers. All clients feel better when their scalp is massaged well, so always ask them if your massage is thorough enough for them.

**POINTS TO REMEMBER**

The three main types of massage used when shampooing and conditioning are shown in Fig. 1.1.1; they are:

- **Effleurage** – a stroking movement to spread shampoo and conditioner through hair and relax the client. Used in shampooing and conditioning.
- **Rotary** (friction) – circular massage movements to clean the hair and scalp. It encourages blood flow to the hair roots; this feeds the hair and makes it healthy. Used in shampooing.
- **Petrissage** – deep, kneading movements. Slower than rotary massage but also encourages blood flow and makes hair healthy. Used in conditioning.

### How to shampoo

1. Cover the client's clothing with a gown and towel. This will help to stop their clothing getting wet or splashed.

2. Check with the stylist which shampoo to use and check for any other instructions. For example, is a conditioner needed? Does the client want a front or back wash?

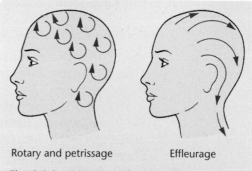

Rotary and petrissage          Effleurage

**Fig. 1.1.1**   Direction of rotary, petrissage and effleurage massage movements

3. Carefully comb through the client's hair to make sure it is free from tangles and check for any infectious or contagious conditions.

4. Make sure the client is comfortable, then turn on the water tap. Thoroughly wet all the hair.

5. Apply the correct shampoo for the type of hair. Use **effleurage** (stroking), massage movements to spread the shampoo through the hair.

6. Next use **rotary** (friction) movements from hairline to crown across the whole head (Fig. 1.1.2). This will loosen the dirt and grease from the hair.

7. Rinse the hair in plenty of warm water then apply more shampoo.

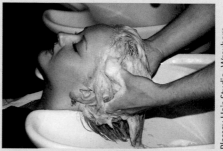

Plassey Hair Studio, Wrexham

**Fig. 1.1.2**   Rotary massage movements during shampooing

8. Use effleurage and rotary massage movements again, then rinse the hair until it 'squeaks' under your fingers. If the hair doesn't squeak or it still feels greasy, then shampoo the hair again.

9. Towel-dry the hair then comb it through carefully.

10. Wrap the client's hair in a towel to stop water dripping onto the face and to keep the head warm until the stylist is ready.

## Conditioning hair

Keeping hair in good condition is very important. Healthy hair is shiny and easier to manage while hair in poor condition will look dull, dry and lifeless and be difficult to handle.

Hair conditioning is carried out on wet hair after shampooing. Not all hair needs to be conditioned, so you must check with the stylist before you put any conditioner on the hair. Using conditioner when it is not needed can make the hair limp, greasy or even too flyaway.

### Conditioners and why we use them

Most conditioners contain oils and waxes as well as various other ingredients. There are many different types of conditioner and each manufacturer will have their own range.

You need to make sure that you know the range used in your salon. Reading the manufacturer's instructions will help you to understand the type of hair the different conditioning products should be used on. Always follow the instructions that are given to you, either from the stylist or the manufacturer.

When used correctly, conditioners will make the hair:

- Shiny
- Easy to brush or comb
- Soft and with more body
- Pliable and more elastic

### The surface condition method

1. Shampoo the hair as you have been told by the stylist.

2. After the final rinse, pour the correct amount of conditioner into the palm of your hand. Put both hands together, then stroke the conditioner on the hair.

3. Use **effleurage** stroking movements to smooth the conditioner through the hair and relax the client.

4. Next use a **petrissage** (kneading massage) movement to stimulate the scalp. A petrissage massage is a rotating movement like the rotary massage used in shampooing, but it tends to be slower (see Unit 2.2).

5. Unless the stylist tells you otherwise, rinse the conditioner from the hair with plenty of warm water.

6. Check that all the conditioner has been removed from the hair. Any conditioner left in the hair could make it limp, flyaway or greasy.

7. Towel-dry the hair then comb it back from the face.
8. Wrap the hair in a towel. Fill in a record card with details of the products you have used.

### What to do after conditioning

- Clean the work area.
- Tell the stylist that the client is ready.
- Place used towels in the correct place.
- Clean and sterilise any equipment such as dressing combs and brushes.
- Check the shampoo and conditioner left in the containers; top up or tell the stylist if the stock levels are low.

### Hot oil conditioning treatments

Hot oil treatments are used for dry scalp conditions. Olive, coconut or almond oils are the most common. The treatment will make the scalp more supple and help to stop dry dandruff.

Although you will not usually be expected to carry out the treatment, you may be asked to remove the oil from the client's hair after the treatment. Oil will not mix with water, therefore it cannot be rinsed from the hair like an ordinary conditioner. Instead you must:

- Put a soapless shampoo straight on to the oil; don't wet the hair first.
- Massage *very* thoroughly until the oil looks like white cream.
- Rinse the hair thoroughly.
- Repeat the process until all the oil has been removed. If any oil is left in the hair, it will be left looking very greasy.

## Making good use of resources

- Do not use too much shampoo or conditioner. Check with the stylist how much is needed.
- Turn off the water tap when not rinsing hair. It is expensive and also harmful to the environment to keep water running.
- Long hair will need more shampoo, conditioner and rinsing than short hair.
- Always tell the stylist if you are running out of shampoo or conditioner. This means that the stock level is getting too low.
- Be organised: plan and think about what you have to do and the best way to do it. Remember, 'time is money'!

## Health and safety points

- Make sure that the client's clothing is *completely* covered by the gown and towel.
- Give the client a face cloth to protect their eyes if carrying out a front wash.

- Do not put hot water onto the head before testing it is the right heat. Do this by running it over the back of your hand or wrist before letting it go onto the client's scalp.
- Do not let shampoo or conditioner go into the client's eyes.
- If any water spills on the floor, mop it up immediately.
- Use the right shampoo and conditioner for the type of hair – always ask the stylist.
- Check that there are no infectious or contagious hair or scalp conditions *before* you begin to shampoo. Tell the stylist immediately if you think there may be. (See Unit 2.2.)
- Always keep your work area clean and tidy. This helps to prevent germs spreading (cross infection) through the salon.
- Be aware of the **Control of Substances Hazardous to Health** (COSHH) Regulations and the proper use of shampoos and conditioners.

## Client care

- Tuck all towels well into the nape of the neck.
- Apply thick, creamy shampoo or conditioner to the palm of the hand and runny, liquid shampoo to the back of the hand before putting on the client's head. This stops it feeling too cold!
- Always ask the client if the water is the right heat for *their* scalp – some clients can stand the water hotter than others.
- Keep checking that the client is comfortable.

**SAFETY TIPS**

- Never shampoo if a client has an infectious or contagious condition – it could spread the condition to other clients and also the staff.
- Always use barrier cream on your hands before shampooing or hand cream after shampooing. When used a lot, shampoos can dry out the skin and cause inflammation (dermatitis).
- Make sure that the right amount of shampoo is used and at the right strength. Otherwise it may cause skin problems to both you and the client.
- Make sure that all shampoo and conditioner is rinsed from the hair. Any left in the hair could cause skin irritation or dandruff.
- Look at the scalp to see if the client has any cuts or breakage in the skin. If they have, tell the stylist.
- When you use a shampoo or surface conditioner, always follow the instructions from the stylist or the manufacturer.

## Blow-drying hair

Blow-drying is a way of drying the hair using brushes instead of rollers. It is done on damp hair and the size of brush that you use will depend on how the client wants the finished hairstyle to look.

The smaller the brush, the smaller the curl. Longer, one-length hair usually needs a larger round brush, otherwise there may be too much curl for you to cope with when you have to dress the hair out. What happens to the hair when it is blow-dried is covered in Unit 2.3.

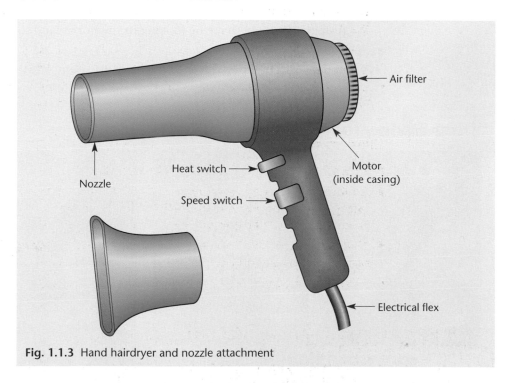

**Fig. 1.1.3** Hand hairdryer and nozzle attachment

## How to blow-dry longer, one-length hair

1. Ask the stylist which products and equipment to use. Set them out on your work area.

2. Ask the stylist and client how the finished blow-dry needs to look. Make sure that you understand what you are supposed to be doing, and how to do it, before you start.

3. Check that the client is well protected with a gown and towel. Check that the electrical equipment is safe to use.

4. Shampoo the hair and towel-dry so it is not too wet.

5. Apply any blow-styling products evenly on to the hair. Comb through thoroughly then comb the hair in the direction of the finished style.

6. Section the hair if necessary. Some salons do not use sectioning but prefer to dry the roots in the opposite direction to the style; this is to give it lift. Ask the stylist which method they would like you to use.

7. If you have dried the root area, section off the top hair.

8. Begin blow-drying at the nape of the neck. Wrap fine sections of hair around the brush and angle the jet of air away from the scalp to prevent burning. The air jet should help to blow the hair around the brush.

9. Make sure the section is dry by allowing it to cool slightly or give it a short blast with a cool air jet. Dry the next section in the same way.

10. Work up the head to the front. But remember, hair will dry in the position it's placed. Always work in the direction of the finished dressing.

11. When the whole head is finished, make sure the hair is completely dry. Check the finished shape by looking in the mirror and look at the style from all angles.

12. Tell the stylist you have finished the blow-dry. Complete a client record card.

## Blow-drying long, one-length hair

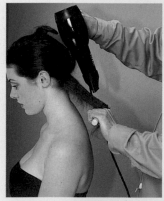
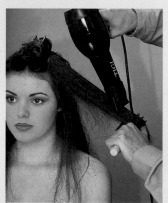
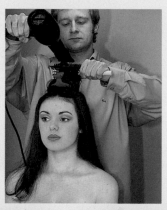
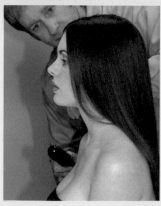
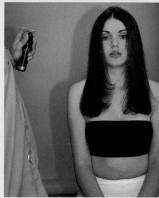
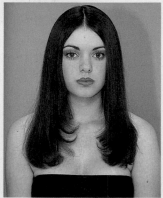

Hair has been blast-dried at the roots and sectioned off. The blow-dry begins at the nape working up towards the top of the head. When the back hair is dry, continue with the sides and finally the top sections. The hairdryer always points away from the scalp to prevent burning. When the hair is completely dry, brush into style then spray with a light hairspray; remembering to stand the correct distance away.

**What to do after blow-drying**

● Show the stylist the finished blow-dry.

● Advise the client on how to keep the style looking good.

● Place any used towels and gowns in the correct place.

● Clean and sterilise the brushes and combs you have used.

● Clean the work area.

**After-care advice for the client**

● Show the client how to brush the hair into its style.

● Tell the client that steam or damp weather will make their style drop (or go curly if they have naturally curly hair).

● Remind the client to cover their hair with a cap if they go swimming or have a shower.

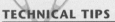

**TECHNICAL TIPS**

● If hair is not completely dry the style will not last.

● Using blow-styling products will help the style last longer.

● Moisture from steam or the atmosphere will make the style 'drop'.

● Wind up the hand dryer wires from handle to nozzle. This helps to prevent them from cracking and breaking.

## Making good use of resources

● Plan what you are going to do and the best way of doing it before you begin.

● Work methodically; it will save you time in the long run.

● Do not use too much blow-styling lotion or mousse; it will leave the hair 'sticky' and cost the salon money.

● If the hair is long or thick, dry it off until just damp before you start the blowdry.

● Drying the hair at the roots, in the opposite direction, will give it extra lift and save time.

● Don't use faulty tools or equipment; it is unsafe and the blow-dry will take longer.

● Keep your work area clean and tidy; it will help you to work more efficiently.

## Health and safety points

● Protect the client's clothing with a gown and towel.

● Using too high a heat may burn the client's hair.

● Blow-drying too close to the client's skin may cause burns as well as discomfort.

- Make sure that all electrical equipment is safe to use. Check for any frayed wires or loose parts.
- Wires from the hand dryer that trail on the floor could cause an accident.
- Stooping while you are blow-drying could give you future back problems.
- Not following the stylist's instructions could create problems for you, the client and the salon.
- Always tell the stylist immediately if you run into any difficulties – they are there to help you.

## Client care

- Adjust the client's position while you are blow-drying so that they are always seated comfortably.
- Set the dryer at a comfortable heat and direct the airflow on to the hair, not the skin.
- All tools and equipment must be clean and sterilised.
- Follow the stylist's instructions.

### Things to do

1. Make out record cards for the clients that you have shampooed and conditioned. Ask the stylist and clients to write comments about how well you carried out the task. Keep them in your portfolio as supplementary evidence of your competence in this unit.

2. Look at your salon's COSHH risk assessment book – ask the stylist if you don't understand how it works. Make a list of the COSHH requirements for shampoos and conditioners.

3. Write to (or ring) your local Health and Safety department. Ask them to send you information on COSHH.

4. Read about the infectious and contagious conditions that a hairdresser needs to know about (see Unit 2.2). Make a list of the conditions with a brief explanation of what they look like.

5. Make a list of all the tools and equipment used for blow-drying in your salon. Briefly describe what each one is used for and how you could prevent damage to each.

6. Read about the Electricity at Work Regulations 1992. Make a list of *your* responsibilities under these regulations.

7. Find out about as many types of hairbrushes as you can. Collect pictures of them. Cut out the pictures and stick them on a plain piece of paper. Underneath each picture write down the type of hair and the style you would use them for. You can find the information in trade magazines, retail or wholesale outlets.

## What do you know?

- Name the **three** main hair types.
- Why should the client's head be wrapped in a towel after shampooing?
- Name the **three** massage movements.
- Which **two** massage movements are used when shampooing hair?
- List **six** health and safety points when shampooing and conditioning hair.
- What do the letters **COSHH** stand for?

- Why should the jet of air from the dryer be angled away from the scalp?
- What should you do when you have finished blow-drying the whole head?
- List **five** health and safety points when blow-drying hair.
- List **three** after-care advice points that you could give the client to help their style stay in longer.

### Keywords

You need to know what these words mean. Go back through the unit or look up what they mean in the glossary at the back of the book. You can also ask a tutor or senior staff member.

**advise, contagious, effleurage, elastic, faulty, infectious, manufacturer, methodically, petrissage, pliable, process, product, resources, rotary, sterilise, stock level**

# Unit

# 2

In this unit you will learn about:

- Neutralising perms.
- Neutralising relaxers.
- Applying temporary colour to the hair.
- Removing colouring and lightening products from the hair.
- Working safely and effectively without wasting either your time or products.

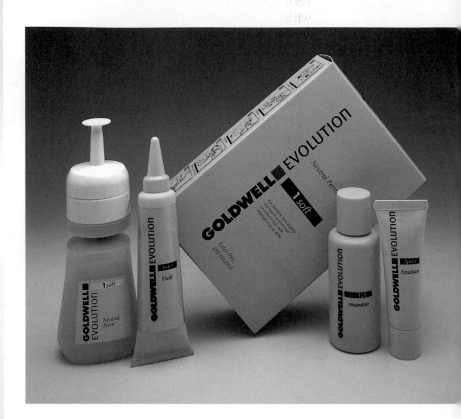

# Introduction to perming, relaxing and colouring hair

## Neutralising hair

Perms make straight hair curlier. Neutralising is part of the perming process and without it the perms would not work.

**POINTS TO REMEMBER**

- Neutralising fixes hair into the new shape created by the perm rods or straightener. Because neutralising is such an important part of the perming and relaxing process, *always* make sure that you understand the manufacturer's instructions or the instructions given to you by the stylist before you start.
- **Hydrogen peroxide** and **sodium bromate** are the chemicals used in neutralisers for perms.

### How to neutralise a perm

1. The stylist will tell you when the perm is ready. Check with the stylist which neutraliser to use. Usually this will be the same brand name as the perm and specially produced to go with it. Make sure that you understand the instructions given to you.

2. Protect the client's skin and clothing with enough clean, dry towels and a face cloth if necessary. Protect yourself with an apron and rubber gloves or barrier cream on your hands.

3. Collect the tools and products you will need. Place them so they will not spill or cause an obstruction or accident.

4. Rinse the hair thoroughly in warm water, usually for five minutes, or according to the instructions given to you.

5. After rinsing remove most of the water by blotting thoroughly with cotton wool. Leaving the hair too wet will dilute the neutraliser and stop it working properly. To check that enough water has been removed, press the palm of the hand onto the perm rods – if the palm is wet when it is removed from the head then the hair needs reblotting.

6. Wrap a strip of cotton wool round the hairline to protect the face and neck.

7. Apply the neutraliser to the wound rods starting at the nape of the neck, working forwards. Make sure that each perm rod is completely covered.

8. Leave for the correct length of time, usually five minutes.

9. Carefully take away the cotton wool and remove the rods and endpapers from the hair. Do this very gently without pulling the hair. The hair must *not* be stretched as the curl is still not fixed at this stage.

10. Apply fresh neutraliser to the ends of the hair. Remember not to drag the hair as this could loosen the curl. Check that all the hair has been covered with the neutraliser. Leave for five minutes or as instructed by the stylist or manufacturer.

11. Rinse the hair thoroughly in warm water and apply a conditioner if instructed.

12. Gently comb through the hair. Wrap the head in a towel. Complete the client's record card.

# Neutralising

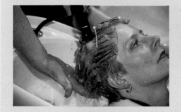
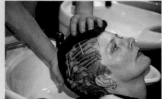
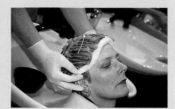
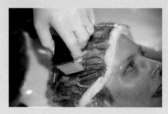
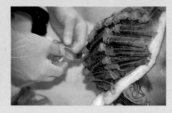
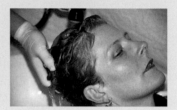

The hair is thoroughly rinsed in warm water then blotted almost dry. Cotton wool is placed around the hairline to protect the client's skin and eyes. Wear rubber gloves to protect your hands then apply the neutraliser. Leave the neutraliser for the correct length of time before *carefully* removing the rods and applying more neutraliser to the ends of the hair. Finally, make sure all the neutraliser is rinsed from the hair before applying any conditioner.

## TECHNICAL TIPS

Look at the perms used in your salon. What types are there? Do they have special conditioners or moisturisers to use on them afterwards If they don't, use an **acidic** conditioner or one specially for permed hair. These conditioners close the cuticle scales on the outside of the hair – this makes the hair look shiny.

## How to neutralise for curly perming Afro-Caribbean hair

### First neutralise the curl rearranger

The curl rearranger is used without any perm rods as the hair is combed straight instead. The stylist will tell you when the hair is ready for this first neutralising stage. Remember that the hair will now be fragile and you must be very careful not to rub or tangle it in any way else you could damage it.

1. Ask the stylist for advice on the length of time you should rinse the hair.

2. Seat the client at a backwash basin and make sure that they are well protected with gown and towel. Some salons also use a protective face cloth for the client's eyes.

3. Rinse the hair thoroughly in warm water for the correct length of time (usually five minutes). If the hair is not rinsed thoroughly, some of the curl rearranger will be left in the hair and this could damage it. Set a timer to make sure that the hair is rinsed long enough – the time always seems longer than it is!

4. When you have finished rinsing, blot the hair thoroughly, to remove the excess water. If the hair is left too wet, the water will dilute the perm lotion used in the next stage and the perm may not take.

5. Gently comb through the hair; it is still in a fragile state and rough handling could damage it. Place a clean towel around the client's neck.

6. Make sure the client is seated comfortably then tell the stylist you have finished. The hair will now be wound on perm rods by the stylist before the next neutralising stage.

**Then neutralise the curl booster**

This is the second stage of the neutralising process. The hair will have been rewound on perm rods by the stylist and left to develop until the hair has just the right amount of curl for the client. It is important to neutralise the hair immediately the stylist tells you to, or the hair may become overprocessed and damaged.

1. Ask the stylist which neutralising product to use. Always use the correct product or the perm may not take.

2. Seat the client comfortably and make sure that they are well protected as before.

3. Rinse the hair, making sure that each perm rod is well rinsed. If any rods are missed the finished curl may be uneven. Set the timer for the correct length of time (usually five to ten minutes).

4. When rinsing is completed, blot the hair thoroughly with a clean towel or cotton wool.

5. Place a clean towel around the client's shoulders and tuck well down at the neck. Place strips of cotton wool around the hairline to stop the neutraliser running onto the skin and face.

6. Apply the correct neutraliser very carefully to each perm rod; if you miss any the perm will not take evenly. Push the neutraliser well into the wound hair – it has a lot of layers to soak through! Leave the neutraliser to develop; the stylist will usually tell you how long but if you are unsure then check the manufacturer's instructions.

7. When developed, carefully remove the perm rods, making sure not to pull or drag the hair as this will alter the curl. Apply fresh neutraliser gently to the ends of the hair. Do not pull or stretch the hair, treat it very carefully or you could spoil the curl. Leave it to develop for the correct length of time, usually five minutes, but check with the stylist or the manufacturer's instructions.

8. Rinse all the neutraliser from the hair very thoroughly using lots of warm water.

9. Condition or moisturise the hair as directed by the stylist. Towel-dry the hair, taking care not to rub or tangle it, then comb through gently.

10. Place a clean towel around the client's shoulders. Wrap the head in a towel and complete a client record card.

**POINTS TO REMEMBER**

- The hair is not fixed in its new shape until it is dry, so it must be treated carefully at all times while you are neutralising.
- If the neutralising is not carried out correctly, all the hard work of the stylist will be undone. This is very bad publicity for the salon and clients will not want to come back.

**TECHNICAL TIPS**

- Long hair will need more rinsing and blotting than shorter hair. Rather than blotting you may be asked to use a dryer for a few minutes on the client's hair.
- You will need to use more neutraliser on long hair.
- The ends of long hair may be dry after a chemical process. Using a deep, penetrating conditioner on these ends will help to keep the hair shiny.
- Take extra care when combing through long hair after neutralising. It is often porous and fragile and the curl could be easily loosened.

## Possible problems

- If all traces of perm lotion are not rinsed from the hair, the neutraliser will not be able to work properly. Because hair is wrapped in an end paper, then perhaps many times round the perm rod, you need lots of rinsing to make sure the water reaches inside the hair.
- Not blotting the hair enough after rinsing. If the hair is left too wet, the water will dilute the neutraliser and stop it working.
- Not rinsing all the neutraliser out of the hair. Neutraliser left in the hair could make the colour lighten and cause breakage of the hair through internal damage.
- Not pushing the neutraliser well down onto the perm rods. Some hair may be missed and not fixed, making it straighter where it has been missed.
- Pulling, dragging or stretching the hair while it is still wet will loosen the finished curl.
- Letting the neutraliser run onto the client's skin may cause irritation of the skin.
- Not organising products and equipment safely. This could cause spillage and wastage, or an obstruction to other staff. It may also be a safety hazard.

## Health and safety points

- Always make sure the client's skin and clothing are well protected before you begin.
- Make sure you understand and follow the manufacturer's or stylist's instructions.
- Mop up any spillage immediately to stop any harmful effects. Wet floors can be dangerous.
- Test the heat of the water on the back of your hand before rinsing the hair.
- Don't let any neutraliser go in the client's eyes. If this happens, rinse immediately with lots of water. Tell the stylist what has happened.
- Letting neutraliser run onto the face or neck could irritate the skin.
- Use the correct products. The lotions you are using may be very strong and using the wrong one could harm the hair or burn the skin.
- Be aware of the **Control of Substances Hazardous to Health** (COSHH) Regulations and how to use neutralisers safely.

**SAFETY TIPS**

Neutralisers contain harsh chemicals, so it is important to:

- Wear protective gloves to avoid skin contact.
- Use hairline cotton wool strip on the client to prevent product running onto the client's skin.
- Check for cuts and abrasions on the client's scalp.

## Neutralising relaxers (straighteners)

Relaxing products are very strong and work on the hair in a different way to perming products. They are also neutralised in a different way. The chemicals used to relax or straighten the hair can burn the skin. They can also *dissolve* the hair if they are not used correctly! *Always* follow the stylist's or manufacturer's instructions *very carefully*.

**SAFETY TIPS**

The relaxer will burn *your* skin too. Always wear rubber gloves and do not touch the relaxer cream without them.

## How to neutralise hair after relaxing

1.  Check with the stylist which products to use and how. Collect all your equipment and the correct products. Always refer to the manufacturer's instructions if you are unsure or have forgotten what to do.

2.  Take the client to a back-wash station. Make sure that the client is well protected with towels tucked well down at the nape and that the client is seated comfortably.

3.  Wear protective rubber gloves. Rinse the hair thoroughly with plenty of warm water. Use the force of the water to remove the relaxer and handle the hair as little as possible. Make sure that *all* the relaxer has been removed.

4.  Apply the correct acidic neutralising shampoo to neutralise the alkalinity of the relaxer. Use gentle stroking massage movement; do not rub the hair or scalp as the scalp may be tender and the hair is in a fragile state.

5.  Rinse the neutralising shampoo from the hair then repeat the process. The stylist or technician will tell you how many shampoos will be needed. Always follow their instructions carefully.

6.  Apply a reconditioning or moisturising agent and leave for the correct time. Remove from the hair by rinsing thoroughly.

7.  Blot the hair gently to remove the excess water; do not rub the hair. Place clean towels around the client. Tell the stylist you have finished.

8.  Clean the workstation and clear away equipment. Fill in a record of what you have done, as directed by the stylist.

## Possible problems

- Letting the relaxer go in the client's eye. This could blind the client, so be extra careful when rinsing the hair. Rinse the eye with lots of water and tell the stylist *immediately*. The client may need medical aid.

- Not wearing protective rubber gloves. The relaxer will burn the skin, including yours!

- Not rinsing the relaxer from the hair thoroughly. Relaxers will carry on working if not removed and will break the hair.

- Rubbing the hair and scalp. This could cause skin irritation and hair breakage.

- Using the wrong product. Always use the neutralising shampoo produced for the type of relaxer used otherwise the hair may be damaged.

- Not protecting the client's clothing. If the products damage the client's clothing, the client can legally claim new ones from the salon.

- Not reading the manufacturer's instructions. If you do not follow instructions correctly, you could cause a great deal of damage to the client's hair and also the image of the salon.

### What can go wrong

*Problem*
Curl drops out completely by the next shampoo.
*Cause*
- Not rinsing hair thoroughly for the correct length of time.
- Not applying neutraliser correctly.
- Not leaving neutraliser on hair long enough.
- Neutraliser is off; it may be old stock, or the neutraliser bottle may have been stored incorrectly.

*Problem*
Curl looser than expected after neutralising.
*Cause*
- Leaving hair too wet before applying neutraliser.
- Too much tension when pulling out the perm rods.
- Dragging the hair when applying the neutraliser.
- Massaging the neutraliser into the hair and scalp.

*Problem*
Uneven curl at the next shampoo.
*Cause*
- Not rinsing hair evenly all over the head.
- Not applying the neutraliser evenly over the head.

*Problem*
Curly root hair, straight ends
*Cause*
- Not rinsing thoroughly for the required time.
- Not leaving neutraliser on hair long enough.
- Not applying neutraliser to the ends of the hair.

*Problem*
Skin irritation around hairline.
*Cause*
- Neutraliser being allowed to run onto hairline.
- No cotton wool placed around hairline.
- Cotton wool saturated in neutraliser and not removed.

## What to do after neutralising

- Clean the work area.
- Make sure the client is comfortable then tell the stylist the client is ready.
- Place any used towels and protective gowns in the correct place.
- Dispose of any cotton wool and leftover chemicals safely, in the correct place.
- Thoroughly rinse and dry any perm rods you have used, then put them away.

- Clean and sterilise any tools and equipment you have used
- Check the stock levels of any products you have used, cotton wool, endpapers and towels. Tell the stylist if any of the stock you have used is getting low so that it can be reordered

## Record cards

Always complete a client record card when you have finished neutralising. Check with the stylist that it has the following information:

- Date
- Hair condition
- Product used, including the strength of the lotions
- Size of rods (if used)
- Development time
- Any precautions necessary
- Finished result and any comments necessary
- Recommended after-care treatment

## After-care advice for the client

- Advise the client to use a special conditioner for permed or straightened hair each time they shampoo their hair.
- Remind the client to cover their hair if they go out in the rain or a damp atmosphere.
- Remind the client to keep their hair covered when out in the sun.
- Tell the client not to shampoo the hair for 48 hours after perming, curly perming or relaxing.

## Making good use of resources

- Only use as much cotton wool as you need to go round the hairline once.
- Turn off the water tap when not rinsing the hair.
- Never leave the top off the perm or neutraliser bottle.
- Use the correct amount of product. Too little could stop the perm or relaxer working, but too much is wasteful.
- Use the correct neutraliser. Using the wrong one could stop the perm or relaxer taking. The perm will drop or the straightened hair will go back to being curly. The hair will then have to be repermed or restraightened.
- Work in an orderly, neat manner – make good use of your time.
- Do not pour any leftover perm or neutraliser back into the bottle. It will be diluted and may not work on the next client.

## Temporary rinses

Temporary rinses add colour to the hair. They coat the outside of the hair and are shampooed out at the next shampoo. But if they are used after each shampoo, over a long time there will be a build-up of colour and this means they will not wash out as easily.

**POINTS TO REMEMBER**

Temporary rinses are made of pure colour and they do not offer the variety obtainable with permanent dyes. They will not lighten the hair and will not usually show if used on hair that is a darker colour than the rinse. Temporary rinses can have these effects:

- Make dull hair more shiny.
- Brighten up faded, tinted hair after perming or between permanent tints.
- Make brassy, blonde hair a softer colour (toning).
- Darken hair.
- 'Mingle in' grey hair.
- Give bright, unusual colours (pink, orange, green, etc.) when used on bleached or lightened hair.

### Temporary rinses for wet hair

- Coloured setting lotion
- Coloured blow-dry lotion
- Coloured mousse
- Coloured gel

### How to apply a temporary rinse

1. Shampoo and towel-dry the hair. If a conditioner is used, make sure it is thoroughly rinsed from the hair otherwise the rinse will not stick to the hair.
2. Ask the stylist which type and colour of temporary rinse to use.
3. Protect the client's clothing with a dark gown and towel. Do not use light towels as they will be stained by the colour rinse. Protect yourself with a tinting apron and full gown.
4. Apply the rinse straight from the bottle, tube or aerosol can. Apply to the roots of the hair then rub through the hair lengths. Comb through the hair with a wide-toothed comb to make sure the rinse coats the hair evenly.
5. When using coloured mousses or gels, apply them to the wide teeth of the comb before applying them to the hair. Again, comb through the hair thoroughly to make sure they coat the hair evenly.
6. Remove any staining to the skin with a piece of damp cotton wool.
7. Check with the client and stylist that they are pleased with the application. Complete a record card.

- Don't leave the hair too wet after shampooing – it could dilute the rinse.
- Always take care which rinse you use on white hair. An auburn rinse will turn white hair bright orangey red!

## What to do when you have applied the rinse

- Make sure the client is comfortable and tell the stylist that you have finished.
- Clean the work area and wipe over the surfaces.
- Place any used towels and gowns in the correct place.
- Put the used cotton wool and any waste products in a suitable bin.
- Rinse and sterilise the comb you have used.
- Check the stock levels of the products you have used; tell the stylist if the stock level is low so that it can be reordered.

## Possible problems

- If the rinse is not applied evenly, it will give a patchy result.
- If the hair is very porous, it may grab the colour on the porous parts. This will give a patchy result.
- Using too much rinse will leave the hair sticky. It could also drip and stain the skin or the client's clothing.
- Not towel-drying the hair enough could dilute the rinse.
- The rinse will not be visible if its colour is lighter than the client's hair colour. Not all shades of temporary colour are suitable on white hair. Always check with the stylist and read the manufacturer's instructions.
- The rinse will stain your hands and clothing if you do not wear rubber gloves and a tinting apron.
- The rinse may stain the client's skin and clothing if they are not protected well enough.
- If you do not follow the stylist's or manufacturer's instructions correctly, you could use rinse of the wrong type or colour, or you could apply it incorrectly. This will give a bad result which is very bad publicity for the salon and will stop the client and the stylist trusting you in future.

## Making good use of resources

- Use only as much rinse as you need – long or thick hair will need more than short or fine hair.
- Use the right product in the right way.

- Use a dark towel and gown on the client – the rinse will stain light towels and gowns.
- Work methodically so that you do not waste time.
- Follow any instructions carefully so that you do not have to reapply the rinse.

## Health and safety points

- Make sure that both you and the client are well protected.
- Do not use too much rinse; it could drip and stain the client's skin or clothing
- Do not let the rinse splash on the floor or work surfaces; someone may slip or become covered with the rinse.
- Use the correct type and colour of rinse in the correct way.
- Do not let the rinse run or splash into the client's, eyes, If this happens, rinse with plenty of water and tell the stylist immediately.
- Follow the stylist's or manufacturer's instructions carefully

## Removing colouring products from the hair

The method used to remove the colouring product from the hair will depend on the type of product that has been used. Different types of materials may also have been used by the stylist and these too will have to be removed from the hair. The most common materials that may have been used could include:

- Foil strips
- Plastic streaking cap
- Cling film
- Easi-meche or packets
- Pots

The colouring products you will be asked to remove from the hair are:

- Semi-permanent colours
- Permanent colours
- Lightening products

**SAFETY TIPS**

When you are taking colouring materials out of the hair, work from behind the client if possible; this will be help to prevent any product going onto the client's face or into their eyes.

## How to remove colouring materials from the hair

1. Seat the client at the washbasin. Make sure that they are well protected.
2. Keep the client sitting upright. Starting at the back and neck area, gently slide any foilstrips, easi-meche, pots, cling film or other similar materials out from the hair.
3. Work up and forwards towards the front of the head.
4. If a plastic streaking cap has been used, rinse the product from the hair then apply a small amount of conditioner before taking off the cap.
5. The hair is now ready for the next stage of removal.
6. Put all the waste materials in a suitable bin.

**POINTS TO REMEMBER**

- **Temporary colour** – washes out at the first shampoo.
- **Semi-permanent colour** – lasts for 6 to 8 shampoos.
- **Permanent colour** – will not shampoo out; it has to grow out.
- **Lightening colour** – has to grow out.

## How to remove semi-permanent and permanent colours

The same method is normally used for removing both semi-permanent and permanent colours. However, some semi-permanent colours contain shampoo. If they do contain shampoo, you will not have to use any extra shampoo after rinsing.

Always check with the stylist and the manufacturer's instructions to find out which type of semi-permanent colour has been used before you begin.

1. Make sure the client is well protected with dark towels and gown. Some salons also give the client a face cloth to protect their eyes.
2. Protect yourself with a tinting apron and rubber gloves.
3. Check with the stylist on the products they want you to use.
4. Put a small amount of warm water onto the hair.
5. Massage well to loosen (emulsify) the colour.
6. Rinse thoroughly until the water runs clear.
7. Apply shampoo if needed – check with the stylist.

**TECHNICAL TIPS**

Colour will last longer if you use a shampoo and conditioner specially formulated for coloured hair. If you do not have these specialised products use a shampoo and conditioner for dry hair. Lightening products and permanent colours can have a drying effect on the hair.

## How to remove lightening products

1. Make sure that you and the client are well protected. Ask the stylist which products they want you to use.
2. Check that the client is comfortable. If the hair has been lightened (high-lighted) using materials such as foil, easi-meche or a cap, make sure they have all been taken out.
3. Rinse all the lightening colour and/or bleach thoroughly from the hair.
4. Shampoo the hair with a suitable shampoo, then rinse again thoroughly.
5. Apply conditioner as instructed by the stylist. Massage gently then rinse thoroughly.
6. Gently towel-dry the hair. Wrap the head in a clean towel.

## What to do after removing colouring products

- Make sure the client is comfortable then tell the stylist they are ready.
- Clean the work area and surfaces.
- Place any used towels and gowns in the correct place.
- Put any used and unwanted materials and products in a suitable bin.
- Clean and sterilise any tools and equipment you have used.
- Check the stock levels of the materials and products that have been used. Tell the stylist if any of them are getting low so that they can be reordered.

**POINTS TO REMEMBER**

Hair can be lightened with either bleach or permanent colouring, but these techniques tend to dry it more than just normal colouring. If these products have been used on the scalp they may leave it feeling tender.

If the hair has been lightened a lot, then the lightened hair may be fragile and more porous. This means you need to take extra care not to rub it too hard when you are massaging and you need to treat it gently when combing it through.

## Possible problems

- Longer or thicker hair will need more colouring product. This will require more rinsing and more conditioner (if used).
- Massaging the scalp and hair too much when they are sensitive. This could make the scalp sore and the hair may tangle or break.
- Not removing all the products from the hair. This could make the scalp red and itchy. Leaving conditioner or shampoo in the hair will irritate the scalp and leave the hair dull.
- Using the wrong shampoo and/or conditioner for the hair type or colouring products used. This could leave the hair in poor condition.
- Using too much conditioner. This could leave the hair greasy and lank instead of shiny.
- Water too hot or too cold when rinsing. Too hot and it may burn the client's scalp, too cold and it will be very uncomfortable.

- The colouring products may stain and irritate your skin or the client's skin if they are not properly protected.
- Not following the stylist's or manufacturer's instructions could cause hair damage and a loss of reputation for the salon.

## Health and safety points

- Make sure the client is well protected. Use a face cloth for extra protection to the eyes.
- Make sure you are well protected with a tinting apron and rubber gloves.
- Try to remove colouring products at a back wash. You are less likely to get products in the client's eyes when you are rinsing the hair.
- Check the temperature of the water on the back of your hand before you rinse the hair.
- Put used and unwanted materials and products in the right place. Dispose of them safely.
- Use the correct shampoo and conditioner on the client's hair.
- Don't let any of the products go in the client's eyes. If they do, rinse with plenty of water then tell the stylist immediately.
- Don't let any products or water spill on the floor, over the client or over the working surface. If this happens, mop it up immediately.
- Follow the stylist's or manufacturer's instructions carefully.

## Things to do

1. Find out the COSHH Regulations for perming (or relaxing if it is carried out in the salon). Make a list of *your* responsibilities. Try to think of when the products could be harmful to either you or the client. Make a list of these possible harmful effects and how you could avoid them.

2. Look at the possible problems on neutralising. Explain how you would avoid each of these problems.

3. Organise a file to record the different types of neutralisers you have used. Write a brief description of how each was used, the instructions you were given and any health and safety notes. Collect the manufacturer's information leaflets for these neutralisers and keep them in your file with your written notes.

4. Keep a copy of the record cards for the clients whose hair you have neutralised. Collect and keep with them any written comments made by the client, stylist or your tutor. Put them in your portfolio as evidence of what you have done.

5. Look through recent trade magazines. Cut out any advertisements for new colouring products and techniques. Keep the information in a file to help you follow trends colouring products and techniques.

6. Keep a log of each different type of colour removal you have carried out. Take a copy of the client's record card and any written comments made by the client and stylist about how well you carried out the task. You can use this information in your portfolio of evidence.

7. Make a list of the different types of temporary rinses used in your salon. Write about the good and bad aspects of each type and say which type of hair is the most suitable for each.

8. Read through the possible problems when applying a temporary rinse. Write about how you could avoid these problems.

9. Make a list of the people who work in your salon. Next to their name write about what they do. Include who you would go to if you had a problem and what the salon procedure would be.

10. Find out which temporary rinses are used in your salon. List each shade and the colour of hair it would suit.

## What do you know?

- Why must you always make sure you understand and carry out any instructions correctly?

- How would you protect the client's **clothing** when neutralising?

- How would you protect the client's **skin** when neutralising?

- How can you check that enough water has been removed after rinsing perm lotion from the hair?

- Why is it important never to drag or pull the hair while you are neutralising it?

- Give **five** ways of making good use of resources.

- What action do you need to take if neutraliser went into the client's eyes?

- Explain why the neutralising process is so important.

- What would happen if some of the neutraliser was left in the hair?

- List **six** things you should do when you have finished neutralising the hair.

- List **four** materials that you may have to remove from the hair before rinsing off the colouring products.

- Describe in detail how you would remove a plastic streaking cap from the head.

- How long will a **semi-permanent** colour last?

- What word is used to describe when we add water to the tint to loosen the colour?

- What product can be used to lighten hair as well as a permanent colour?

- List **five** ways you can make good use of the resources for removing colour from the hair.

- Why do you need to tell the stylist if stock levels are getting low?

- List **nine** health and safety points you need to think about when removing colour.

- Why should you not massage the hair and scalp too hard when it has been coloured?

- What would you do if some of the product were accidentally splashed in the client's eyes? Who would you go to for help?

**Keywords**

You need to know what these words mean. Go back through the unit or look up what they mean in the glossary at the back of the book or in the NVQ Occupational Standards. You can also ask a tutor or senior staff member.

barrier, description, dilute, dissolve, hazardous, methodically, mingle in, neutraliser, obstruction, orderly, penetrating, porous, sensitive, spillage, sterilise, substances, temporary

In this unit you will learn about:

- Looking after clients and other visitors.
- Taking messages and seeing to enquiries.
- Asking questions.
- Answering the telephone.
- Making salon appointments.

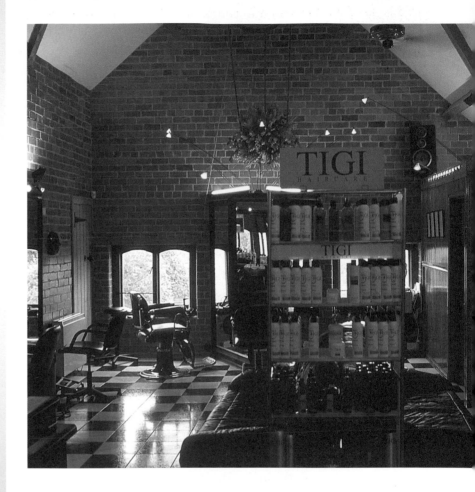

# Introduction to salon reception

## Salon reception

The salon reception is usually the first area of the salon that the client sees and comes into contact with. Working on reception and learning how to behave correctly with clients is very important.

**POINTS TO REMEMBER**

**First impressions count** – if the client does not like what they see or how they are treated they will go somewhere else.

Hairdressing is what is known as a **service industry**. This means that hairdressers give a service to their clients. A client does not have to come to your salon – they will only come if the service is good and they are made to feel special. To give a good service the salon must be:

- **Professional** – treating the client with respect and giving a high standard of work.
- **Safe** – tools, equipment and the actual building should be safe. All staff should make sure their work takes into account the health and safety of the client.
- **Pleasant and relaxing** – every salon visit should be enjoyable for the client. This will make them want to come back again.

### Reception duties

You must take these duties very seriously as they can win or lose clients for the salon. Reception duties include:

- Dealing with visitors
- Dealing with clients (expected and unexpected)
- Dealing with enquiries
- Answering the telephone
- Taking messages
- Making appointments

#### Dealing with visitors

Many types of people visit the salon, but not all of them want to make an appointment. Visitors include sales representatives, trades people (e.g. window cleaner) and training coordinators. No matter who the visitor is or what they want, they must always be greeted and attended to as soon as they come into the salon. Remember that everyone who enters the salon could be a future client. Follow these steps:

- *Smile* then ask if you can be of help.
- Find out the person's name and the purpose of their visit.

- If you cannot help them yourself, excuse yourself then find a more senior member of staff to deal with the visitor.
- If the visitor has to wait, make sure they are comfortable and offer them a drink or magazine.

### Dealing with clients

It is important to let all clients know, by what you say and how you act, that you are genuinely pleased to see them and you wish to be as helpful as possible. One way to do this is to make sure they are not ignored. Welcome them (by name if possible) and attend to them as soon as they walk into the salon.

- *Smile*, then ask if you can be of help.
- Check the client's name. If they have an appointment, mark it off in the appointment book.
- Help the client with their coat; hang it in a suitable place. Your salon may expect you to put a gown on the client when you have taken their coat, so make sure you follow the salon's procedures.
- Seat the client in the waiting area. Tell the stylist that their client has arrived and say which service they are having.
- If the client has to wait, offer them a drink and place some magazines near by.
- If it is a regular client, take out their record card ready for the stylist. You may not have to do this if the salon has a computer system. Follow the salon's procedures.

If the client doesn't have an appointment, you will need to ask them what service they need and when. If you are unable to book the appointment, or there is a problem, then you must excuse yourself to the client and ask a more senior staff member for help.

**POINTS TO REMEMBER**

Reception is all about **communicating** with people. We have to communicate with clients in a way that makes them feel special and welcome. We can communicate with someone in three ways:

- **Verbal** – speaking to people; this is the way that most of us think we communicate.
- **Written** – taking messages and booking appointments.
- **Non-verbal** – how we treat people, our general manner towards them. Using gestures like smiling, shrugging the shoulders or pulling a face will send unspoken messages to other people. Make sure that your unspoken messages are good ones.

### Dealing with enquiries

The general public will sometimes want information instead of booking an appointment. Here are some of the things you may be asked about:

- **Price list** – this should be displayed on the wall in the reception area, where it can be seen. Salons sometimes provide a smaller, printed leaflet for the client to take away.

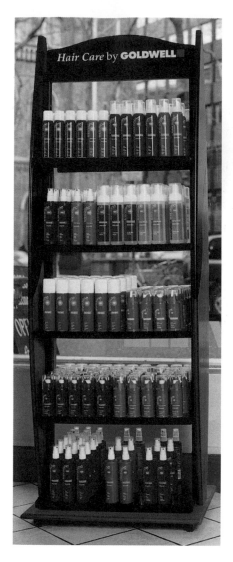

- **Information on salon services** – the services offered by the salon can be found on the price list. Sometimes the salon will have a publicity leaflet that gives a short description of each one and what it does. Even if it does not, you must know what services the salon offers and be able to give some information on them.

- **Information on hours** – you need to know the opening hours of the salon and the working hours of each stylist, otherwise you could make mistakes when booking appointments.

- **Information on products** – the product should be clearly marked with the price. You should also have a good understanding of what each product is and what it does. Read all the information given to the salon by the manufacturer; this will help you to answer questions.

- **Sales and employment** – you will not be expected to deal with sales and employment enquiries, but you must know who to pass them on to.

### Asking questions

Two main types of question can be asked in the salon:

- **Closed questions** – will give you one-word answers.
- **Open questions** – help you to find out more about the client.

Always try to ask open questions if possible. They will help you to get a much fuller answer from the client. Look at the example below. Mr Neale's answer will be yes or no but Mrs Duncalf will have to say much more than one word. You will therefore find out much more about Mrs Duncalf than Mr Neale!

**TECHNICAL TIPS**

When dealing with visitors or clients face-to-face remember that your body language should tell clients they are important and welcome in the salon. Smiling and eye contact are good ways of doing this!

*Closed:*    Would you like a conditioner on your hair, Mr Neale?

*Open:*    How do you usually have your hair styled, Mrs Duncalf?

### Answering the telephone

The telephone is one of the most common ways that a client communicates with the salon. The client cannot see you when you answer the telephone, they can only hear your voice. If you sound offhand and rude, the client will not want to visit the salon, which is very bad for business.

Always answer the telephone in a clear, polite voice. *Smile*; even though the client can't actually see you, your smile will come through your voice. You will also look good to any other clients who may be watching. Remember:

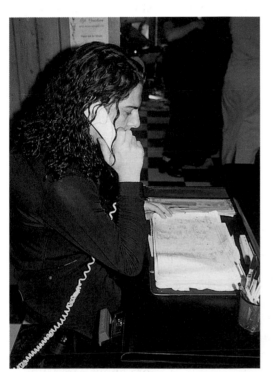

Dealing with telephone enquiries

- Answer the telephone within three rings if possible.
- Give the name of the salon, your own name and ask how you may help.
- Listen carefully to what the caller is saying.
- When a client makes an appointment or leaves a message, always repeat the details back to them to make sure that you and the client have understood correctly.
- If the client has made an appointment, let them know that you are looking forward to seeing them.

| What not to say | What to say instead |
| --- | --- |
| Mornin' | Good morning |
| Hiya | Hello |
| Dunno | No |
| Yeah | Yes |
| Okay | All right Fine |
| Ta | Thank you |
| Seez ya | Goodbye Look forward to seeing you soon |

### Emergency calls

Emergency telephone calls are free of charge at any time of day or night. No matter where you are, ring 999 or 112 and this will connect you to whichever of these emergency services you need: police, fire or ambulance.

When the telephone is answered, you will be asked which you require. You then need to:

- Tell the operator very clearly which service you need.
- Give your telephone number, the address and any easy directions.
- Listen carefully to the operator; you will be guided through questions.
- Answer the questions you are asked as clearly and fully as possible.
- Replace the telephone receiver when you have finished the call.

**POINTS TO REMEMBER**

When you are making an emergency telephone call:

- Try to stay calm.
- Speak slowly and clearly.
- Give as much information as you can.
- Replace the receiver when you have finished.

### Taking messages

Always **write down** a spoken (verbal) message (Fig. 1.3.1). If you don't, you may not remember exactly what has been said. Writing down the message will also act as a **reminder** to pass it on later. You may have to fold the message in two if it is private. Put the person's name on the outside and mark it 'urgent' if it needs to be dealt with quickly. Include these details when you write down a message:

- Date and time
- Name of the person giving the message
- Name of the person taking the message (your name)
- Exactly what the message is

---

## TELEPHONE MESSAGE

For the attention of: *Janet*

*Please phone Mrs Butterworth (0207 935 0121) about her appointment tomorrow.*

Message received by: *Karen*

Date: *24 May*      Time: *11.20 am*

---

**Fig. 1.3.1**   Written telephone message

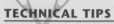

**TECHNICAL TIPS**

When you have written down a message, always repeat it back to the caller to make sure that you have got it exactly right. Getting the message wrong can be as bad as no message at all.

**POINTS TO REMEMBER**

Forgetting to give a message or getting a message wrong could have terrible consequences for the salon or whoever the message was for. Think how you would feel if someone forgot to give you an important message.

### Making appointments

Booking appointments correctly is very important. Not booking an appointment carefully can lead to all sorts of problems in a busy salon. It can waste the time of both the stylist and the client, making them irritable and cross. Before being able to book any appointments you will need to have a good understanding of the salon's **appointment system**. If you have any doubts when you are booking an appointment, always ask a more senior member of staff. Find out before you go on reception:

- Which days of the week each member of staff works.
- The hours each day that each staff member works.
- Any days during the week that the salon is closed.
- Which members of staff specialise in any particular area, e.g. perming or tinting.
- Any abbreviations used in the appointment book.
- The timings for each service and treatment that the salon carries out.

**TECHNICAL TIPS**

- Always book appointments in pencil so they can be easily rubbed out if the client has to cancel.
- If the time or date that a client wants is not available, offer the nearest alternative; never say no.

Here are some abbreviations that your salon **may** use. Not all salons use exactly the same abbreviations, so you need to learn the ones for your salon.

- S/S – shampoo and set
- B/D – blow-dry
- P/W – permanent wave
- Tint – permanent colour
- Semi – semi-permanent colour
- H/L – highlights
- Cond – conditioning treatment

**TECHNICAL TIPS**

If possible, check with the client's chosen stylist that the appointment is all right. Remember that making a mistake can make the salon:

- Look disorganised
- Seem unprofessional
- Lose money

### Confidentiality

Clients will often tell stylists or other staff members things that are personal and confidential. If this happens to you, you must keep it confidential; don't tell anyone else about it and **don't gossip**. If you do it will get back to the client and you will lose their custom; you might even lose your job.

Arrangements to do with work such as wages, tips, appraisals, one-to-one discussions, private disagreements or supervisory sessions are all confidential and should not be discussed with anyone else.

If a client tells you that they, or anyone in their family, has a contagious or infectious condition, you must tell your supervisor or manager immediately and in private. Although this information is also confidential, it could affect the health of other clients and needs to be dealt with by a senior staff member.

## Possible problems

### Answering the telephone

- Telephone cannot be answered within three rings. When you do answer, apologise for the wait before giving your name and the name of the salon.
- You are busy with another client. Excuse yourself to the client then answer the telephone. It can be very off-putting if the telephone keeps ringing.
- The caller wishes to speak to another member of staff. Ask who is calling then ask them to hold while you get the person they need.
- You have to leave the caller. Ask them to hold for a moment, excuse yourself and apologise. Do not keep them waiting too long.
- You mishear what the caller has said. Ask the caller to repeat their request.

### Scheduling appointments

If mistakes happen when an appointment is booked, it can make the salon look unprofessional or disorganised and it could be very costly. Here are some possible mistakes:

- Client booked with the wrong stylist.
- Client booked for the wrong service.
- Client booked at the wrong time.
- Two clients booked at the same time with the same stylist.
- Not enough time scheduled for the service the client wants.
- Overbooking a stylist, so they get behind and clients have to wait.

## Things to do

1. Make a list of the services and treatments carried out in your salon. Keep this information safe in your file for future reference. Next to each service and treatment, write down how long it takes and how much it costs.

2. Collect a copy of the different messages you have taken in the salon (not confidential messages). Put them in your portfolio as part of your evidence for this unit.

3. Draw up a memo pad which could be used in the salon. Read through the section on taking messages in this unit to find out what headings you will need. Make sure the headings will give you all the information for a complete memo.

4. Write out a step-by-step guide on what your salon expects you to say when you answer the telephone. Keep it for future reference or put it in your portfolio as part of your evidence for this unit.

5. Read the following case study then answer the questions.

   You answer a telephone call from a client who wishes to speak to the salon owner about a perm she has had at the salon. The salon owner will not be in the salon until the following day. The client will not speak to any other member of staff about her problem.

   (a) Explain what you think you should do.
   (b) Write down your salon's procedure for summarising an important telephone conversation. Remember to include any important points.

## What do you know?

- What are the **three** ways you can communicate with someone?
- What is meant by non-verbal communication?
- List **five** things that people may ask you about.
- Why is it important to smile at the client even when you are talking on the telephone?
- Give **five** possible problems when answering the telephone.

- What does **confidential** mean?
- Name the two types of question. Give your own example of each.
- What **four** main things should you remember when making an emergency telephone call?
- Why is it important to book appointments correctly?
- List **six** possible problems when booking appointments.

### Keywords

You need to know what these words mean. Go back through the unit or look up what they mean in a dictionary or in the glossary at the back of the book.  You may also find the meaning of some of the words in the NVQ Occupational Standards, or you can also ask a tutor or senior staff member.

**abbreviations, appraisals, confidentiality, contagious, coordinators, impressions, irritable, operator, reminder, service, urgent**

# 4

In this unit you will learn about:

- The reason why it is important to look after clients.
- How to communicate in the best possible way with clients and the people you work with.
- When to involve other people working in the salon in client care.
- Why it is important to be careful with information about clients.

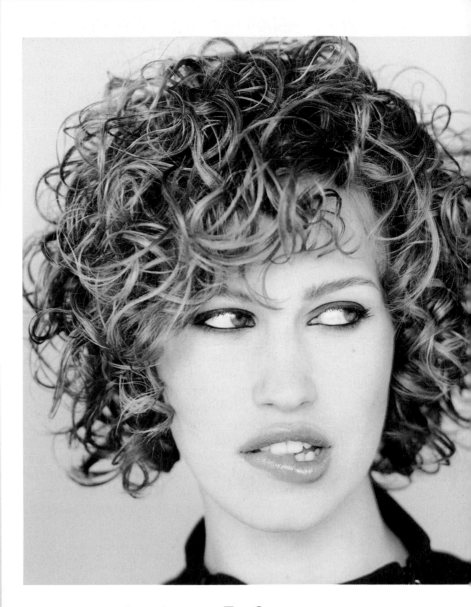

# Working together

## Looking after clients

Client care involves making sure that clients feel **comfortable** and **satisfied** with the services and the way they have been treated. Why is this important? A salon is a business and it cannot keep going without clients. Client care is very important for two reasons:

- It determines whether clients come back to the salon.
- It affects what clients tell other people about the salon.

# Activity

Make a list of the things that are important in producing a feel-good experience in a salon. Try to do this from the client's viewpoint.

A client's experience of a salon starts with their first contact, often by phone. This is covered in Unit 1.3. When a person comes into the salon they like to be greeted in a friendly manner. They also like to feel looked after or valued. But there is a point though where this can be a bit too intense; if the salon appears to be trying too hard, many clients begin to feel uncomfortable.

Try to develop an awareness of client comfort. Look around and think, 'Are they alright?' You can tell by facial expression and body posture. Are the clients relaxed and being looked after?

If they are carrying things, if they have a coat or other outer clothing, ask if you can help them with this. Take care of their personal belongings. Put them where they will be safe. If not sure, *ask* other salon staff.

We will now look at the main aspects of client care in more detail.

## Communication

Effective working relationships are very important in the salon, both for client satisfaction and so that you can make a worthwhile contribution to the salon team. A key factor in forming and keeping a relationship with someone is **communication**.

Communication is the passing of information from one person to another. Most people think of this as spoken (verbal) communication but body language (non-verbal) communication is also involved. We show our interest, attitude and how we feel by non-verbal communication and this is often more important than what is actually said.

### Who are the clients?

The clients are the customers of the salon. They may be:

- Known clients who have used salon services before.
- New, unknown clients.

Any of these clients may have some kind of disability and may require special consideration. Clients can also be difficult and it is important to tell your supervisor if you have any difficulties.

## Verbal communication

The verbal communication with a client is very important. All members of staff should be pleasant, polite and helpful at all times. Remember that the client is entitled to the best possible service.

## Good communication

There is an old saying about treating others as you would like to be treated yourself. This means putting yourself into the other's place and listening carefully to them. It also includes being reasonable and polite to them. Here are some points:

- If someone asks you to help, respond positively.
- If you need help, ask for it politely even if you feel pressurised.
- Try to be clear and accurate in what you say. People respond positively to this. Think about what you need to say before saying it. Clear and precise messages get you what you want.
- Make sure you show the appropriate non-verbal signals. You show your feelings in this way. Be interested, keen to find out, positive. As you listen to someone, show that you *are* listening.

## Non-verbal communication

Non-verbal communication can be just as expressive as speaking. Postures, distances and the way in which we hold our bodies are all ways in which we express ourselves. Indeed, many psychologists believe that a person's non-verbal behaviour can have more bearing on communicating feelings and attitudes than their words. Thus, the client must always be treated in a pleasant and polite manner not only verbally but also by the body language that is used. There are four main areas to consider.

### Distance

Everyone requires their own space. Touching and moving too near to the client can make them feel uncomfortable as usually only intimate relationships are allowed such close contact.

### Facial expression

An expressionless face which lacks emotion will appear cold and hard. However, too much emotion can make the person appear neurotic! When working in the salon, try to maintain a positive facial expression, e.g. smiling, so that the client feels they are in a pleasant, happy environment.

### Body posture

Body posture is believed by psychologists to provide clues as to what people really think or feel. Lounging around the salon in a slovenly manner does not create a businesslike impression and will make the client question your professionalism and therefore your practical ability even if this is unfounded.

### Eye contact

Eye contact with the client is extremely important as it is believed to be the basis of trust. Looking elsewhere when talking to the client will not only make them feel uncomfortable but will also make them doubt your sincerity.

## How to manage a difficult client

Everybody encounters a difficult client at some time. It is not an easy situation to be in, but make sure you stay calm and polite. There is no point in getting involved in an argument. If necessary, explain carefully and calmly that you are going to get your supervisor involved and will only be a moment. Often other people will be alerted by the client's actions and behaviour, but make sure you ask for assistance.

# Activity

Draw two posters; one on how to look after salon clients and the other on how not to. Which ones are about communication?

Ask an experienced member of the salon team to role-play a difficult client; see how you handle the situation. Swap roles and try it again. Discuss what happened in the two role plays.

## When to seek help

A lot of communication with clients involves confidence, good training and practice. There will almost certainly be times when you need help. How will you know when this is? If this is after some problem with a client then it is too late. If in doubt, ask your supervisor for help.

Many trainees are reluctant to ask a supervisor. But remember there is a balance between asking for help too often and not often enough. The best rule is to err on the side of caution. If in doubt of any kind, ask for help.

As your experience grows, this help will be needed less and less.

**POINTS TO REMEMBER**

There are five aspects to dealing with clients:

- Be courteous.
- Be clear and precise.
- Offer help and assistance.
- Have good body language.
- Clarify any uncertainties.

## Confidential information

A key factor in any successful salon operation is communication which encourages trust both between client and salon staff and also between the staff. Just as a client trusts a salon to deliver a good, safe and cost-effective service, they also expect information about themselves to be treated as confidential. Some of this information is deliberately gathered and entered onto record cards – either on paper or by computer. These records contain personal information yet can be accessed by other salon staff and by the clients themselves. It is therefore necessary to be careful what information is entered in these records. There have been cases of salon personnel putting insulting remarks about a client and then, at the next appointment, the client seeing it.

There is also the common situation of clients chatting to stylists and others about all sorts of things. They forget that other people may be listening, such as someone tidying up or helping with the treatment. It is very important not to pass any information on. The key thing to remember here is: See all, hear all, say nothing.

If situations arise where you feel uncomfortable about something you have overheard or you feel that others in the salon are breaking the rule of confidentiality, have a talk about this with your supervisor. Breaking rules of confidentiality is wrong and can lose the salon clients.

# Activity

What should a salon have as rules of confidentiality? Write down your ideas. Find out from a salon what their confidentiality rules are. How do your ideas compare with the actual example?

## Working as part of the salon team

Getting on well with who you work with depends on forming and keeping a good working relationship. When there is a good working relationship the salon atmosphere is positive; clients and staff feel this positive atmosphere and people react well to it. There is nothing worse than a salon where problems are unresolved and where obvious tension and bad feeling exist between the staff. Some people are easier to work with than others but there are some basic things everyone can do to help develop and keep effective working relationships.

**POINTS TO REMEMBER**

- You are an important member of the team.
- Treat people as you would want to be treated yourself.
- Help willingly.
- Be positive about assisting others in the salon.
- Don't be afraid to ask for help or for clarification about what you're to do.

### Who are your colleagues in the salon?

Colleagues are the people you work with These may be:

- Other trainees
- Stylists
- Supervisor and/or manager
- Other people who work in the salon, e.g.
  - receptionist
  - beauty therapist

### What to do if things go wrong

There will always be problems between people working in the salon. These problems may be small or large, short-term or long-term, easy to sort out or difficult. The most important thing is to discuss any difficulty. Try to resolve it with the person concerned. Stay calm and polite.

If you feel you cannot discuss the problem with those concerned, or if you have discussed it and the problem is still there, take the matter to your supervisor. Most things can be sorted out if there is a will to do so, and this is much easier if problems are resolved at an early stage.

## Activity

Design a poster about good working relationships in the salon team. Include some ideas on how to achieve them and explain the advantages for both people and business.

## Helping the salon team

Your activities (your role) in the salon will depend on a variety of things, e.g. the type and size of the salon and your own experience. The key thing is to be **clear** about your role and where the **limits** of your responsibilities lie. This should be set up with you and reviewed regularly. Communication is very important, both listening and talking, as is a positive attitude to your job and a willingness to learn.

## Activity

Make a list of what you do (your role) with the following:

- Clients
- Technical services in the salon
- General duties, e.g. the work area

## Preparing yourself to help the salon team

The main factors here are your **experience** and **knowledge**. Are you clear on when and how to help members of the team? If you are not sure, then **ask**. Clarify anything that you are not sure about.

# Activity

Write a short story about an incident where someone **does not** follow instructions properly. What happens?

The technical services offered by most salons will include:

- Perming (permanent waving)
- Colouring and bleaching
- Setting
- Cutting
- Blow-drying
- Dressing hair

Giving skilled assistance in carrying them out is very important as they are key salon operations and generate most of the salon's earnings. Here are the basics.

### Before

- Get the information needed.
- Gown the client.
- Choose the products, tools and equipment needed and arrange them in a suitable way.

### During

- Pass the products and tools to the stylist and remain on hand to help when needed.

### After

- When, the stylist has finished, make sure that the products, tools and equipment are taken away, cleaned and stored.
- Inform the stylist.

## Preparing for technical services

You need to know exactly what kind of service you will be assisting the stylist to carry out. Make sure you are very clear about this. You cannot prepare things properly if you are not clear. If you are not sure then ask. Get clarification from the stylist.

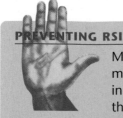

### PREVENTING RSI

Muscles do two kinds of work – dynamic and static. Dynamic work, when the muscles are moving, keeps the blood pumping through the muscle, carrying in oxygen and nutrients and carrying out waste products. Static work, when the muscles are holding a position, restricts the blood flow so the waste products accumulate and cause fatigue, which is felt as pain. This is why it is essential that muscles are kept as relaxed as possible and that you alternate holding tasks by using a variety of techniques. Experiment with different ways of doing each task.

### Before

Gowning is carried out before starting any hairdressing procedure. It protects the client's clothing from chemical spillage or cut hairs. Adequate care *must* be taken when gowning the client as any damage to the client's clothing will be the responsibility of the salon, and the client has every right to expect a replacement of any clothing which has been damaged through negligence.

You will then need to look at **record cards** and the **appointment book**. You will learn from experience which products, tools and equipment are needed and if particular stylists like doing things in a particular way. In addition, you will soon know how best to arrange things.

### During

Whatever the technical service, the stylist will operate much more effectively with efficient help. Make sure you are polite and courteous. If anything is not clear, ask for clarification. Be careful in passing things. Scissors can be stabbed into someone. Chemical products can be spilled.

### After

When the service has been completed, tell the stylist that the client is ready for the next stage (if applicable), throw away disposables, clean any tools and arrange them in a tidy way. Clean any equipment. Wipe down the working surfaces and chair.

Generally tidy up the dressing station and put things away.

### Safety

Health and safety issues are covered in detail in Unit 1.5, both in terms of what to look out for and what to do. But always remember these points:

● Do not allow products to get onto skin or into eyes.
● Take care to avoid cuts when using sharp instruments like scissors.
● Be aware of the chances of infection.
● Look out for problems with electrical equipment.

# Activity

Design a poster on each of these subjects. You could use Unit 1.5 to help you.

(a) Preventing infection

(b) Electrical safety

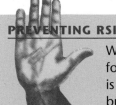

**PREVENTING RSI**

When a dispenser has a very small hole for the solution to come out, you are forced to squeeze hard, straining the wrist and forearm, especially if your wrist is bent in any direction. Make sure the hole is the right size for the proper flow but have it as large as possible so that you won't have to squeeze hard. Keep the bottles quite full for the same reason. Experiment with different hand grips as you apply solution and alternate them.

## Personal health

The standard of the salon depends on the standards of its staff members. Taking care of your personal health and appearance will not only help you to function more efficiently, it will also make you feel more alive and energetic. Eating a sensible diet which includes plenty of fresh vegetables and a balance of vitamins, minerals, fats and carbohydrates will prevent tiredness and give a glow to the skin.

### Posture

Hairdressing may not seem like it, but it is a physically tiring profession and most hairdressers have to stand on their feet for a long time. Tired, irritable staff cannot give their best service to the client, so it is very important that they stand and walk in ways that avoid too much strain on the body. Strain reduces your ability to work efficiently and sometimes it leads to long-term problems, e.g. back strain.

Posture is the correct placing of the body in relation to the feet. If it is correct, staff will be able to work more efficiently and feel less tired. The major points for a good posture are:

- **Stand upright** – stooping causes backache, tiredness and makes it difficult to breathe correctly.
- **Balance** – the weight of the body should be evenly distributed on both feet. This reduces strain on the back of the muscles.
- **Correct footwear** – shoes should be comfortable, attractive and heels should be a sensible height. Avoid open-toed shoes as hair fragments can enter under the skin and cause infection.

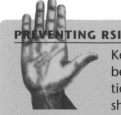

**PREVENTING RSI**

Keep your feet as cool and comfortable as possible. Open-toed shoes should be avoided because hair falls as it is being cut and may cause itching or infection. Many stylists develop calluses and corns so take precautions with your shoes – make sure they are lightweight, have padded insoles, are a perfect fit, and have a sensible heel height for balance and comfort. Make sure you won't slip in them – there will often be water on the floor. Tend to blisters promptly and use corn plasters as needed. A pumice stone will remove hard skin and lotion will keep the skin soft.

## Personal appearance

Personal cleanliness is important in any walk of life but particularly in the salon, where assistants very often work physically hard, in warm surroundings (which increases sweating), and in close proximity to the client.

Body odour and bad breath can be offensive to both the client and other members of staff, and steps should be taken to ensure personal freshness at all times. Here are a few basic guidelines which can be adapted to suit your needs:

● Bathe regularly and always use a deodorant when necessary – at least once a day.

● Regular brushing of teeth and correct diet help to prevent bad breath. It is also advisable to have a dental check-up every six months.

● Avoid eating foods with an unpleasant odour, such as onions or garlic. They may taste delicious when eaten but they are very unpleasant second-hand.

● Always look neat and well groomed. Hair should be kept clean and well cut and if possible it should be coloured and/or permed – this encourages the client to do likewise. Stylists with long hair should keep it off the face but in a fashionable style.

● Nails and hands should be well cared for. Where possible, use a hand cream at night before going to bed; this will help to counteract the drying effect of degreasing shampoos, styling aids, etc., and reduce the chances of developing dermatitis. Nails must be kept clean and of reasonable length to prevent scratching the client's scalp. Nail polish should be unchipped.

● Overalls or salon uniform must be spotlessly clean and fresh. Make use of tinting aprons to prevent staining when colouring or perming. Any clothes worn beneath the overall should not be allowed to show and woollen cardigans or jumpers should be avoided as they provide good conditions for skin bacteria to thrive. Cotton or a cotton/polyester overalls are durable, they are easy to launder and they do not increase perspiration. Nylon overalls do increase perspiration and can therefore be uncomfortable during busy periods.

- Avoid wearing excessive amounts of jewellery, particularly jangling bracelets; excessive jewellery is disconcerting to the client and it hinders efficiency. A watch or a ring can be worn, but it may be damaged by the chemicals used in the salon so it is not usually worth the risk.

## Non-metallic tools: care and maintenance

### Brushes

Brushes should be kept as clean and sterile as possible. When not in use they should be kept in a sterilising cabinet.

#### Method of cleaning

1. Comb any hair from the brush using a wide-toothed comb and remove any other loose particles from the bristles and base.
2. Fill a basin with lukewarm water and add a cleaning fluid (not too strong or it might damage the brush).
3. With the bristles pointing downwards, swish the brush about on top of the water. Do not immerse wooden brushes as the water will crack the protective varnish and split the wood.
4. Rinse carefully in clean water to which some disinfectant has been added.
5. Towel-dry the handle and base of the brush and pat the bristles on a towel to remove excess moisture.
6. Leave the brush to dry face downwards on a clean towel.
7. When dry, place in an ultraviolet disinfecting cabinet.

### Combs

Combs should be thoroughly cleaned regularly to prevent loose flakes of skin and other debris lodging between the teeth of the comb at the base. When not in use and after use on each client, combs should be kept completely submerged in an antiseptic solution of the correct strength or in the sterilising cabinet.

#### Method of cleaning

1. Brush combs with either a nail brush or a special comb brush to remove loose debris.
2. Fill a basin with lukewarm water and cleaning fluid, as for cleaning brushes.
3. Immerse combs for several minutes to loosen any grease or oil particles.
4. Scrub combs on each side individually with a nail brush.
5. Rinse in lukewarm water to which some disinfectant has been added.
6. Dry thoroughly and place in a sterilising cabinet or an antiseptic solution.

It is not always necessary to use disinfectant in the rinsing water if the brushes and combs are being placed immediately into the ultraviolet disinfecting cabinet.

## Metallic tools: care and maintenance

### Scissors

Scissors should be carefully looked after and always kept sharp. Remember the following points to make sure they are always in good working order:

1. Always dry scissors after use on wet hair.
2. Keep scissors away from strong chemicals, e.g. permanent wave solution and bleach.
3. Scissors should not be dropped as this can alter their balance and it could loosen the pivot or screw.
4. Each pair of scissors should be used by only one person. If the same pair of scissors is used by everybody, it blunts the blades very quickly.
5. Never use scissors for anything except cutting hair.
6. Scissors should only be sharpened by experts.
7. Sterilise scissors by wiping them carefully with spirit then placing them in the sterilising cabinet for the recommended time.
8. The pivots should be treated with lubricating oil from time to time to prevent stiffness.
9. Store away from dust as this is a source of possible infection.

### Razors: safety and open

Open razors must be kept sharp by **stropping** on a leather strop, or by **honing** on a special stone known as a hone. Safety razors must have the blades changed regularly to make sure the razor is always sharp.

- Always dry razors after use, otherwise the metal will rust.
- Keep razors away from permanent wave solution, bleach or any other strong chemicals.
- Wipe razors with spirit after use then place them in a sterilising cabinet for the recommended time.

## Clippers

Hand clippers and electric clippers are cleaned in the same way but electric clippers should also be checked for frayed wires, faulty plugs, etc.

### Method of cleaning

1. Remove all loose hairs with a tissue or piece of flannel.
2. Remove any grease with surgical spirit.
3. Lubricate joints with a lubricating oil.
4. Place in a sterilising cabinet for the recommended time.

## Styling irons and hot brushes

Remove any grease or stains with surgical spirit. Electrical styling irons and hot brushes should be checked for frayed wires and faulty plugs.

## Pressing combs

Rub the teeth of the comb with an emery board to remove any grease and stains then wipe over with surgical spirit. Check electrical pressing combs for frayed wires and faulty plugs.

**Summary of tools**

| Tools | Type | Use |
|---|---|---|
| Brushes | General-purpose<br>Styling<br>Neck | For dressing and everyday brushing of hair<br>When blow-drying the hair<br>To remove cut hair from face and neck |
| Combs | Tail comb<br>Dressing comb<br>Cutting comb<br>Setting comb<br>Afro comb | Sectioning, lifting, weaving, never disentangling<br>Disentangling and dressing the hair<br>More pliable than other combs, used when cutting<br>When setting and finger waving<br>To style and dress curly hair, e.g. Afro-Caribbean |
| Scissors | Plain straight edge<br>Very fine serrated edge<br>Wide-spaced serrated edge (aesculap) | For all cutting techniques<br>For all cutting except slither-cutting techniques<br>To thin hair, usually on dry hair only |
| Razors | Open<br><br>Safety razor | Used mainly in men's hairdressing to cut wet hair and in shaving<br>Same use as the open razor but has changeable guarded blade |
| Clippers | Hand (manual) and electric | In men's and ladies, hairdressing to cut hair close to scalp |
| Hot brush | | To temporarily curl dry hair |
| Styling irons | Electrically heated | To temporarily curl, straighten or crimp dry hair |
| Pressing combs/<br>straightening irons | Electrically heated and non-electrical | To straighten Afro-Caribbean or curly hair |

## Development within the job role

There are many things which influence job satisfaction. Most of them have been mentioned in this unit. They include relationships with and attitude towards clients and the salon team.

It is very important to believe that you make a valued contribution through your role in the salon. There is little or no satisfaction in working well below your capabilities or when far too much is being demanded of you. Both are frustrating, and feelings of being undervalued or held in too little regard are very damaging to the team's operation. Most people like to feel they are in an interesting, challenging (but not overwhelming) job and that a reasonable amount of trouble is taken by managers and supervisors to keep in touch with staff feelings and needs.

Good management includes reviewing salon staff's current levels of expertise and competence then setting up processes to develop them further. One way of doing this is to have a **staff appraisal** system. Although an appraisal may sound threatening it can be a very positive experience when carried out properly.

### Defining your job role

Is there a detailed description for your job in the salon, including duties, responsibilities and accountability? If yes, is it available today? Is it accurate? If no, why not? A list of what is expected of you should be central to your development review.

### Appraising your job role

Appraisal has two aspects: review and self-appraisal. Self-appraisal is where you look at your own strengths and weaknesses, you consider your own achievements and suggest where you may need to develop. Review is carried out by your supervisor. Appraisal should be:

- Positive.
- Identify strengths as well as weaknesses.
- Set realistic and attainable targets within a specified time period.
- Provide support, including development opportunities to help achieve the target.
- A regular, supportive occurrence in the salon's operation.

To conduct appraisals, it requires a list of **development activity targets** which can be discussed between you and your supervisor after a certain time has elapsed. This will deepen and broaden your skills and experience, and it will ultimately improve your career in hairdressing.

Appraisal can be informal or more formal, with a written record of the targets agreed and the timescale for achievement and review. The system is much better if a written record is kept.

Here is one possible way to operate an appraisal system:

1. Look at the job description and think about your role in the salon. Are there areas for development? What are your strengths and weaknesses?

2. Meet with the persons who will carry out the appraisal. Discuss the appraisal, agree what should be reviewed and talked about. This is called **setting the agenda.**

3. Carry out the appraisal of those items agreed in step 2.

4. Complete a written record of agreed targets, how they are to be achieved and by when. This is called the **development action plan**.

## Development activities

Several methods can be used to learn:

- **Watching** other people in the salon.
- **Asking** for help and guidance when you need it.
- **Training** in the salon or elsewhere.

Training may take place on a course or it may be on training nights. You should be given a reasonable time for your development and you should be given realistic targets to achieve. Nothing succeeds like success, and achieving realistic targets provides genuine encouragement to continue in a positive way.

### Things to do

1. Working in pairs or small groups discuss and write down:
   (a) Reasons why client care and consideration are important.
   (b) Some examples of good and bad practice. Explain why they are good or bad.
   (c) The difference between verbal and non-verbal communication.
   (d) Examples of non-verbal signals, both good and bad, which a client can receive.

2. Discuss how you should fill in your personal diary or logbook to cover this unit.

3. (a) Make a list of all the tools and equipment that are used in your placement and/or training salon.
   (b) Collect illustrations or photographs of a selection of each type of tool and equipment, including any extra or new equipment which may be available.
   (c) Cut out and mount the illustrations. Print a brief summary under the illustration giving the use of each.
   (d) Present your work neatly in the form of a portfolio.

4. Self-appraise yourself in your job role. Make a list of **strengths** and **weaknesses** then show this to someone whose opinion you would trust. Do they agree with your assessment?

5. Are there areas of the salon's activities that you would like to take part in? List these areas and discuss them with your supervisor.

## What do you know?

- What is meant by verbal and non-verbal communication?
- Why is customer care important?
- Explain the responsibilities of the people working in the salon.
- List the line of command in the salon.
- List the methods of verbal and non-verbal communication.

- Why is it important to have good working relationships with colleagues in the salon?
- Why is it important to follow instructions?
- What can happen if the rules of confidentiality are broken?
- List the opportunities by which staff in the salon can develop themselves in their jobs.

### Keywords

You need to know what these words mean. Go back through the unit or look up what they mean in the glossary at the back of the book (or ask a tutor or senior staff member).

**appointment, appraisal, colleagues, communication, confidential, courteous, development action plan, honing, hot brushes, hygiene, infection, non-verbal communication, pressing comb, record card, sterile, stropping, styling iron, technical service, valued**

In this unit you will learn about:

- Fire (and how to evacuate the salon).
- Accidents, emergencies and how to report them.

You will also cover the main health, safety and security factors important in the salon.

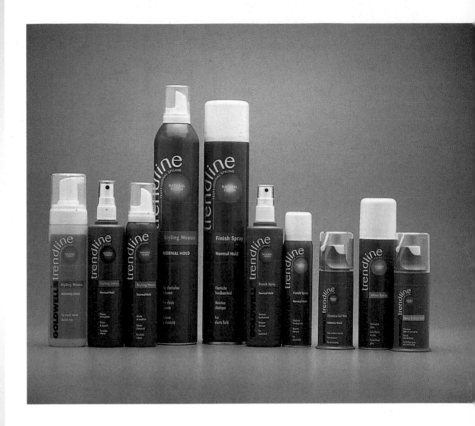

# Salon health and safety

## Dealing with accidents and emergencies

### What to do

- Stay *calm*.
- *Report* the event immediately to:
  - your supervisor
  - the first aider
- *Assist* if you are competent to do so.

## Activity

1. Find out who in you salon is responsible for:
   (a) Fire evacuation
   (b) First aid
2. Draw a plan of your salon. Using coloured arrows, indicate the ways in (access) and the ways out (egress).
3. Where is the fire assembly point?

## Fire and evacuation procedures

There are two main causes of fire in salons: smoking and electrical faults. Fires due to **smoking** can be caused by:

- Lighted cigarettes falling on to the floor, into seating, etc.
- Ashtrays with still smouldering cigarettes being thrown into rubbish bins.

There is also a risk of fire if people smoke near a client whose hair is being sprayed with lacquer. Never allow a client to smoke when using any kind of aerosol spray on their hair.

### Salon policy

A well-run salon will have as a matter of policy:

- Prominent signs indicating fire exits.
- Notices stating the evacuation procedure and the assembly point. Active encouragement of staff to report potential hazards, be they direct fire hazards or obstructions to speedy evacuation of the salon. Examples could be blocked staircases, entrance halls, salon equipment in front of fire doors.
- Familiarisation of new staff with fire and evacuation procedures and the location of emergency and fire-fighting equipment in the salon as part of new staff induction.
- Regular review of the policy to take into account new developments.

In addition, it is good practice to have a fire drill, a simulation of a real emergency, so that all staff know clearly what to do and any weaknesses in procedures are shown up.

## What to do

- Stay calm.
- Make sure everybody gets out of the salon and goes to the assembly point.
- Depending on the nature and extent of the fire, decide whether or not to tackle it, if in doubt, *do not* tackle it. Remember that aerosol spray cans and hydrogen peroxide containers will explode if sufficiently heated.
- Try to turn off the main electrical supply. If this is not possible (or you are uncertain), do not use water to try to put out the fire. Water is a good conductor of electricity and electricity flowing through it could deliver an **electric shock**. The salon should have at least one suitable fire extinguisher. Use it to put the fire out if it can be used without putting anyone at risk.

# Activity

Make a list of situations where the salon may need to be evacuated. What could happen if this were not properly organised?

## Salon hygiene

Hygiene is important in many industries but particularly in hairdressing when staff are dealing directly with the general public. Indeed, there is **legislation** on health and hygiene in the workplace, which means the salon is required by law to make sure it is a safe place for both clients and staff. It is a good idea to look at leaflets published about this, and they can be obtained through the local Environmental Health Department.

Each salon will have its own preferences and procedures for making sure that it is kept clean and tidy and that the tools and equipment are sterilised after use (Unit 1.4).

Everyone who works in a salon has a responsibility both to themselves and others to work in a healthy and safe manner. Much of good health and safety practice needs to be routine so that people in the salon are protected from the most likely hazards. Handwashing and sterilisation help to prevent cross-infection in the salon.

## Personal hygiene

Details of personal appearance and hygiene are given in Unit 1.4, p. 50. But here are three main points:

- Keep up a smart and businesslike appearance
- Look after your health.
- Wash your hands and sterilise equipment.

## Routine health and safety

Salon staff should be able to:

- Recognise potential or actual hazards.
- Prevent a hazard developing and/or rectify the problem.
- Use the system for reporting hazards.

Many salons have developed a set of health and safety procedures for staff to follow, based on government legislation such as:

- Health and Safety at Work Act 1974
- COSHH Regulations 1990
- Workplace (Health, Safety and Welfare) Regulations 1992
- Manual Handling Regulations 1992
- Personal Protective Equipment at Work Regulations 1992
- Provision and Use of Work Equipment Regulations 1992
- Electricity at Work Regulations 1992

### Health and Safety at Work Act 1974

The Health and Safety at Work Act 1974 puts a duty on all salon workers to act in a safe and responsible way. It also lists recommendations for **first-aid kits** and also requires that: a written record be kept of all accidents in an **accident record book**. This lists the sex, age and occupation of the victim, the nature of the accident and the date of first absence from work (if this applies).

### COSHH Regulations

The COSHH Regulations took effect from January 1990 and have been reinforced by the Health and Safety Framework Regulations of January 1993. They embody the important idea of **risk assessment**. This involves answering the following questions:

- **Tasks** – what do we do in the salon?
- **Hazards** – what are the hazards?
- **Risks** – how likely is a problem to arise?
- **Actions** – what appropriate precautions need to be taken?

In order to work this out, information is needed on the content of hairdressing products and what potential hazards these could be. This information has to be supplied by the manufacturer of the hairdressing product, using chemicals taken from a list of substances whose risk assessment has already been worked out.

## Other regulations

- **Workplace (Health, Safety and Welfare) Regulations 1992** – cover a range of hairdressing practices and the surroundings in which they take place.
- **Manual Handling Regulations 1992** – cover the reduction of risks due to lifting or touching objects. *Everyone* must do all they can to reduce these risks.
- **Personal Protection Equipment/Provision and Use of Work Equipment Regulations 1992** – cover training for use of equipment and require suitable protective equipment is to be supplied.
- **Electricity at Work Regulations 1992** – require electrical equipment to be kept in a safe condition and require regular safety testing.

## Local by-laws

- Local by-laws often involve registration of the salon with the local Environmental Health Department so that periodic checks by environmental health officers can be made.
- Local by-laws often overlap with other regulations in requiring adequate ventilation in toilet and washing facilities, general cleanliness, etc.

# Activity

Design a health and safety pamphlet to be given to new salon staff. Make sure it contains:

(a) The names of people who supervise first aid and salon evacuation
(b) A list of dos and don'ts.
(c) An explanation of why health and safety is everyone's responsibility.

# Potential hazards in the salon

Health and safety is about **recognising** the potential hazards in the salon to know which ones can be **rectified** easily and when and how to **report** their occurrence. This section concentrates on the major points only and it divides them into four categories.

## Physical injuries

### Scissors and razors

Scissors and razors are designed to be sharp. Scissors can cause nicks or puncture wounds if pushed in points first. Scissors should always be carried with points inwards and razors should never be carried open. Both scissors and razors should be cleaned by wiping them in a direction away from the body. Make sure scissors and razors are out of the reach of children in the salon.

### Tripping and falling

- Loose or broken floor coverings should be reported and repaired immediately.
- Trailing electric flexes are a trip hazard and tugged flexes can cause electrical faults. Tugging its flex can topple the attached appliance, perhaps injuring staff or clients.
- Beware of slippery surfaces; mop up any spillages immediately.
- Do not obstruct evacuation routes or access routes.

### Knocks

Knocks can be caused in a variety of ways, often as a result of another accident, e.g. someone collapsing after an electric shock. They can also be due to:

- Equipment collapsing onto a client, e.g. infrared octopus or steamers, when someone bumps into them or trips over the flex.
- Equipment being cleaned; there is a risk of pushing it over while cleaning it. Many salon dryers have strong springs in their stands and if the dryer is removed for cleaning and the spring released, the stand flies upwards with considerable force. This may strike someone cleaning the stand.

## Electricity

Many of the accidents that occur when using electricity are simply due to thoughtlessness, carelessness or downright bad practice. People can be at risk for two different reasons:

- **Overheating cables and apparatus** – this could cause a fire. Fit the correct fuse, plugs and fuse boxes. Arrange for regular and expert checks on plugs, cables and electrical equipment. It is important not to overload a circuit.
- **Electric shock** – this can happen when electricity flows through a person's body.

### Do

- Make sure plugs are wired correctly and have the correct fuse for the appliance.
- Have electrical equipment checked on a regular basis. All equipment checks and repairs and all changes to the electrical supply should be carried out by a competent electrician.
- Make sure that staff are trained to know what to do if a person receives an electric shock.

### Don't

- Handle electrical appliances with wet hands or allow water to splash onto appliances.
- Overload sockets or other circuits by running too many appliances from them.
- Fit a larger fuse into a fuse box or plug if it keeps blowing.
- Run flexes under floor coverings or place them where there is a chance of someone tripping over them.
- Pull a plug by tugging at its flex.

## Chemical

Hairdressing services often involve the use of chemicals on the hair and some of them are sprayed onto the hair using **pressurised containers**, e.g. hair lacquers. The chemical hazards in the salon come from the following three main sources.

### Skin or eye contact

Be aware of the risk involved in carrying out any hairdressing operation (even shampooing) that involves chemicals, and handle chemicals with care. Chemicals can be swallowed, especially by children, so care should be taken to put them out of reach.

### Storage and disposal

Accidental spills can be avoided by replacing caps and stoppers on containers immediately after use. If a spill does occur:

- Wipe it up immediately.
- Avoid skin contact.
- Report the event promptly to your supervisor.

It is very important that products are stored and used in accordance with manufacturers' recommendations and that warnings are noted and followed.

Do not use caustic soda (sodium hydroxide) to clear blocked drains – get a plumber to do it. Caustic soda can cause severe skin burns.

### Dermatitis (eczema)

Dermatitis involves the body overreacting to a substance it has been exposed to. Many of the chemicals used in hairdressing may cause dermatitis. Both the hairdresser and the client are at risk, with the hairdresser at greatest risk due to repeated and long-term exposure to hairdressing chemicals. The hairdresser can be protected by using rubber gloves for any hairdressing service that involves chemicals, including shampooing.

## Biological

Biological hazards consist of infections and infestations caused by living organisms. Anything that is either **infectious** or **contagious** can be passed between people or transmitted in the salon. This is called cross-infection and more details can be found in Unit 2.9.

## Routine hygiene procedures

The salon should always be kept clean and tidy. Well-trained staff should automatically tidy any dirty areas. A salon which has hair all over the floor and dirty towels strewn about the place is very off-putting to the client and looks inefficient. A strict code of hygiene should exist, even during busy periods – bacteria thrive in the salon's warm, moist atmosphere, and risk to the client must be minimised.

Hairdressers work with hair and are therefore used to handling it and seeing it about. Clients feel differently – other people's hair in the wrong place can make them feel a little sick. Try to see things from the client's viewpoint.

# Activity

Design a poster for salon staff entitled 'Salon hygiene – What it means to you'. Make it lively and colourful. Your poster should explain why hygiene is important both to clients and to salon workers.

## Good habits

- **Shop floor** – the floor should be swept and mopped each day and never left untidy. Cut hair should be swept up immediately. Check.that all floor coverings are sound. Any loose tiles, lino, carpet, etc., can be dangerous to staff and clients.

- **Reception area** – this should be kept clean and tidy with a cloakroom or rack for the clients' coats, away from the main salon. If there is a retail sales area, the items for sale should be attractively displayed with the prices clearly marked and the display dusted regularly.

- **Worktops** – these should be kept free of litter, e.g. empty setting lotion bottles, and tidied up after each client. They should be wiped over regularly and kept free from dust.

- **Chairs** – these should be kept clean and free from hair. A vinyl covering makes cleaning easier. They should be wiped down every day, including the backs and the legs as these tend to get splashed with lotions. Any splitting or tearing of the material must be reported immediately.

- **Mirrors** – they should be cleaned every day and lacquer stains removed immediately with a lacquer solvent, such as methylated spirit or alcohol, e.g. surgical spirit. Back mirrors also need cleaning regularly to remove any lacquer stains or fingerprints.

- **Towels and gowns** – dirty towels should be placed in a linen basket after use and should not litter the salon. Clean towels only should be used on the client and any towels with holes in them should be discarded or recycled as cleaning cloths, etc.

- **Brushes, combs and rollers** – every client should have a clean brush and comb used on their hair. Combs should be kept in antiseptic and brushes in a sterilising cabinet. Rollers and brushes should be washed and disinfected regularly.

- **Trolleys** – trays and trolleys should be cleaned at the end of each working day and the feet of the trolleys should be checked to make sure that loose hair has not been caught in them.

- **Magazines** – keep all magazines tidy and throw away any that look tatty.
- **Wash bowls** – wash bowls and fittings should be kept clean and wiped over after each shampoo. Front wash bowls must be disinfected regularly to prevent unpleasant smells. Hair traps can be used to help prevent blockage, but the hair should be removed from these traps after each shampoo.
- **Equipment** – steamers and infrared lamps should be cleaned after use. Always make sure that the water bottle on the steamer has enough water in it before use (distilled water should be used) and the steamer should be cleaned out regularly. Infrared bulbs should be checked before use and any faulty bulbs reported.
- **Vapour and ultraviolet cabinets** – make sure the vapour steriliser cabinet is checked each day and refilled with sterilising solution. Keep cabinets clean inside and out.

## Fire safety quiz

1. How do staff and clients get out of the salon?
2. What would you do if you noticed a fire exit, corridor or a doorway blocked by something that would hinder a rapid evacuation of the premises?
3. Where are the fire extinguishers in the salon? What types are they?
4. List the fire extinguishers that are suitable for an electrical fire. List those that are unsuitable.

## Things to do

1. In small groups try to describe an accident you know about or have come close to in the salon. What caused it? What action was taken?
2. Design a safety poster for display in the salon.
3. Outline a salon's health and safety policy (establishment rules).
4. Briefly list legislation (national and local) covering health and safety, and describe what to do if:
   (a) you can see a potential hazard
   (b) an accident happens
   (c) there is any spillage, breakage or waste

## What do you know?

- Which local **by-laws** affect your salon?
- What does **legislation** mean?
- Why is it important to **brush** teeth and **bathe** regularly?
- Why is personal **hygiene** important?

- Suppose you were to stand **incorrectly**, what would be the long-term effects on your health and appearance?
- How does your employer expect you to **dress** when working in the salon?

### Keywords

You need to know what these words mean. Go back through the unit or look up what they mean in the glossary at the back of the book (or ask a tutor/senior staff member).

accident, aerosol spray, cross-infection, emergency, fire evacuation, health and safety at work, legislation, personal hygiene, personal protective equipment, pricing, products, profit, resources, security, stock, stock control, sundries

# Level 2

# 1

In this unit you will learn how to:

- Assess the client.
- Use good communication skills.
- Carry out tests on the hair and scalp following the correct procedures.
- Protect information about the client in order to ensure confidentiality.

You will also look at:

- Advising clients on salon services.
- Maintaining records.

And you will gain experience in advising clients on the use of after-care products.

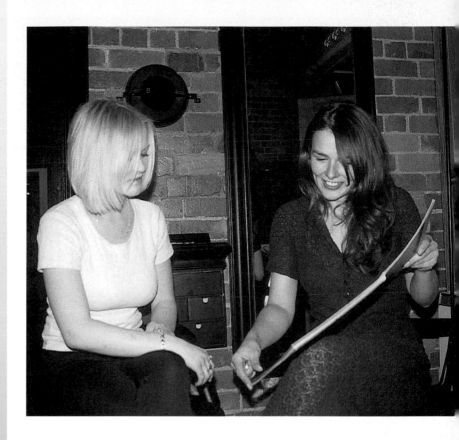

# Client consultation

## Assessing the client

Client care starts at reception – as soon as the client enters the salon. Take the client's coat and any other belongings that will not be needed and put them in a safe place. Be prepared to return items to the client if they require them during their time in the salon or as they leave (Unit 2.7).

Client assessment involves gathering information and that needs two-way **communication** with a client. To do this properly, the hairdresser needs to:

- **Look** carefully at the hair and scalp to see if any chemicals have previously been used.
- **Listen** carefully to the client's wishes and how they reply to your questions.
- **Feel** the hair to judge the condition, porosity and texture.
- **Assess** whether there are any potential problems and whether the client's wishes match up to what is actually possible.
- **Question** the client to gather more information.

To carry the assessment further a number of factors need to be considered. These include:

- Hair growth patterns
- Face shape
- Age, lifestyle and hobbies
- Conditions of the hair and scalp
- Various tests on the hair and skin

This information can then be used to judge whether the client can receive the service they are asking for, and advice can be given about whether the treatment or service is appropriate for them. These aspects are now considered in more detail.

### Communication skills

Good communication skills are required to ask a client **tactfully** for the information needed to make decisions about the appropriate service or treatment. Two important areas for good communication skills are active listening and questioning.

#### Active listening

Some people are naturally good listeners, others need to learn how to do it well. Listening skills include:

- Listening to someone without thinking about yourself or planning how you are going to reply. If you are thinking about other things, you cannot listen to what the client is saying.
- Using eye contact, nods and smiles to show you are paying attention.
- Checking that you have understood. Use phrases like 'So what you are saying is...'. This gives the person the chance to clarify things to you.

Listening attentively will help the client describe their requirements as precisely as possible and it will make sure that you fully understand the client's needs.

## Questioning

Questioning is used to get further information from the client. Questioning should not be carried out so as to put the client on the defensive. Good questioning, like good listening, makes the client feel valued and therefore adds to client satisfaction. Here are some important types of question.

*Negative*  Negative questions should be avoided if possible as they usually elicit a negative response from the client. For example:

*Trainee*:    You didn't want a conditioner on your hair, did you?

*Client*:    No.

The trainee is inviting the client to say no.

*Positive*  These questions are asked in such a way as to elicit a positive response from the client. They are phrased so that it is very difficult for the client to say no. For example:

*Trainee*:    I notice that your hair is very dry. Would you like me to use a conditioner to make it silky again?

*Client*:    Yes.

The client will almost certainly wish to have silky hair again.

*Closed*  A closed question usually elicits a one-word response from the client. For example:

*Trainee*:    Is your hair dry?

*Client*:    Yes.

*Open*  An open question will usually elicit a much longer response and encourage the client to give a lot more information or an opinion. Open questions are useful for finding out a lot of information about the client and their hair before deciding which product to recommend. For example:

*Trainee*:    What other treatments have you had on your hair over the past few months?

*Client*:    Now let me think a moment … it was permed before my holidays and tinted when I got back.

The client will then disclose more information to help the stylist to diagnose the hair condition and suggest a suitable treatment.

# Activity

Make a list of dos and don'ts when advising a client.

## Client care: personal information

It is good salon practice to keep information about clients stored on a card or on computer. However, it is very important that this information is:

- Accurate
- Up to date
- Relevant

Ask yourself, 'If the client saw this record, would they be completely happy with it?' Another source of information is what the client tells you or may be passed to you by other salon staff. Anything the client tells you should be treated in the strictest confidence. Only that information directly related to salon services should be passed on to other salon staff. A client overhearing or being told gossip about other clients will wonder if their confidence will also be betrayed.

## Data protection: computer records

Many salons use information technology to help run the business. This includes keeping personal information, names, addresses, etc., on the salon's clients. The Data Protection Act 1984 regulates the use of all computerised personal information relating to living individuals and places obligations on those who record and use such information (technically called data).

Broadly speaking, the Data Protection Act grants individuals three basic rights, which may be described as the right of access to personal information held on computers; the right to compensation, through the courts if necessary, for inaccuracy, loss, destruction or unauthorised use of data; and the right to correction or erasure of inaccurate data.

### Seven principles of data protection

The act is administered by a data protection registrar in accordance with the following principles, which are embodied within the act and are the standards by which the salon can be judged.

Personal data shall:

- Be collected and processed fairly and lawfully.
- Only be held for specified, lawful, registered purposes.
- Only be used for registered purposes or disclosed to registered recipients.
- Be adequate and relevant to the purpose for which it is held.
- Be accurate and, where necessary, kept up to date.
- Be held no longer than is necessary for the stated purpose.
- Have an appropriate security surrounding it.

It is now an offence to hold personal data without being registered. The register entries describe the types of data subjects to which each purpose applies, the classes of personal data held for each purpose, the sources from which any of the data may be obtained by persons or organisations to whom the data may need to be disclosed, and also the countries outside the UK to which it may be intended to transfer the data. These entries are contained in a register which the data protection registrar has made widely available for public inspection through local libraries.

## What is your responsibility?

As a salon employee you may have to handle personal data during the course of your work. You may receive a computer-printed form which contains personal details or you may be involved in the collection of personal information that will eventually be processed by computer. There are very few employees who will not at some stage come into contact with sensitive personal data which has been computerised. In this situation the act now says that you can be legally responsible for the confidentiality of the personal data, which *must only be used* to assist you to carry out your job; it must not be given to people who have no right to see it.

The importance of security measures in relation to personal data cannot be overemphasised. Here are some example:

- Physical security of equipment such as computers, terminals, magnetic tapes, disks, etc.
- Data security, including password protection and the storage and disposal of output materials such as printouts.

# Activity

Make a poster listing **all** the information that a salon could hold on an individual client. Show why it is important that this information remains confidential.

## Face shape, age, hobbies and lifestyle

### Face shape

The client's face shape is a key factor in the design of the completed style. For details of styles that are suitable and unsuitable see Unit 2.3. A client suggesting an inappropriate style is a good example of where to use tact and care in subtle ways to convince them that another approach would be better.

It is important to question the client closely; they may know exactly what they have in mind but have great difficulty in describing it. If this is the case, it is often useful to keep a book of fashionable hairstyles available in the salon to show the client. The hair stylist will then have a visual description of the style or look that the client is aiming for.

### Age, hobbies and lifestyle

The age of the client is a very important consideration. A middle-aged person cannot always wear the same style as a teenager, although a current fashion trend can often be adapted to meet the needs of both, as long as it is not too extreme.

The general lifestyle and hobbies of the client also need to be considered. When assessing a client's personality, clothes, etc., it is important not to gown up until starting the procedure. Also find out how much time the client will be able to spend on maintaining their hairstyle; they may have time for something elaborate or they may prefer something that requires minimal attention. These and many other questions need to be asked to find out exactly what the client expects and requires of the salon service.

## Testing hair and skin

Various tests can be performed on the hair and skin to make sure there will not be any problems when carrying out further treatments or when a treatment is completed.

Always explain to the client why you are carrying out the tests – it will increase their trust in your expertise and encourage them to accept any of your recommendations. Remember to record all test results for future reference. Table 2.1.1 is a summary of tests.

# Activity

Using the rightmost column of Table 2.1.1, find out how the tests are carried out. Draw up a three-column table. Put the name of the test in the first column, its purpose in the second column, and briefly explain how to perform it in the third column.

**Table 2.1.1  Summary of tests**

| Type of test | Use of test | More details |
|---|---|---|
| Curl test | To find out the amount of processing that has occurred | Unit 5a |
| Elasticity test | A general test of hair condition and strength, particularly of the cortex. Hair is stretched | Unit 5a Unit 5b |
| Incompatibility test | To check for the presence of metallic dyes on the hair | Unit 5a Unit 6 |
| Porosity test | To check the hair cuticle for damage and/or being open | Unit 5a Unit 6 |
| Strand test | To follow the development of the colour during tinting | Unit 6 |
| Skin (allergy) test | Carded out before a para dye is used, it checks for any allergic reaction to the tint | Unit 6 |
| Test curl | To check the correct rod size and lotion, and to find out the processing time | Units 5a, 5b |
| Test cutting | To check whether a chemical treatment is suitable | Unit 5b Unit 6 |

## Incorrect use of chemicals

A client may come into the salon showing the signs of a previous incorrect chemical treatment or they may ask for a service which would produce the effects of overapplication or overprocessing. The incorrect uses of chemical treatment are summarised in Table 2.1.2.

**Table 2.1.2  Summary of incorrect treatments**

| Chemical treatment | Main effects of incorrect use on the hair | More details |
|---|---|---|
| Bleaches | Overlapping application onto previously bleached hair may weaken hair or produce uneven colouring. Uneven application will cause more bleaching in some areas than others, producing a patchy look | Unit 6 |
| Neutralisers | The curl will not last long-term | Unit 5a |
| Perm lotions | Uneven application will lead to uneven curl. Lotion on the scalp can cause irritation and chemical burns | Unit 5a |
| Relaxing chemicals | Uneven application produces uneven straightening or relaxing. Can easily cause damage | Unit 5b |

## Advising clients on after-care procedures

An important feature of client care (and the client's feelings of satisfaction with the salon) is the after-care advice they receive. This includes the salon services they may wish to use in the future and products they may wish to buy and take away with them. After-care procedures may include:

- Advice on the use of shampoos and conditioners.
- Whether to use styling and finishing products and, if so, which ones.
- Any practical tips or precautions on using home haircare appliances, such as curling tongs.

This advice is clearly to the client's benefit but it also serves the purpose of helping to promote (or sell) the salon services and products. Never underestimate the power of perception (how people see things). If the client perceives you as an expert, they will take your advice. However, they will not wish to attend your salon or buy goods if they do not like what they see. First impressions are important and a prospective client/buyer can be encouraged to enter the salon by its smart and clean exterior and to keep returning because of its welcoming interior and the attitude of the staff employed there. Thus, promoting the salon and selling goods can be divided into three main areas:

- Promoting the salon image
- Promoting salon services
- Selling retail goods

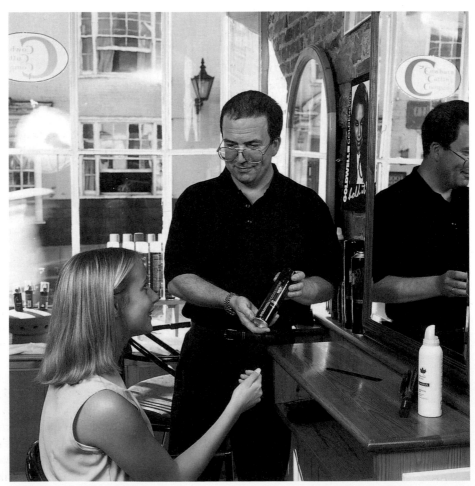

Goldwell/Michael Balfre Photography

## Promoting the salon image

It is important to attract the client through the salon doors. New clients will attend the salon because it has been recommended by someone else or because they like the look of the salon from the outside. This means the exterior of the salon must always project the salon's image and the type of work it does. It should always be kept clean and if there is a window display, this must be regularly changed to attract attention.

The type and standard of work that is produced by the salon will also present a certain image. The standard of work should be as high as possible and can be improved by regular training nights for both junior and senior staff.

The appearance of the staff will also contribute to the image of the salon, so looking neat, smart and professional is very important. For example, if you were to find yourself in hospital surrounded by nurses wearing shorts and T-shirts, you would not be filled with confidence. This is because they would not be projecting the image of what you perceive that a nurse should look like. Although their attire will make no difference to the standard of their work, it will influence how capable you think them to be. The same applies to hairdressing; if the staff look the part, the clients will believe they are competent.

# Activity

Draw up a chart with two columns headed:

Good image     Poor image

Under each heading list all the relevant factors you can think of. For example, smart appearance might go in the good column whereas dull window display might go in the poor column.

## Promoting the salon services

Before you can sell any salon service, you must have a thorough knowledge of what these services are, how they work and what benefits they will bring to the client. Often staff are reluctant to use or recommend new products as they are unsure of these points. However, most manufacturers have trained technical staff who will demonstrate their products at the salon. And manufacturers will usually run short courses at their own training centres to give further tuition. These courses are very useful as they also give background knowledge and usually offer ways in which to promote the products. Always remember that the manufacturers are also in business and it is in their best interest to help you as much as possible; the more of their products you use, the more profit they make.

Many stylists feel uncomfortable about recommending further treatments to their clients. But this reluctance is misplaced because the client relies on the experience of the stylist to make their hair look its best. Very often the client is totally unaware of the range of services available. Perhaps they realise that the salon does tints, but they could be unaware of how the effects range from the most dramatic shade to the very subtlest sheen. It is the responsibility of the stylist, as the expert, to guide and advise the client as to what treatments would be the most suitable and beneficial. After all, the worst that can happen is that the client will say no. The conversation below gives an indication of how a treatment can be advised to the client without giving offence:

*Client:*   I like my new haircut but the top keeps going flat. I know I should have a perm but I hate curls, and besides, the back is now too short to curl.

*Stylist:*   Your hair is rather fine so it really needs extra bounce. A body wave or root perm would be ideal as it will only give root lift and will not make it too curly. In fact, it will not give any curl at all but it will make the blow-dry hold for longer and give your style the height you like. I only need to wind the top so that the other hair will be unaffected.

*Client:*   That sounds ideal. I hadn't realised it was possible to have a perm without curl and without having the whole head done. When can I book my appointment?

Using a variety of techniques in the salon also creates interest, particularly if they are visually different from the norm. When clients see something unusual, their curiosity is aroused and they will want to know all about it. For instance, when Molten Browner perm rods first came onto the market, clients wanted a perm just to try the rods.

When selling salon services, keep to the golden rule of knowing your products and what they are capable of. Never promise something that is impossible to achieve. If a particular product or service is unsuitable for the client's hair, tell them so and recommend something else. In time, when clients find that your recommendations improve their hair, they will learn to trust you and it is highly unlikely they will take their custom elsewhere.

# Activity

Choose **three** products or services offered by a salon; it is a good idea to choose products with which you are **fairly unfamiliar**. List some ideas on how you could sell these products or services to the client.

## Selling retail goods

When selling retail goods it is essential that the products are attractively displayed in a prominent place. Unless they are on show, clients will not know exactly what is for sale. Large stores know the value of a good display stand where people can touch and try products. Remember, if a prospective buyer holds something, they are more likely to buy it. The next time you go shopping, look at how the goods are arranged and see what type of arrangement makes you stop and want to buy the products displayed.

The best place to display retail goods is in the reception area so that when the client is paying the bill, they can buy the goods at the same time. Clients waiting in the reception area will also be able to look at what is displayed, and people passing the salon can easily call in to purchase whatever they wish without having to go into the main body of the salon. For this reason it is a good idea to make sure the retail display is visually attractive from the outside of the salon as well as inside.

All retail goods should be clearly marked with the price. Many people are put off buying products if they have to ask how much they are. The display should always be well stocked and clean; it is surprising how dusty goods can become in a very short period of time and nothing is more off-putting to a prospective buyer than to see goods which look soiled or as if they have been on the shelf a long time. Human nature being what it is, we believe that if nobody else wants them then they cannot be any good!

There are a multitude of products available for use on the hair and skin, and it can be very confusing to be confronted by a vast range. Clients buying their hair products from other stores are often ignorant of what they should buy and this is where the stylist's expertise comes into its own. The stylist knows the client's hair and can

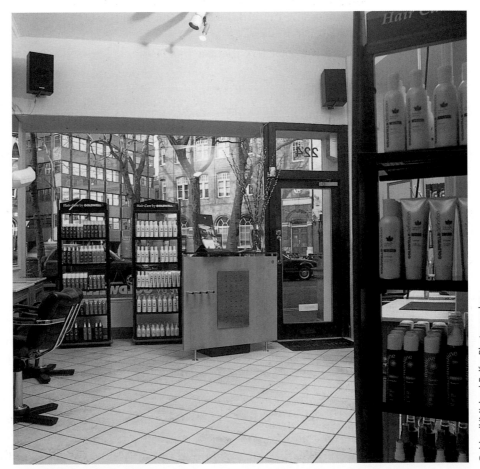

Goldwell/Michael Balfre Photography

therefore recommend a suitable product. They also know the effects that the various products will have on the hair, and these can then be explained to the client. If making a purchase at another store, the client must make a more uniformed choice as the assistants will not have the same amount of professional knowledge.

Often the best way to sell retail products is to use them in the salon, explaining their use when they are being put on the hair. A stylist might say something like this:

> I am just going to put some wax onto the ends of your hair to make it fall into strands and give a more tousled effect. I find that this particular wax is excellent for your type of hair as it counteracts any dryness and is very economical to use. In fact, we sell a great deal of this product and it is extremely popular with our clients.

This stylist has covered several points here:

- **Introducing** the client to a new product – wax.
- Telling the client **where to apply** the wax for a certain effect – onto the ends of the hair.
- Explaining to the client the **effect** it will have on the hair – make it fall into strands and give it a more tousled effect.
- **Personalising** the product – excellent for your type of hair.
- Giving some **benefits** of using the product – counteracts dryness and is very economical to use.
- **Informing** the client that the wax is for sale – we sell a great deal of this product.
- **Showing** that it must be effective because so many people buy it – it is extremely popular with our clients.

Using the products in the salon has an added advantage in that the client has tried the product on their hair and therefore has an indication as to its benefits. In this way many of the products almost sell themselves.

Promotions are also an ideal way of boosting sales and there are many different ways this can be done. For example, instead of promoting cheaper perms, why not keep the price the same but include a free specialised shampoo for home use? This will prolong the life of the perm by ensuring that the client uses the correct shampoo as well as introducing them to a new product. And when the client requires more shampoo, they will be more likely to purchase it from the salon than anywhere else. Other examples include selling small travel packs of the products during the summer months, or gift sets which are popular over the Christmas period. Other ideas for increasing sales:

- Take one product line and sell two for the price of one.
- Take two different product lines and sell them at a discount when they are purchased together. For example, shampoo and mousse together is cheaper than buying the shampoo then buying the mousse.

## Selling techniques

If you look around your salon, you will probably notice that some stylists make far more sales than others. Watch carefully how they deal with the client about what they are selling and how they believe firmly in the products. This brings us back to the point that good product knowledge is essential and the best way to find out about the products is to use them yourself.

Some people seem to be born salespeople who are able to communicate easily and persuade others as if by magic. For those who find it more difficult there are certain strategies which can be used to help overcome any initial nervousness and ask questions in the most beneficial way.

To overcome initial nervousness make sure you have enough product knowledge; this will give you confidence. Then take a deep breath and speak calmly. Remember to sound enthusiastic and positive when you talk – you will be surprised at how well the client will respond.

# Activity

Carry out a role play where you try to sell an after-care service or product to a client. Get some feedback from your partner on how you did.

## Providing information to clients

If a client wishes to return to a salon, they need a basic set of information to help them. Many salons provide clients with attractive pamphlets or cards giving information about the salon such as:

● Telephone and fax number
● Contact name (or names)
● Opening hours
● Dates, times and prices of any repeat appointments
● Price list of services

With this ready to hand on a business card or pamphlet, a client who is pleased with a salon's services will find it easy to return.

## Things to do

1. Write out some guidelines on active listening and types of questioning for use in the salon.

2. Make a poster on breaches of confidentiality. In other words, explain what can happen if the rules on confidential information are broken.

3. Design an illustrated pamphlet to give to clients explaining how and why their scalp and/or hair can be tested.

4. Choose an after-sales service or product which you genuinely feel is well worthwhile. Outline how you would convince someone else of its worth.

5. Design a poster 30 cm × 60 cm (12 in × 24 in) for promoting a special offer in your salon. The special offer can be on retail goods or on salon services. You may use any medium you wish, e.g. pastel, paint, crayon, ink, pictures and letters cut from magazines, stencils, etc. Sketch your ideas in rough before you start your final piece of work; this will help you to organise your ideas.

## What do you know?

- List the **four** main features of good communication during an assessment.

- Outline the factors about a client which need to be considered during an assessment.

- Describe the **main** types of questioning.

- What are the **main** provisions of the Data Protection Act?

- List the **eight** types of test that can be used on hair. Explain the purpose of each one.

- Take **four** chemical treatments regularly used in the salon. For each treatment, describe the **main** effects if it is used incorrectly.

- With regard to hairdressing, into which **three** areas can selling be divided?

- How can the standard of work in a salon be improved and maintained?

- Why is it important that salon staff look neat, smart and professional?

- Why are staff often reluctant to use or recommend new products?

- How can using a variety of hairdressing techniques in the salon, which are visually different, help or promote the selling of salon services?

- What is the best place to display the retail goods and why?

- What advantage does the stylist have over the shop assistant when selling products for the hair?

- Name **three** ideas which could be used to promote and boost retail sales.

- What strategies can be used to overcome nervousness when selling?

In this unit you will learn how to shampoo and condition hair, including:

- Client consultation.
- Stock levels.
- Health and hygiene considerations.
- The practical techniques of scalp massage and types of shampoo to use.
- The practical techniques of conditioning treatments.

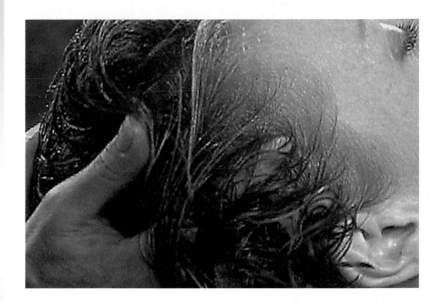

# Shampooing and conditioning hair

## Cleaning the hair and scalp

### Three factors

#### The dirt on a hair shaft

Hair (or skin) is made dirty by a wide range of materials like skin flakes, dust particles of many types, salt from dried sweat and so on. These materials could easily be dissolved or removed using water, except they are also mixed with the oily sebum which coats the hair and skin. This combination will not dissolve easily in water and therefore water alone is not able to clean the hair or skin efficiently.

#### The surface of hair and skin

Skin, when viewed closely by the unaided eye, shows pits and small wrinkles. When seen through a microscope, the outer cornified layer of the skin appears as a rough, flaking surface. Similarly, the outer cuticle of the hair shaft, with its overlapping scales presents a rough surface, even when the hair is in good condition.

Rough surfaces, like those of skin and hair, present a large number of places where dirt can lodge. So in order to remove the dirt, the water must be able to penetrate into these microscopic hollows and cavities.

#### The final condition

After they have been cleaned, it is important that hair and skin have their outer layers left undamaged and that some natural oil remains. Sebum has an important function in preventing skin and hair from becoming dry and brittle. A cleaning action that is too efficient will strip the hair and skin of all the sebum. With hair, the hair shaft is dead and the hair can be coated with a controlled amount of oil from a conditioner. With skin, the drying and cracking of the cornified layer allows micro-organisms and chemicals to penetrate to the living cells of the germinative (basal) layer just underneath. The chemicals may cause dermatitis, and the micro-organisms may cause infections.

### Cleaning action of shampoo

#### Shampoos reduce the surface tension of water

Surface tension results from the attraction of molecules at the surfaces of a liquid (i.e. where the liquid is in contact with other materials) towards the molecules in the rest of the liquid. This means that a liquid surface will tend to contract to cover the smallest possible area. The surface of a liquid in a tube is called a meniscus and it looks rather like a thin film. The minimum area principle explains why water droplets are spherical, and the surface of water in a basin can be seen more clearly by dropping a hair onto it. Surface tension also occurs when water forms a surface against hair and skin, and it prevents the water from penetrating into the rough surface of the skin's cornified layer or into the hair cuticle.

Shampoo reduces the surface tension of water, which allows it to penetrate into all parts of the surface of hair and skin. The process of bringing the water and surface to be cleaned into more intimate contact is described as surface activity. Because of this, soap and shampoo are sometimes described as **surfactants** (short for surface active agents).

### Shampoos help water to remove dirt

Water cannot properly dissolve oily materials like sebum, but it can break them up into tiny droplets, i.e. emulsify them. Shampoos will attach to the oily dirt on hair and skin, removing them as tiny droplets, i.e. emulsify the oil (Fig. 2.2.1) and prevent the droplets from going back on to the hair in two ways:

● The shampoo molecules surround the oil droplets and keep them separate from one another.

● The shampoo molecules coat the surface of the skin or hair and prevent the oil droplets from being redeposited.

To summarise, shampoos help water to clean hair and skin by:

● Reducing surface tension in the water, allowing the water to wet or penetrate the surface of hair and skin more effectively.

● Acting as an emulsifying agent, causing the oily dirt to break away in tiny droplets, which are then prevented from redepositing on the hair or skin.

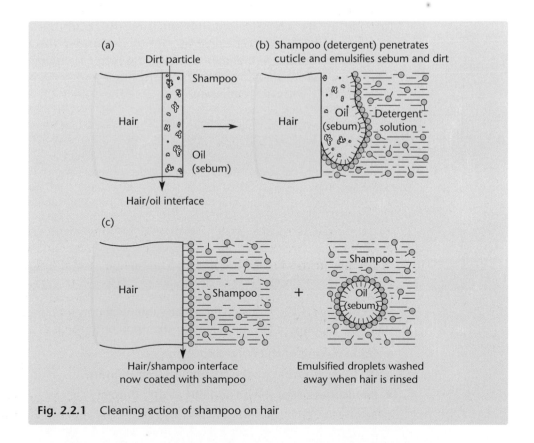

**Fig. 2.2.1**  Cleaning action of shampoo on hair

## Action of conditioners

Conditioners and conditioning treatments are covered in detail later in this unit, but in summary:

- Conditioners are designed to leave hair with a good shine, smooth and easy to brush or comb.
- Some conditioners just coat the hair surface, others go into the cortex of the hair.
- Many conditioners are pH-balanced and leave the hair slightly acidic (pH 5.5 to 6.5); this closes the hair cuticle scale and makes the hair smooth and shiny.

## Health and safety points

Shampoos and conditioners contain chemicals which have a relatively low hazard rating when carrying out risk assessments under COSHH (Control of Substances Hazardous to Health) Regulations. But there is still some risk. Here are some things to avoid:

- Running shampoo or conditioner into the client's eyes.
- Long-term exposure of the hairdresser's unprotected skin if protective gloves are *not* worn.
- Exposure of sensitive skin, cuts or rashes for both client and hairdresser.

In addition the electrical equipment used for conditioning treatments, e.g. streamers, needs to be checked as safe to use under the Electricity at Work Regulations. Finally, remember to check the water temperature on the **back of your hand** before spraying onto the client's hair and scalp. Make sure the client is comfortable with the temperature.

**SAFETY TIPS**

Never pull on the cable connecting a piece of electrical equipment to the plug. If this does happen by accident, check the cable carefully where it goes into the plug and into the piece of equipment. If in doubt then report it to your supervisor so that a check can be made by a qualified person.

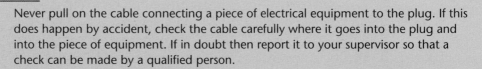

## Scalp massage

Scalp massage is the name given to the rubbing action involved in cleaning hair or skin. The rubbing or the massaging of shampoo onto the hair and scalp causes:

- Good mixing of the water and shampoo.
- Good penetration by the shampoo/water mixture.
- Emulsification of the oil and dirt as tiny droplets.

There are three scalp massage techniques used in shampooing hair. They are used to work the shampoo well into the hair and to encourage emulsification of the oil and dirt.

## How to carry out hand massage

Hand massage should be carried out with sure, firm movements. Nails should be kept to a reasonable length to prevent scratching the scalp, and the hands and wrists should always remain flexible.

There are three main types of hand massage used in hairdressing:

- Effleurage
- Petrissage
- Rotary (friction)

**SAFETY TIPS**

Jerky, uncontrolled movements can be uncomfortable or even painful to the client.

**Effleurage** is a slow stroking movement applied to the scalp with the fingers and palms in a slow rhythmic manner. It is used at the beginning and end of each massage treatment to relax muscles and relieve tension; it also distributes the shampoo or conditioner through the hair.

Both hands are held at the centre, front of the head and then pulled firmly down the back of the head to the nape (Fig. 2.2.2). The hands are then placed at either side of the head at the temples and again pulled firmly back round the contours at the sides of the head down to the neck and easing out to the shoulders, thus relieving any tension in the neck muscles.

**Petrissage** is a slow, firm kneading movement in which the skin is gripped by the fingers and rotated over the skull. It increases the blood circulation and gives deeper stimulation of the glands and muscles.

Place both hands in a claw-like position on the scalp then rotate the skin over the skull without moving the fingers over the scalp.

The right hand moves in a clockwise direction while the left hand moves in an anti clockwise direction.

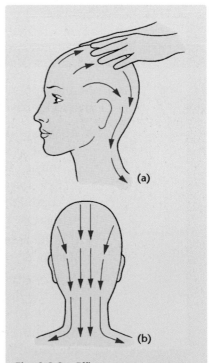

**Fig. 2.2.2**   Effleurage massage movements

The hands are lifted from their position one at a time and replaced elsewhere on the scalp until the whole scalp has been massaged. Always leave one hand in contact with the scalp when removing the other; this ensures continuity of the massage. If both hands are removed together, the massage becomes jerky and unpleasant.

**Rotary** (friction) is the most well known of all hand massage movements as this is the movement used when shampooing the hair. Friction is also a kneading movement and the fingers are still rotated in opposite directions for each hand. But unlike petrissage, the movements are quite quick and vigorous, with the fingers moving over the surface of the skin.

The hand is held in a claw-like position and the pads of the fingers are moved firmly over the scalp in circular movements away from the hairline up to the crown, then from the nape up to the front of the head and back down to the nape again.

Table 2.2.1 gives a summary of the hand massages.

**Table 2.2.1 Summary of hand massages**

| Movement | Description | Use |
|----------|-------------|-----|
| Effleurage | A gentle stroking movement | To relax muscles and relieve tension. Used at the beginning and end of each treatment |
| Petrissage | Slow, firm, kneading movement | To increase circulation and to stimulate glands and muscles |
| Friction | Quicker kneading movement with pressure applied | To improve circulation and glandular activity, used when shampooing |

## Shampoo ingredients

In addition to a soapless detergent, e.g. sodium lauryl ether sulphate, many shampoos have the following ingredients:

- **Auxiliary detergents** – these are weak detergents which alone are not very effective at removing oil from the hair, but which:
  - thicken the shampoo
  - help to keep a rich lather
  - condition the hair
  - increase the solubility of the main soapless detergent.

- **Common salt** – common salt (sodium chloride) is often added to thicken the shampoo.

- **Acids** – citric acid (e.g. lemon juice in lemon shampoo), and othe acids condition the hair by leaving it slightly acid after shampooing. Shampoos that contain acids are often called pH balance or acid balance shampoos.

- **Antiseptics** – shampoos may contain antiseptics and chemicals which inhibit the early stages of dandruff. Zinc pyrithone has both properties and is found in medicated or anti-dandruff shampoos.

## Special shampoos

### Dry hair

Dry hair results from either insufficient sebum being produced by the scalp or too much sebum being removed during chemical processes like bleaching and perming. The aim is to replace the natural oils in sebum with other oils:

- Lanolin is used in cream shampoos.
- Olive oil and other plant oils are used in oil shampoos.

Oil shampoos are for very dry hair. Shampoos for greasy hair have a higher proportion of soapless detergent to remove the surplus oil.

### Damaged hair

The aim is to coat damaged hair and, if possible, fill in the missing particles of cuticle. Here are some shampoos for damaged hair:

- **Egg shampoo** – where a raw egg is added. The egg proteins coat the hair and the scalp and act as a barrier on the scalp to other chemicals in the shampoo. For this reason, it is recommended for sensitive scalps.
- **Beer shampoo** – where beer is added. The coating slightly thickens each hair and so adds body to the whole head.
- **Protein shampoo** – contains proteins which have been broken down into a mixture of single amino acids and short chains of amino acids. There is some evidence that the amino acids will be absorbed by the porous regions of the hair, i.e. they are substantive to the hair, but this is not entirely accepted.
- **Herbal shampoo** – may contain one or a variety of herbal extracts. Whether these substances condition the hair is far from clear, but they are normally used to add sheen and gloss to the hair. Examples of herbal extracts are rosemary, sage and camomile.

### Brightening shampoo

Brightening shampoo is a mild bleach containing a soapless detergent with 10 vol. (3 per cent) hydrogen peroxide.

### Colour shampoo

Colour shampoo contains a temporary dye in addition to the soapless detergent. The dye belongs to the azo group and coats the hair cuticle but is easily washed off after a few shampoos.

### Dry powder shampoo

Dry powder shampoo is used where it is difficult to carry out a wet shampoo; e.g. when a person is bedridden. It contains a mild alkali mixed with an absorbent powder like starch. The alkali breaks down (or saponifies) a little of the sebum on the hair, so making a soap. This soap then cleans the hair during the thorough massage that follows. The powder absorbs the soap/oil mixture.

Table 2.2.2 gives a summary of the main types of shampoo and their uses.

### Table 2.2.2  Summary of shampoos

| Type | Use |
| --- | --- |
| Cream | Dry, brittle hair, bleached, tinted, permed, Afro-Caribbean hair |
| Oil | Extremely dry, bleached, tinted, permed, Afro-Caribbean hair |
| Medicated | Mild dandruff |
| Egg | Sensitive scalps, children's hair |
| Beer | Lank, fine hair |
| Lemon | To adjust pH to 4–6 after hair has been bleached, tinted or permed |
| Protein | Limp, chemically damaged hair |
| Herbal | To add sheen |
| pH balance | To adjust pH to 4–6, useful on chemically damaged hair |
| Dry powder | Invalids, in between wet shampoos |
| Brightening | Mild bleach, e.g. to highlight dull hair |
| Colour | Temporary tints |

## Precautions when shampooing

1. The client must be adequately protected: clothes should be completely covered by a gown and towels tucked well down at the nape. If a front wash is to be used, the client should be given a face cloth to protect their eyes.
2. Hair must be thoroughly disentangled prior to shampooing.

### TECHNICAL TIPS

Always follow the manufacturer's instructions for shampoo type. Some conditioning-type shampoos may need to be left on the hair for a few minutes.

3. The temperature of the water should be checked on the wrist or the back of the hand before allowing the water to run on the scalp.
4. Use the correct shampoo for the client's type of hair.
5. Liquid shampoo should be allowed to run over the back of the hand then on the scalp to minimise coldness.
6. Cream shampoo should be applied to the palm of the hand before being evenly distributed over the whole head.
7. Effleurage movements are used to distribute the shampoo then rotary hand massage is used in circular movements from hairline to crown, throughout the whole head.
8. Take care to make sure the hair is thoroughly rinsed after each massage.
9. After shampooing, the hair should be towel-dried and disentangled away from the face.

## Shampooing and surface conditioning

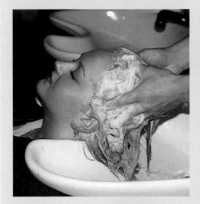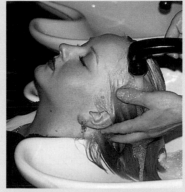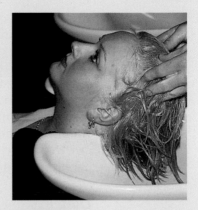

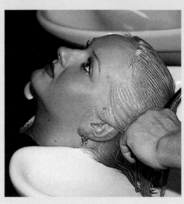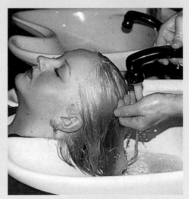

After shampoo has been applied, the hair is massaged using rotary massage movements to stimulate the scalp and emulsify the dirt and oil. The hair is then rinsed thoroughly before applying surface conditioner and massaging with effleurage then petrissage massage movements. Some salons prefer to comb the conditioner through the hair at this point before rinsing for a second time.

10. Make sure you tidy and wipe down the work area.

11. If you notice that you are running low on shampoo or clean towels remember to report this to your supervisor. This will help to make sure nothing runs out.

**POINTS TO REMEMBER**

- Hot water taps should be turned off during massage unless a mixer tap is used, in which case the whole tap is turned off. This is to conserve hot water.
- Never allow the client to leave the shampoo area with hair dripping on to the face. Always wrap hair in a towel to keep the head warm.

## Greasy hair

Greasy hair is caused by the overactivity of the sebaceous glands which produce far more sebum than is necessary to coat the skin and hair. This excess sebum forms a sticky coating on the skin and hair, allowing dirt and bacteria to adhere to it easily. Without regular attention the bacteria can cause dandruff, and if a fringe is worn, it can also be the cause of spots and blackheads on the forehead

Young teenagers, particularly during puberty, are especially prone to this condition and, unfortunately, the overactivity of the sebaceous glands is not confined to the scalp area alone. The skin on the face is often affected and this can give rise to common acne (*acne vulgaris*). It is possible to give help and guidance for this in three important areas.

### Diet

It is not clear whether a high level of fats or sugars in the diet is linked to excessive sebum production. There is conflicting evidence for and against each view. As the majority of people take in far more fat and sugar than is necessary, there is no harm in erring on the side of caution and suggesting their intake be reduced.

### Drying aids

There are many products which are now manufactured especially for greasy hair. They include shampoos, setting lotions and special conditioners without the addition of oils or waxes. Common salt also has a drying effect on the hair. However, it is well worth remembering that bleaching, tinting and perming are all processes that dry the hair and can be used to combat oiliness. They also have the added advantages of making the hair look better and increasing trade in the salon.

### Shampooing

There is no evidence that frequent shampooing results in the excess production of sebum. Most oily hair needs washing every two or three days. A dry shampoo used between shampoos is often useful to absorb some of the unwanted sebum, but vigorous brushing of the hair should be avoided at all times as this stimulates the sebaceous glands and distributes the excess sebum along the entire length of the hair shaft.

Shampoos containing oils or creams should be avoided. A soapless shampoo with no additives is the most effective, but it should not be used at too high a concentration, particularly if the hair has to be shampooed frequently.

## Conditioning the hair and scalp

### Hair condition

The hair shaft is dead and cannot repair itself in the way that living parts of the body can.

In the average life of a typical scalp hair, it may have been:

- Brushed and combed nearly 10,000 times.
- Washed (using a shampoo) about 600 times.
- Blow-dried (after the shampoo) about 600 times.
- Permanently waved about 16 times.
- Tinted 40 times (perhaps with a bleach included).

It says much for the toughness of the hair structure that it can stand up to all this punishment without disintegrating. Hair does age, however, and the oldest hair is at the hair points; this hair has usually suffered more damage than hair near the scalp. The different amounts of damage need to be considered when deciding the processing time in bleaching, tinting and perming hair.

Hair condition is considerably affected by the degree of **cuticle damage**. Cuticle damage can result from a number of factors which will be classed here as internal and external.

## Internal factors

### Age

General slowing down of hair growth and production of the natural sebum results in dry hair and scalp. Unpigmented white hair may have a coarser texture than pigmented hair.

### Diet

A well-balanced diet is essential for healthy hair. It has been suggested that there is a link between high sugar and oil intake and greasy hair and skin. However, expert opinion tends to be divided on this.

### Drugs and illness

Drugs and illness can have a profound effect on the hair, and even an illness as simple as the common cold can alter hair condition. With more serious illnesses, the drugs and treatment used can cause rapid thinning and even baldness, e.g. chemotherapy. A hormone imbalance or fever illnesses, e.g. glandular fever, can also cause thinning of the hair.

Internal reasons for hair in poor condition are largely beyond the control of the hairdresser. However, even if the hairdresser is only able to improve the hair superficially, there are still psychological benefits to the client by improving the hair visually.

## External factors

External factors can be physical (or mechanical) damage, caused by brushing, combing and heat, or chemical damage, caused by chemical treatments and the ultraviolet rays in sunlight.

### Physical damage

When the hair is in good condition the cuticle scales of the hair shaft are tight into the hair. This makes the hair smooth and shiny. When combing or brushing hair, especially backcombing or backbrushing, the cuticle is roughened by the mechanical scraping of the brush bristles or comb teeth. This leaves the hair dull and liable to further mechanical or chemical damage. The increased friction caused by roughened hair can lead to the production of static electricity in the hair and this can cause hair fly, making the hair less manageable.

Tight rollers, pins or clips on the hair can cause physical damage, especially on chemically treated hair. The hair normally contains some water, chemically bound to the cortex fibrils, and some of this water can be lost from the hair by blow-drying or by the drying effect of the atmosphere. Reduction in the water content of hair reduces its elasticity and this influences the movement of the hair.

### Chemical damage

Chemical damage includes the damage caused by the ultraviolet rays in sunlight and the damage caused by the chemical treatments used in hairdressing.

## pH and hair condition

The pH scale is a 14-point scale which measures acidity or alkalinity:

- pH 7 is neutral, neither acid nor alkaline
- below pH 7 is acid
- above pH 7 is alkaline

Hair is in its best condition if slightly acid (pH 5.5) but many hairdressing processes upset this pH balance, as can be seen in Fig 2.2.3.

Details on how conditioners are used to restore or balance hair pH are given in the section on acid conditioners.

## Conditioners: the three types

### Oil-based conditioners: external or surface conditioners

Sometimes called **emollients** or **conditioning creams**, oil-based conditioners are the simplest method of conditioning. The oil added to the hair, in a measured dose, replaces the natural oils removed by shampooing, perming, tinting or bleaching. The oils used are often in the form of an **emulsion** in water, which makes them easier to spread onto the hair, and they are left coating the hair when the water evaporates. **Lanolin** (from sheep's wool) or slightly altered forms of lanolin are good substitutes for human sebum and they are often used.

To make sure the conditioning effect lasts beyond the next shampoo, moist heat (e.g. hot towels or a steamer) can be used to swell the cuticle, allowing the conditioner to penetrate deeper into the hair shaft. As the hair cools. the cuticle scales close, trapping some of the conditioner between them, thus preventing complete removal at the next shampoo.

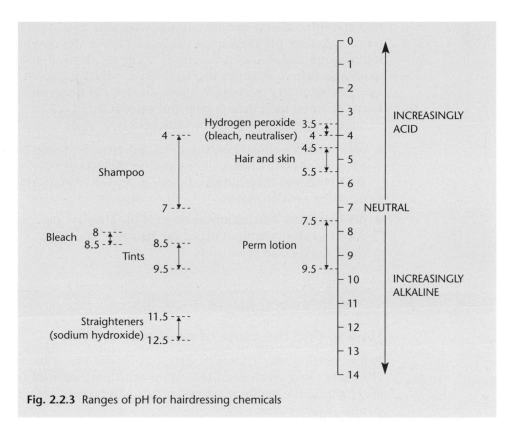

**Fig. 2.2.3** Ranges of pH for hairdressing chemicals

## Substantive conditioners: internal conditioners

Substantive conditioners become fixed to, or absorbed into, the hair shaft, mainly due to the **electric charge** on the conditioner molecule and the hair shaft. This category includes some soapless detergents and **polyvinyl pyrrolidone** (PVP), which acts as both a setting agent and a conditioner.

Other materials which appear to be absorbed by the hair include the protein conditioners sometimes called **restructurants**. Because the hair is dead it cannot be fed, but it does have the ability to absorb small polypeptide chains and single amino acids. These are produced by breaking down animal or plant proteins and the evidence is that some are deposited on the cuticle and some pass through the cuticle into the cortex. The amount absorbed by the hair seems to increase in the more damaged areas of the hair shaft, which is a very good property for a conditioner to have. But the evidence does show that this type of conditioner is most effective at protecting the hair from damage, so it is best applied before a perm, tint or bleach is carried out. It is not clear whether protein conditioners used after the treatment in any way increase the tensile strength or elasticity of the hair, although it seems likely that they do.

## Acid conditioners

Acid conditioners are based on the natural skin and hair secretions (sebum and sweat) having a pH of between 4 and 6. They produce an **acid mantle** over the hair and this makes it smooth and shiny because at acid pH the cuticle scales are flat. At alkaline pH the cuticle swells and the scales open slightly, so the hair looks rough and dull and it is more liable to physical and chemical damage. Acids also help to hold the water-soluble products produced by perm lotion and peroxide attacking the hair. Without an acid pH these products can be washed from the hair during shampooing and weaken it.

There are two types of acid conditioner:

- **pH restorers** – contain organic acids, e.g. citric acid, and have a pH of about 3. They are used to chemically neutralise the alkaline deposits left on the hair after perming, bleaching and tinting, and they are formulated to leave the hair with a pH of about 4.
- **pH balancers** – are mildly acidic (pH 6). They are used in pH balance shampoos to ensure the final pH of the hair is acidic. Organic acids are used, e.g. citric, tartaric and lactic acids.

## Conditioning treatments

### How to find the cause of poor hair condition

Before starting any treatment, first look at and touch the hair and scalp. This assessment will give a good indication as to the extent of the damage and will also indicate the depth of treatment that will be needed to restore the hair to a natural, healthy state.

Question the client about the possible reason for the damage. Very often the client will have a good idea as to the cause of the hair's present condition, particularly if prompted with suggestions from the hairdresser. However, always remember to question the client tactfully and sympathetically – they obviously know their hair is not at its best otherwise they would not want the treatment. Consider the following areas when assessing the hair and scalp.

**Hair assessment**

- **Hair types** – is the hair dry, brittle, greasy or wiry?
- **Hair texture** – is the hair fine, medium or thick?
- **Hair porosity** – is there a high degree of porosity? If so, has this been caused by chemical or physical factors such as bleach, tint, straighteners, permanent wave solution, sunlight or heat? Or is it because the client's hair has above average porosity?

**TECHNICAL TIPS**

Know the products and treatments available, their uses and their limitations.

- **Hair abnormalities** – are there any of the following present: fragilitis crinium (split ends), monilethrix (beading), alopecia (baldness)? If so, what has caused them?

Scalp assessment

- **Skin type** – is the skin dry, greasy or normal?
- **Skin abnormalities** – are any of the following present: psoriasis, pityriasis capitis (dry dandruff), seborrhoea (greasy dandruff)?

## Choosing the treatment

Before choosing any treatment, the stylist must have a sound knowledge of the products available and must be aware of their limitations. Never promise the client instant results if the hair is badly damaged; instead, explain what the treatment will do, how many treatments will be needed and why. Hair can be so badly damaged as to be almost beyond repair and the only real remedy would be to remove it by cutting until new, undamaged hair takes its place. However, even this type of hair can be made more supple and therefore easier to handle by careful and thorough use of restructurants, conditioners, oils, etc. Knowing which product to use and how to make it more effective is essential if the client is to have confidence in your judgement.

The intended effect of any hair or scalp treatment is to make the hair more supple and to improve the circulation of the blood. An improved blood supply brings more food and oxygen to the hair and scalp, which encourages hair growth and makes the sebaceous glands more active.

Heat and massage increase the blood supply to the scalp by causing the blood capillaries in the skin to dilate so that more blood flows into the skin; this can be clearly seen when the scalp turns pink in colour.

## Heat treatments

A heat treatment can be carried out in various ways depending on the source of heat.

Sources of heat

- **Steamer** – produces warm, moist heat.
- **Hot towels** – produce warm, moist heat. Their temperature should be 60°C.
- **Accelerator or infrared** – produces heat only, therefore has a more drying effect.

**TECHNICAL TIPS**

Use distilled water in the steamer kettle to prevent any limescale deposit reducing the efficiency of the equipment.

- **Rollerball machine** – this produces infrared radiation and has a fan to speed up the processing. These machines have two advantages:
  - the source of heat moves around the machine so hair is heated evenly
  - hairdressing operations can still be carried out while the client is sitting under the rollerball.
- **Climazone** – produces even, warm heat.

## Massage treatments

Massage is a form of manipulation which can be achieved either with the hands or mechanically with the vibro machine. The psychological value of massage has been very underrated in the past and this is one area in hairdressing that salons have not exploited to the full. Very few salons provide treatments which include the use of all the forms of massage, particularly when carrying out oil or conditioning treatments.

**POINTS TO REMEMBER**

A good massage, expertly carried out, not only benefits the hair and scalp but also gives the client a feeling of well-being.

### Uses of massage

- To soothe and relax the client.
- To stimulate the sebaceous glands of the scalp to produce the natural oil, sebum.
- To increase blood circulation in the skin capillaries and therefore to help nourish the hair and scalp.
- To soften and improve skin texture by making it more pliable.
- To ease contracted tissue, e.g. in the neck muscles.

### Hand massage

The three types of hand massage are covered earlier in this unit:

- Effleurage
- Petrissage
- Rotary (friction)

### Vibro massage

Vibro massage is a mechanical massage that uses electricity as its source of power. The scalp is stimulated by friction between the vibrating applicators and the scalp. Do not be tempted to use added pressure when massaging with the vibro machine as this could be uncomfortable for the client. There are three main rubber applicators for use with the vibro machine (Fig. 2.2.4):

- Spiked applicator.
- Sponge applicator.
- Rubber-domed bell

The spiked applicator is the most common attachment for hairdressing as its rubber prongs will move through the hair quite easily. It is used on the scalp in either circular or straight movements.

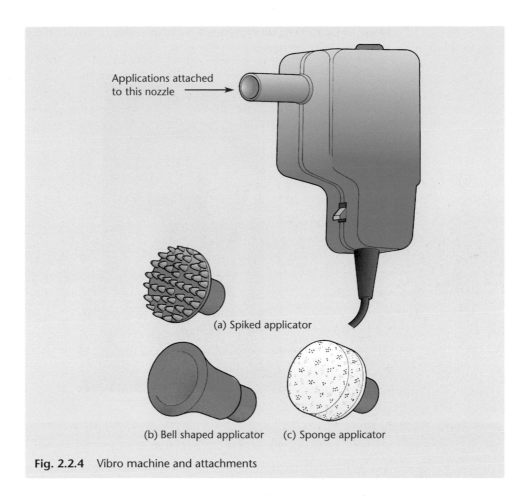

Applications attached
to this nozzle

(a) Spiked applicator

(b) Bell shaped applicator

(c) Sponge applicator

**Fig. 2.2.4** Vibro machine and attachments

## Conditioning products

Before advising any client about conditioning products, the stylist should be familiar not only with the range available but also how they work.

Hairdressing manufacturers spend a lot of money and research to produce whole ranges of haircare products for particular hair types and common hair or scalp disorders, the choice of which depends largely upon personal preference. However, before buying a whole new range of products, try them first to assess the results. Most manufacturers are only too willing to provide a sample of the product before you buy.

It is very important that you have every confidence in the product and know exactly its limitations. Remember that the client will be disappointed if the results are not as good as they were led to expect. Explain to the client how a course of treatments may be necessary to achieve a good result – if the hair or scalp has been mistreated or neglected it is unfair to expect it to be miraculously transformed overnight.

It would be virtually impossible to list every kind of hair or scalp disorder and give a full account of each treatment. However, the two most popular types of treatment will be dealt with in more detail as they can be adapted to meet a variety of needs.

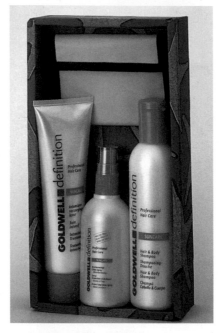

Goldwell/Michael Balfre Photography

## A basic conditioning treatment

A conditioning treatment will have a more lasting effect on the hair than a conditioning rinse. Any types of conditioning agent may be used for the treatment, either a pH balance or the more traditional type, depending upon the requirements of the hair.

### Uses of a conditioning treatment

- To replace the natural oil of the hair and scalp.
- To make sure the hair has the correct pH.
- To lubricate and moisten dry hair, thus making it more supple and easier to handle.
- To soften and improve the texture of the skin by making it more pliable.
- To relax the muscles and relieve tension.
- To increase the blood circulation and stimulate the glands and muscles of the scalp, allowing them to be more effective.

## Hot oil treatment

Oil treatments are of maximum benefit to the client who suffers from a dry, tight scalp and dry brittle hair due to the inactivity of the sebaceous glands. Vegetable oil is preferred to mineral oil as it is more easily absorbed into the skin and hair. Deep massage movements with a combination of hand and vibro massage are recommended with this type of treatment to loosen the scalp and stimulate the sebaceous glands, helping them to produce more sebum. The massage also helps to remove any flakes of dry skin that may stick to the scalp.

## Purposes of hot oil treatment

- To lubricate the scalp, making it more supple and elastic.
- To soften brittle hair caused by lack of sebum, giving it a healthier shine.
- To loosen the scalp by relaxing the muscles and relieving any tension.
- To increase the blood circulation and stimulate the glands and muscles of the scalp, allowing them to be more effective.

## How to carry out an oil treatment

1. Protect the client with a gown and towel, making sure the towel is tucked firmly down at the nape.
2. Assemble the equipment and heat the oil by pouring it into a small bowl. Place the small bowl in a larger bowl filled with hot water. This is known as a water bath. The oil should be heated to a temperature of 55 °C.
3. Disentangle the hair and check the scalp for cuts and abrasions.
4. Divide the hair into four sections.
5. Wrap a hot moist towel around the head or steam the hair for five minutes under a steamer. This swells the hair and opens the cuticle scales, which helps absorption of the oil.
6. Check the temperature of the oil. While the hair and scalp are still warm, apply the warm oil to the scalp using a cotton wool swab or brush.
7. Start the application at the nape and continue up towards the front, working from side to side as quickly as possible.
8. When application is complete, draw the oil through the lengths of the hair by massaging the scalp. First use the effleurage movements to soothe and relax, then use the petrissage hand massage to stimulate the sebaceous glands and loosen the scalp.
9. Apply the steamer for 10–15 minutes or use several hot moist towels.
10. Massage the scalp again while the hair and scalp are still warm. The vibro machine may be used but the massage should be finished with an effleurage hand massage.
11. To remove the oil, add soapless shampoo directly onto the hair before applying water. Massage the shampoo into the hair using friction movements until it looks white and creamy and the hair no longer lathers.
12. Rinse the hair thoroughly and shampoo again with soapless shampoo. It may often be necessary to shampoo the hair several times to completely remove

all traces of the oil from the hair. Any oil left on the hair will look lank and greasy when it has been dried.

13. After the final rinsing, towel-dry the hair then distangle ready for setting or blow-drying.

14. Complete a detailed record of the work carried out.

15. Advise the client on the after-care of the treatment.

## Record keeping

A detailed record should be kept of all hairdressing treatments, particularly those that will be carried out over a period of weeks. This builds up a very clear picture of how the hair is reacting and progressing with the treatment, and any modifications to the treatment, e.g. increasing or decreasing the massage time or even changing the product, can be done without getting in a muddle. See Fig. 2.2.5 for an example.

**RECORD CARD**
**HAIR/SCALP TREATMENT**

Name: .................................................................... Tel no: ................................

Address: ..............................................................................................................

.............................................................................................................................

| Hair assessment | Type | | Porosity | | Diseases/abnormalities | |
|---|---|---|---|---|---|---|
| | | | | | | |
| Scalp assessment | Skin type | | | | Diseases/abnormalities | |
| | | | | | | |
| Cause of damage | | | | | | |

| Date | Conditioner/ lotion | Type of massage | Time | Source of heat | Time | Result |
|---|---|---|---|---|---|---|
| | | | | | | |
| | | | | | | |
| | | | | | | |
| | | | | | | |

**Fig. 2.2.5** Example of client record card

## Things to do

1. The following table has been devised to help you recognise various hair types, to choose the correct shampoo and to be aware of necessary safety procedures when shampooing.

   Collect hair cuttings of the following types of hair then attach them to a piece of paper. Select a suitable shampoo for each type, giving reasons for your choice. Complete the table.

| Hair type | Hair cutting | Suitable shampoo | Reasons for choice |
|---|---|---|---|
| Permed<br>Fine textured<br>Coarse textured<br>Tinted<br>Bleached | | | |

   Next take samples of five (or more) different shampoos. Try to choose a variety of types and prices. You may also find it interesting to include your own favourite type.

   On small sections of your own or someone else's hair, try out shampooing with equal amounts of each shampoo. Compare them on these six aspects and make a table of your findings:

   (a) thickness
   (b) colour
   (c) scent
   (d) lathering
   (e) cleaning action
   (f) hair condition after shampooing

   You can set the shampoos a more difficult task by moisturising the fingers with a little mineral or vegetable oil and putting this onto the hair first. This will produce hair which is very greasy. Wash the small sections as before.

2. The condition of the hair has an important effect on all our hairdressing services. This assignment aims to help you identify the characteristics, both visual and tactile, which show whether the hair is in good or poor condition. You will need:

   ● two sheets of A4 card
   ● scissors, pencils, ruler
   ● chosen materials for the collage
   ● glue or cow gum

   Now read the following two statements:

   (a) Hair in poor condition feels rough, dry and brittle; it looks dull, lifeless and without shine.
   (b) Hair in good condition feels supple, bouncy and pliable; it looks shiny, healthy and gleaming.

Using these descriptions of the hair, create two collages: one to illustrate hair in poor condition and one to illustrate hair in good condition.

Each collage must be on an A4 size card with a 2.5 cm (1 in) border. You may work with any medium to create the effect that you want, e.g. silver paper, foil, eggboxes, fabrics, dried pulses or pasta, empty cartons, tacks or nails and/or any other materials which you feel will give the visual and tactile (touch) illusion of the two hair conditions.

Assemble all your equipment and materials then work out your designs in rough before placing the materials on the card. Do not glue or stick your materials to the card until you are completely satisfied with the result. When the design is finished and firmly glued in place, either draw a 2.5 cm (1 in) border around it or mount it on another larger piece of card which will give the same size border.

3. Design a record card similar to Fig. 2.2.5 and fill in the details of a real or imaginary client.

## What do you know?

- What is meant by the term **surface tension**?
- Shampoos **reduce** surface tension. Explain why this is important in cleaning hair.
- What is meant by the term **emulsify**?
- Why should the water used for a shampoo be **run over the stylist's hand** before spraying onto the client's head?
- After shampooing, why should hair be dried and disentangled **away from the client's face**?
- List **three** common additives in shampoo and explain what each does.
- What is a **pH balance** shampoo? How does it work?
- What types of shampoo should be **avoided** if a client has greasy hair?
- List **four** factors involved in hair condition.
- What effect does **heat** have on hair condition?
- Explain why backcombing or backbrushing hair may cause **more** damage than brushing or combing.

- Hair that has been made **alkaline** by chemical treatments, why is it rough and dull?
- In what form are most **oil-based** conditioners applied to the hair?
- Distinguish between pH **restorers** and pH **balancers**.
- Why is a **well-balanced diet** important to maintain healthy hair?
- Why does **age** play an important part in the condition of the hair?
- Which layer of the hair directly affects its **porosity**?
- What is the purpose of a **pH** conditioner?
- Name the layer of the hair which is most affected by **restructurant** conditioners.
- What is the **natural oil** of the hair and scalp called?
- Which type of **vibratory** application is most suitable for use on the head?
- What effect does **massage** have on the blood capillaries?

# 3

In this unit you will learn about:

- Safe and effective styling and dressing, including:
  - basic health and safety
  - client comfort,
  - information on products.
- Identification of client needs.
- Factors influencing the final choice of style.
- Practical techniques of drying, setting and dressing.
- How to handle long hair.

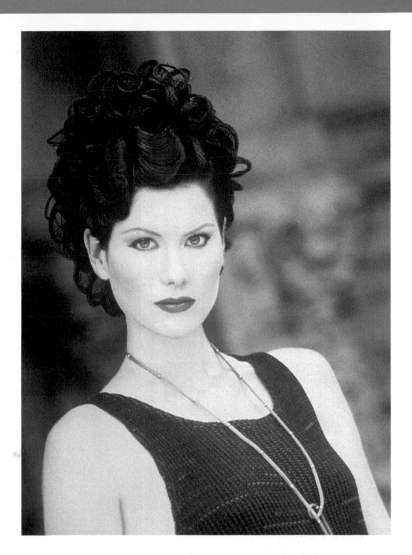

# Setting, drying and dressing hair

## A few preliminaries

Before you begin styling, consider some basic factors:

- **Client comfort** – make sure the client is sitting comfortably and is correctly gowned.
- **Client requirements** – you need to listen carefully and discuss fully with the client their ideas or expectations of the finished style. This type of communication is considered more fully in Unit 2.1, together with the client-based factors such as face shape and problem features.

# Activity

Write down your salon's requirements for gowning before styling hair by drying or setting.

## Health, hygiene and safety

### Heat

Dryers, accelerators, hot tongs, etc., all pose a heat hazard as they can cause **burns**. Make sure to avoid contact with the client's scalp and take care when holding or using equipment that uses heat.

### Electrical equipment

There is a duty under the Electricity at Work Regulations 1992 to make sure that electrical equipment is safe to use and that it is used safely:

- Check that electrical wires on equipment are safe before use.
- Always dry hands before using any electrical equipment.
- Take care not to have trailing electrical wires; either you or the client may trip and be injured.
- Take all necessary precautions when using electrical equipment (see Unit 2.9).

### Chemicals

A large number of substances are used as setting and styling aids; some of them pose a risk to the client and hairdresser, so they are covered by the COSHH Regulations 1992. This is particularly true of sprays, whether mechanically pumped or aerosols. Aerosol sprays produce a mist of tiny droplets which can drift about in the salon and are easily inhaled by client and stylist. Use sprays sparingly and be careful where you direct them. Here are two other important points:

- Aerosol sprays are supplied in **pressurised** containers which must not be punctured or incinerated. Dispose of the containers carefully.
- The propellants used to make the spray are often very **flammable**, hence they are a fire risk. Never use an aerosol spray near flames or allow smoking anywhere nearby.

Avoid chemical contact with the client's scalp or the stylist's hands. Take particular care not to allow anything to run into the client's eyes. Even products containing usually non-hazardous chemicals can cause intense eye irritation.

## Cross-infection

Cross-infection is a biological hazard of passing harmful micro-organisms from one client to another or from client to stylist. It can be prevented by routine hygiene procedures such as:

- Clean gowns and sterile neck strips for each client.
- Sterilising tools and equipment between clients, particularly brushes and combs (see Unit 2.9).
- Using clean towels on each client.

In addition there is a slight chance of small animal parasites being carried between people (technically known as infestation); which will be prevented by the routine hygiene precautions for bacteria and other infectious micro-organisms.

## General good practice

- Be aware of any adverse effects of the products being used.
- Do not splash or spill any products onto the floor or over the client, especially into their eyes. Splashes and spillages create a safety hazard.
- Always follow the manufacturer's instructions for each product.

# Activity

List the reasons why the work area should be kept neat and tidy. Make this into a salon poster.

## How setting works

Hair is **hygroscopic**, which means it is capable of absorbing moisture. When the hair is shampooed, a small amount of water penetrates the outside cuticle of the hair and enters the cortex. Once inside the cortex, the water breaks some of the weak, water-breakable hydrogen bonds that help to hold the polypeptide chains in position (Fig. 2.3.1).

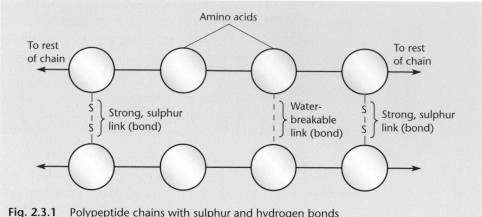

**Fig. 2.3.1**    Polypeptide chains with sulphur and hydrogen bonds

Breaking these bonds allows the polypeptide chains to move slightly past each other, allowing the hair to be moulded into a new position. The action of drying the hair then removes the water from the cortex, refixing the hydrogen bonds in a new position and holding the hair in whatever shape it has been moulded into. This wet–move–fix sequence is the basis of wet set, also called cohesive set.

When hair is in its normal, unstretched state it is known as **alpha keratin**; when it is moulded or stretched and then dried into a new shape it is known as **beta keratin**. Thus, a physical change takes place in the hair when it goes from an unstretched state.

Since hair is hygroscopic, it will gradually absorb moisture from the atmosphere around it. This moisture again breaks the hydrogen bonds, causing the hair to revert back to its natural, unstretched state. That explains why a blow-dry or set appears to drop out.

How quickly drop-out occurs depends on the air humidity; it happens more quickly in damp (humid) air. When the style is washed out, a large amount of water is put directly on the hair either deliberately in shampooing or accidentally, when caught in a rain shower.

When hair is in its natural, unstretched state it is known as **alpha keratin**; when stretched it is known as **beta keratin**. Therefore, when the hair is wetted, stretched and then dried during setting or blow-drying it changes from alpha keratin to beta keratin and it will remain as beta keratin until the cross-linkages revert back to their previous positions.

## What happens during dry setting

No extra water is added during dry setting, and some of the natural moisture in the hair is driven out by heat. Much heat is supplied by the techniques used in dry setting, e.g. heated rollers. The heat is in direct contact with the hair, which means it is carried into the hair with less being lost into the atmosphere.

Some of the water is turned into hot water vapour (steam), some is lost through the cuticle and the rest breaks some of the water-breakable cross-linkages, which allows the polypeptide chains to be moved, e.g. by stretching the hair around a heated roller. Next the cross-linkages re-form, fixing the chains in their new positions as the hair cools. Because some of the water vapour usually present in the hair has been lost during dry setting, the hair ends up with less moisture inside compared to wet setting. The hair will therefore quickly absorb any water vapour from the air around it.

The equipment used when dry setting includes heated curling tongs, crimping irons, straightening irons, hot brushes, marcel waving irons and heated rollers, all of which involve the use of heat very close to the skin of the face and scalp. Extreme care must therefore be taken to prevent skin burns.

With a wet set, it is mostly the water added during wetting that is driven off, so the hair at the end of this process contains only a little less water or the same amount of water than at the beginning. This means it does not usually absorb water as quickly as a dry set and it therefore lasts longer.

**TECHNICAL TIPS**

To make both wet and dry sets last longer, use a setting lotion.

## Products used in drying and setting

A variety of products are used and include:

- Setting aids
  - lotion
  - mousse
  - gel
- Dressing aids
  - wax
  - creams
- Sprays and lacquers to hold the hair
- Moisturisers to add moisture to the hair
- Activators to maintain a natural (or permed) curl

Setting aids are covered in this section; the other products are covered where they are relevant. Remember to tell your supervisor if products are getting in short supply.

### Setting aids

Setting aids coat the hair with a barrier to prevent the absorption of atmospheric moisture; this makes the set last longer. The choice depends on the type of finished style. Gels have the greatest moulding facility. All setting aids contain weak glues which hold the hair in place. Glues are not necessarily sticky; some work by bonding together and these glues are often used in setting aids. The active ingredients of setting aids depend on the type being used. Some use natural gums, e.g. tragacanth and karaya. Many use an artificial gum or plastic called polyvinyl acetate (PVA) which coats the hair. In practice PVA is often mixed with polyvinyl pyrrolidone (PVP) to make it stick to the hair better. The mixture is often 60 per cent PVP and 40 per cent PVA. The three main types are:

- Setting lotions
- Gels
- Mousses

Setting lotions are the most runny of the setting aids. This may cause problems with application due to dripping and running.

**Gels** contain chemicals which stiffen the hair but they become much less viscous when rubbed on the stylist's hands and then the client's hair. Materials which are viscous until brushed or rubbed and then become more liquid are called **thixotropic**. They have the advantage of being non-drip and have a good moulding ability to the stylist.

**Mousses** are foams which contain very small bubbles. The smaller the bubbles, the denser the foam. The bubbles are produced by the **propellant** in the pressurised container when it is released. Mousses are often used for scrunch and natural drying.

## Before the styling: key factors

### Head and face shape

The shape of the hair can alter the shape of the face by emphasising good features and minimising others. The professional stylist needs to be able to recognise the various facial shapes. An oval face shape (Fig. 2.3.2) is believed to be the perfect shape and the stylist should aim to achieve the illusion of an oval shape on their client.

#### Long face

To avoid a long face, create width at the sides using loose soft waves or curls. Medium length hair is best with the fullness around the ears. Fringes can shorten the effect of an overlong face. This is shown in Fig. 2.3.3(a).

#### Round face

Short hair is most suitable for a round face, with height on top of the head and the side hair flat, preferably covering the cheeks. An asymmetrical hairstyle or a parting will minimise the roundness, but a full fringe across the forehead will emphasis the roundness of the lower face. This is shown in Fig. 2.3.3(b).

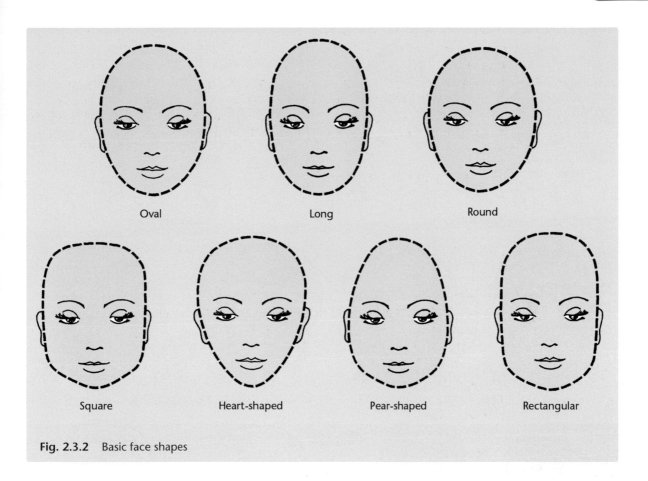

**Fig. 2.3.2**  Basic face shapes

### Square face

A soft design is needed to reduce the angular jawline. Fullness at the temples and cheekbones gives an illusion of roundness and the face shape can be softened by covering the jawline if possible. This is shown in Fig. 2.3.3(c).

### Heart-shaped face

Play down width at the temple and create fullness round the chin. An asymmetrical style or a side parting also looks effective on this face shape, as shown in Fig. 2.3.3(d).

### Pear-shaped face

Hair should be given width above the chin and left soft at the nape to soften the lower part of the face. This is shown in Fig. 2.3.3(e).

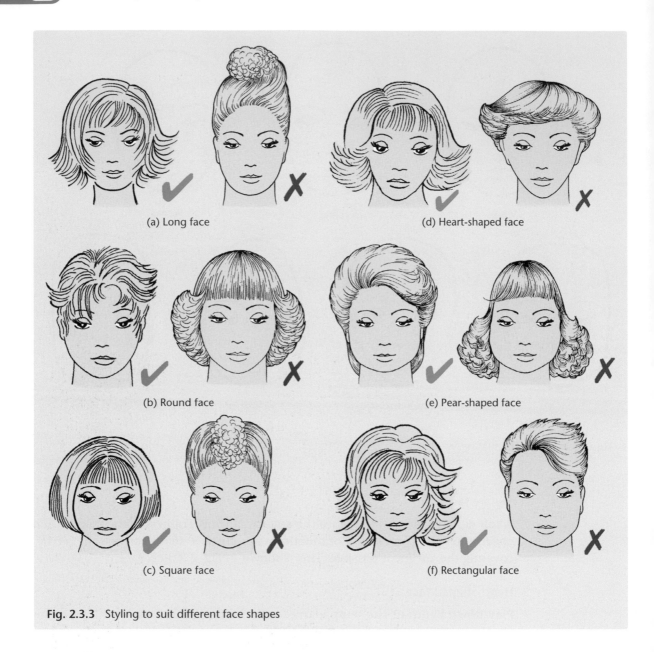

(a) Long face

(d) Heart-shaped face

(b) Round face

(e) Pear-shaped face

(c) Square face

(f) Rectangular face

**Fig. 2.3.3**  Styling to suit different face shapes

### Rectangular face

A rectangular face is longer then a square-shaped face but it has the same strong jawline, which needs to be disguised with softness. A fringe will help to reduce the length of the face and a side parting offsets its angular features. This is shown in Fig. 2.3.3(f).

## Problem features

The hair may be pulled back to reveal good features but problem features should be disguised so that the eye is drawn away from them, focusing attention on the more attractive features. Here are three less attractive features (Fig. 2.3.4).

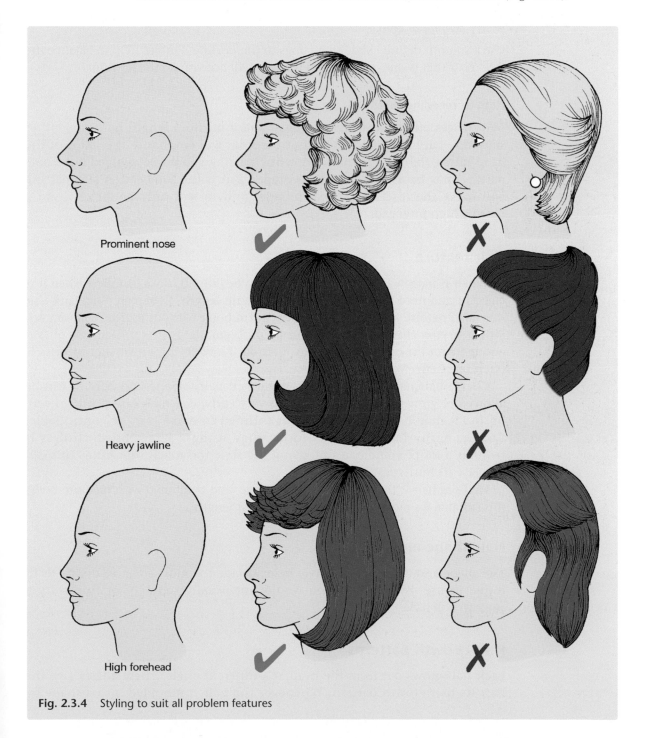

Prominent nose

Heavy jawline

High forehead

**Fig. 2.3.4**    Styling to suit all problem features

### Prominent nose

Emphasise other parts of the face and head with soft curls at the chin line or hair that hugs the face. If a fringe is worn it should be full and loose. Avoid centre partings as this emphasises the length of the nose and draws attention to it.

### Heavy jawline or chin

Use a smooth definite style that clings to the jawline. Fringes help to balance the face. Hair that is drawn back from the face will accentuate the jawline.

### High or receding forehead

Full fringes minimise a high forehead and a medium length hairstyle, either smoothly curving or flicked back at the sides will emphasise the shape of the head rather than the forehead. A centre parting should be avoided but a side parting may be used if the hair is draped across the forehead. A side parting will make the forehead appear broader and so will only be effective on a narrow high forehead.

## Hair texture

Fine hair is narrow in diameter and tends to be limp. It looks its fullest when it is club cut and need to grow no longer than chin length. Extremely fine, lank hair may also require a soft perm to give it extra body without a great deal of curl. Finger drying this type of hair can be problematic as it is difficult to obtain enough root lift or volume by this method. Blow-drying on smaller brushes is often more effective.

Coarse hair has a larger diameter and is usually strong and wiry. It can be allowed to grow longer unless it is also very curly, in which case it will go very bushy. It may have to be layered or thinned to make it more controllable. Coarse, bushy hair may need to be dried using a larger brush. Unless it requires a lot of volume, avoid giving the style too much root lift as this can increase its bushyness.

Medium hair is the easiest type to manage, and combined with medium body, it is suitable for most hairstyles and most hair lengths.

## Hair shape and cut

The shape and cut of the hairstyle helps decide the most effective drying technique to use. For example you would not usually scrunch- or finger-dry a smooth bob style.

## Hair growth patterns

Each hair grows out from the head at a different angle. These angles give the hair its hair growth pattern. Whenever the hair is moulded into a shape by finger, blow or natural drying, the direction of the hair's growth pattern *must* be taken into account before starting the treatment.

Always try to incorporate the natural fall or any movement of hair into the finished style; this will make it last much longer. Any problems such as double crown, awkward hairline, etc., should be carefully camouflaged by the way it is styled.

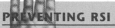

**PREVENTING RSI**

Create mini-breaks (30 seconds or so) to move around and rest your hands and arms. You might use this time to explain to your client how to maintain the style, which conditioners or shampoos to use, etc. Be resourceful – your client will appreciate the special attention, so the time is not wasted. Making the client's next appointment gives you the rest and encourages your client to return.

## Hair elasticity

Hair elasticity is an important consideration in styling because it largely determines the movement and bounce in the finished style. Hair in good condition has a high level of elasticity.

## Personality and lifestyle of the client

The client's finished hairstyle should meet their needs. Sporting hobbies create the need for a sleek, well-cut, easy-to-manage hairstyle, whereas a client who entertains a great deal will probably need a more elaborate hairstyle. Likewise, a quiet, subdued person will not thank the stylist for an outrageous style whereas a person with an extrovert personality probably would.

When the client arrives, look at the style of clothes and the image they currently project, find out if they wish to change their image and what they expect of the style. In other words, look and listen very carefully to the client *before* beginning the treatment. Client consultation is extremely important to allow you to use the correct products, equipment and techniques to give the best results.

## Setting tools

### Brushes

There are many different brushes; the choice depends upon the task and the stylist's general preference. The brush most commonly used to dress out a set is called a general-purpose brush. General-purpose brushes are made in various shapes and sizes and can be half, three-quarters or full round. Natural bristle is recommended because of its more gentle action on the hair.

## Combs

A variety of combs have been engineered to aid the dressing, disentangling or setting of hair. Whichever type of comb is used, it should be made of a sturdy, durable material which will not create static electricity and which must also be easy to sterilise after use. Vulcanite is the material used for most hairdressing combs as it fits all these requirements. The teeth of the comb should have rounded points with a fine taper and there should be adequate space between them where they join the base. Combs can be obtained in many shapes and sizes; here are the most common:

### Tail comb

Tail combs have fine teeth. The tail part of the comb can be made of the same material as the teeth or it can have a thin metal, stiletto tail (known as a pintail comb). Care must be taken when using a pintail comb as the tail is almost like a fine knitting needle and if used carelessly it can stab either the client or the operator. Tail combs are for sectioning, lifting or weaving the hair. Never use the tail comb for disentangling the hair as the teeth are too fine.

### SAFETY TIPS

Combs with broken or irregular teeth should not be used as they may scratch the scalp or tear the hair.

### Dressing comb

Dressing combs have a fine end and a rake end; they can be obtained in various sizes according to individual preference. They are used for disentangling and dressing hair.

The wide teeth of a dressing comb are normally used to smooth and mould the hair. There are many sizes of dressing combs to choose from and the stylist should choose whichever is the most comfortable to handle. Very large dressing combs are more difficult to use but are ideal when there is a lot of volume and for backcombing the hair as it smooths the hair into shape very quickly and easily without flattening or removing too much of the backcombing.

There are various other dressing combs available; some are specially adapted to incorporate larger teeth at one end to smooth the hair, and prongs at the other end to lift the hair if necessary, thus incorporating the duties of both dressing comb and tail comb. Other combs have been designed to aid backcombing by having alternate long and short teeth.

### Setting comb

Setting combs have a fine end and a rake end, usually smaller than a dressing comb. It can also be used by the stylist when finger waving.

### Afro comb

Afro combs are very thick; their large teeth are ideal for creating volume without frizz on extremely curly or Afro-Caribbean hair.

## Practical methods for setting hair

### Rollers (roller setting)

Rollers are used in setting to give lift, height and volume to a hairstyle. To produce a successful style that is durable and lasts well, careful planning is needed. The planning can be divided into two areas:

- Natural hair direction.
- The size of rollers.

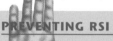

**PREVENTING RSI**

Adjust the chair height to avoid bending and to avoid holding the arms up – both great strains on the arms and shoulders. Headaches are a common result of straining the shoulder muscles – as they are attached to the skull at the back and sides of the neck. Change your position by using a stool to sit on. Turn the chair for further flexibility. Avoid bending your back; bend your knees to keep your spine in its proper position.

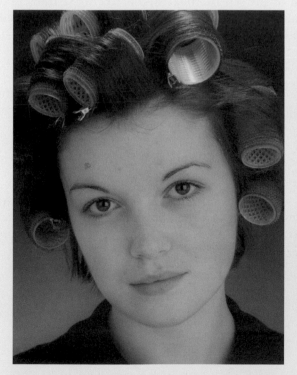
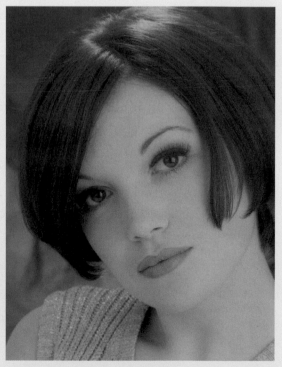

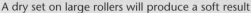
A dry set on large rollers will produce a soft result

### Natural hair direction

The rollers should be placed in the hair in the direction of the finished style, so it is very important to decide beforehand the movements of the finished style. Before placing any rollers in the hair, always comb the hair thoroughly to see which way the hair falls naturally. The growth direction of the hair is known as the hair growth pattern. This growth direction of the hair is built into the hair due to the distribution and angle of the hair follicles in the skin.

Setting the hair against the hair growth pattern may produce a good result when it is combed out initially, but the style will not last very long and will tend to stick out at odd angles to the scalp the following day. As most clients expect their sets to last from one shampoo to the next, it is important to make full use of any natural features like hair growth patterns and incorporate them into the style.

Different results can be achieved depending on how the roller section and rollers are angled from the scalp. Remember that the hair will dry where it is placed, also it is important to angle the roller and roller section correctly to achieve the desired result. Three different effects are shown in Figs 2.3.5–2.3.7.

The placing of rollers in straight, ladder-like rows, particularly at the hairline, should be avoided if possible as it causes breaks in the hairstyle and makes dressing out more difficult. Any wispy hair at the nape of the neck should not be dragged, as this will not curl it tightly enough. If the hair has been correctly set there should be little need for much backcombing when dressing out, as the hairstyle should fall into place when it is brushed.

After planning the direction of the set, the next step is to choose the size of the roller to use in order to achieve the required result. The following factors will influence the size of curler to use.

### Hair texture and density

It is important to check carefully not only the texture of the hair, but also the density, before choosing the roller size to use. The **texture** of the hair refers to its

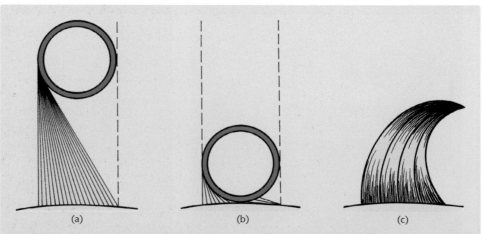

**Fig. 2.3.5**   Roller positioning for normal lift: the hair is wound at right angles to the scalp; the roller should be placed exactly in the centre of its own section

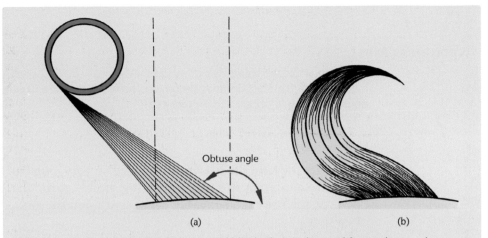

**Fig. 2.3.6**    Roller positioning for increased lift: the hair is dragged forward at an obtuse angle to the scalp

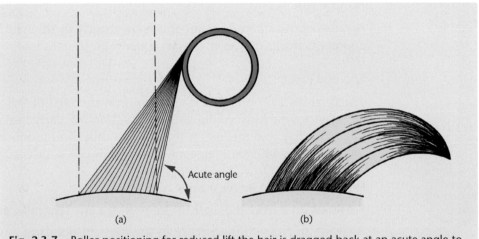

**Fig. 2.3.7**    Roller positioning for reduced lift the hair is dragged back at an acute angle to the scalp

diameter; a large diameter applies to thick hair and a small diameter to fine hair. The **density** refers to the amount of hair on the head. It is possible to have fine textured hair that it very abundant (i.e. a lot of hairs per square inch on the scalp); likewise, it is possible to have thick textured hair that is very sparse (i.e. few hairs per square inch on the scalp).

Fine textured hair usually needs a smaller roller than thick textured hair to produce the same amount of curl, because there are fewer water-breakable crosslinkages in fine hair. But if the hair is very abundant (or dense), this can create too much curl because of the amount of hair.

Thick textured hair usually needs a larger roller, but again the density of the hair must also be taken into consideration. If the hair is very sparse, a larger roller may not be needed.

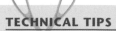

**TECHNICAL TIPS**

The more times the hair is wound round the roller, the more polypeptide chains are moved when the cross-linkages are broken. So when they are fixed in their new positions by drying, a tighter curl is produced.

### Hair length

The longer the hair, the heavier it becomes; so very long hair may need a smaller roller to counteract the hair's dragging effect, particularly for a curly style. However, the size of roller is very dependent upon the amount of curl in the finished style.

Long hairstyles that are very smooth need rollers with an extremely large diameter; a roller that is too small will produce too much wave and curl movement, and this makes dressing the hair difficult.

### Natural curl

Because of the amount of curl and body already in the hair, naturally curly hair and permed hair may need a larger roller than straight hair.

### The end result

The final decision on roller size depends on the type of style the client requires, i.e. whether the finished dressing is to be smooth, curly, wavy or a combination. The main rule to remember is that a small roller will produce a small curl with a lot of bounce, whereas a large roller will produce a large curl with less bounce.

### How to place a roller for normal root lift

1. Divide off a section of hair the same width and length as the roller.
2. Comb the hair thoroughly from the roots to points at a right angle from the scalp.
3. Place the points of the hair in the centre of the roller, making sure the tension is even on either side of the section. Then turn the roller, using the thumbs to hold the points in position until they are locked round the roller.
4. Wind the hair and roller evenly down to the scalp. The wound roller should be in the centre of the section when wound.

Note the position of the securing pin if one is used. It should hold the roller firmly in position without marking the hair and it should never be secured in a way that marks the client's scalp or causes the client discomfort.

Once the skill of correctly placing a roller in the hair has been mastered, it is possible to experiment with different roller positions to create different effects. Combing the wet hair into the direction of the finished style before setting, then placing the rollers in this direction, leads to more interesting styling and also produces a more durable hairstyle for the client.

## Mistakes and precautions when roller setting

- Hair section too wide. This causes drag at the roots, either in front of the roller or behind the roller.
- Hair section too narrow. The roller will overlap onto the next hair section so that the root hair of this section will be dried completely flat to the head (Fig. 2.3.8(a)). If all the hair sections are too narrow, the root lift will be uneven throughout the head.
- Hair section too long. This causes loose hair at each end of the roller when winding (Fig. 2.3.8(b)).

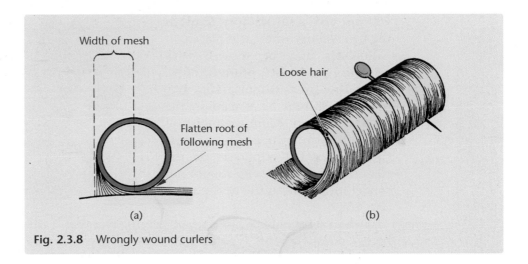

**Fig. 2.3.8**    Wrongly wound curlers

- Hair section too short. This creates the same problem as the hair sections which are too narrow, i.e. the roller will overlap and flatten the hair at the sides of the roller and can also cause difficulties when placing the other rollers.
- Roller pin pressing onto the scalp. This will leave marks on the skin and will cause the client discomfort.
- Roller pin not securing the roller properly. The roller will drop or become displaced while drying, which will spoil the finished style.
- Roller pin marking the hair. This can create kinks in the hair when dry.
- Hair points bent back or not wound completely round the roller when winding will create fish-hook ends, which when dressed make the hair appear frizzy on the ends.
- Uneven tension or winding. This leads to uneven movements in the hair.
- Placing rollers in straight, ladder-like rows causes breaks in the style and creates difficulties when dressing the hair.
- Wispy nape hairs should not be dragged or the napeline of the finished style will be uneven.
- Never underestimate the importance of the natural direction of hair growth. A well-placed set not only helps the dressing of hair but also gives a long-lasting style.

## Pincurls

To style the hair with pincurls the hair should be thoroughly wet to allow the stylist to mould the hair correctly. It is important to use any natural hair growth patterns and movements to give durability to the style. As with roller setting, the hair should be combed in the direction of the finished style and the pincurls placed in that direction. A pincurl is usually taken from a square section and the curl must be kept as round at the points of the hair as it is at the roots. The durability of the pincurl depends on its degree of roundness and how smoothly it is wound from the roots. Twisting or buckling the hair, either at the roots or along its length, will not give a satisfactory result as the hair will dry where it is placed.

Pincurls may be secured with one-pronged or two-pronged clips, depending on personal preference, but they should be placed so the ends of the clip secure the points of the hair firmly in position while the head of the clip rests on the stem of the curl; the clip should not hinder formation of the next pincurl (Fig. 2.3.9).

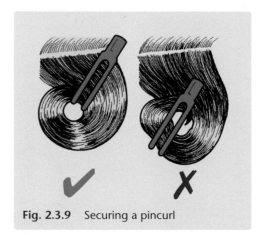

Fig. 2.3.9    Securing a pincurl

Special care should be taken when securing hair that is either fine, bleached or highly porous as this type of hair marks easily. Pincurls are best suited to medium textured hair with a slight natural movement. Very thick or extremely curly hair is difficult to pincurl and buckles easily, whereas very fine, straight hair usually needs extra lift and body.

The size of the pincurl is determined by the hair texture and the finished style. Thick hair usually needs a larger pincurl than fine hair to achieve the same result. The pincurl will loosen and drop slightly when it is dressed, so allowance should be made for this by making the diameter of the pincurl slightly smaller than the required result. There are several different types.

### Clockspring (Fig. 2.3.10(a))

The clockspring pincurl is small and tight with a closed centre which produces a tight curl on the ends and a looser wave at the root – A clockspring pincurl is usually used at the nape of the neck when a curly effect is required.

### Flat barrel spring (Fig. 2.3.10(b))

the flat barrel spring is an open-centred curl which is formed flat to the head. This is the most common type of pincurl and is also used when reverse pincurling to form wave movements.

### Barrel spring or stand-up (Fig. 2.3.10(c))

The stand-up pincurl also has an open centre and is formed to stand up from the head. It is secured by passing a clip through the curl at the base. Its stem direction is directed up and away from the direction of the finished dressing, creating lift and volume in the same manner as a roller. If it is used in conjunction with rollers, the pincurl must be the same diameter as the rollers.

### Stem curls (Fig. 2.3.10(d))

Stem curls are open-centred pincurls with a long stem. A section of hair is taken from a square base and wound either from root or point. The curl is then placed above, below or to either side of the base, depending on the direction of the finished style; this produces a long stem to the pincurl and can be used to accentuate hair growth direction at the nape or sides of the head.

### Sculptured curls (Fig. 2.3.10(e))

To create sculptured curls, the hair is combed thoroughly and moulded in the exact position for its dressing; it is then secured by either tape or clips. Tape is usually used in preference to clips as it does not mark the hair and it holds the moulded hair more securely in position. A sculptured curl produces a soft effect at the nape, sides or fringe area, especially on very short hair.

### Reverse pincurls (Fig. 2.3.10(f))

Reverse pincurls are formed in one direction and then reversed back around the head in the opposite direction. On looking closely at a wave movement, it reveals an S–shape, which bends in one direction and then bends back in the opposite direction. By reversing the pincurls one way and then another, it is therefore possible to achieve wave movements in the hair.

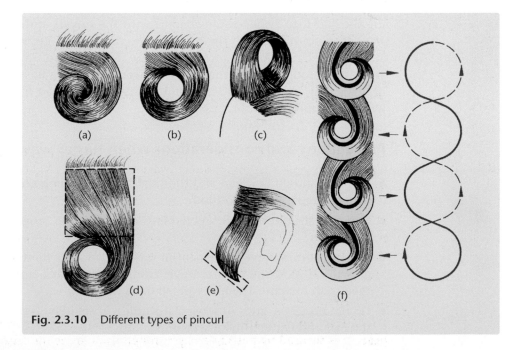

**Fig. 2.3.10**    Different types of pincurl

## Precautions and considerations when pincurling

- Hair should always be thoroughly wet when pincurling.
- Carefully consider the hair and its growth patterns before starting to pincurl.
- Use any natural wave movements.
- Work to the shape of the head, i.e. in curved movements not straight lines.
- The durability of the curl depends on its degree of roundness; a perfect pincurl should be as round at the points as it is at the roots.
- Do not twist or buckle the hair, either when forming the pincurl or when securing it.
- Special consideration should be given to permed, tinted, bleached or highly porous hair, as these hair types are often more difficult to pincurl and can mark or buckle more easily.
- The hair should be kept flat when forming the pincurl unless it is a stand-up pincurl.
- The diameter of the pincurl determines the size of the final curl, so take care to wind the correct size of pincurl for the desired effect. Bear in mind that the set will drop slightly when dry.
- When reverse pincurling, the pincurls along each row should be wound in the same direction but in the opposite direction to the previous row. The curls should be a uniform size and arranged in a brickwork pattern to eliminate unwanted partings.

## Finger waving

Also known as flat waving or water waving, finger waving is a method of moulding the hair into S-shaped movements with the fingers and comb, producing a wave. The point at which the hair changes direction is known as the crest (Fig. 2.3.11); the height of the crest, hence the depth of the wave, depends on the amount of moulding with the fingers. Finger waving can be achieved on straight or wavy hair, but naturally tight curls, coarse or permed hair will not usually wave successfully.

## Precautions and considerations when finger waving

- The hair should be clean and thoroughly wet. A thick gel setting lotion will help to keep waves in position.
- The hair should be well tapered and of reasonable length, particularly on the crown.
- Use any natural wave movement in the hair – do not fight against the natural growth. To find the natural wave, comb all hair back from the client's face then push forward. The hair will fall in its natural line.
- Do not use clips, grips or wave claws unless absolutely necessary as they mark the hair and flatten the wave centres.

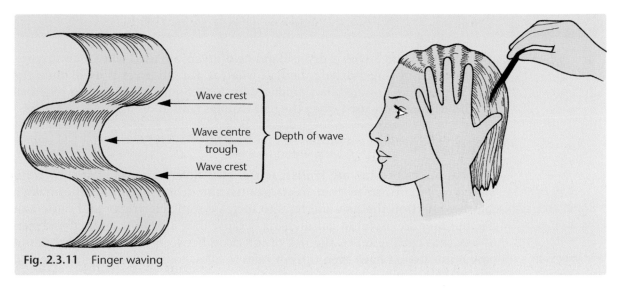

**Fig. 2.3.11** Finger waving

- Use the coarse end of the comb and avoid scratching the scalp by leaning the comb slightly towards you.
- All waves should be the same width and slightly smaller than the required result to allow for slight loosening.
- Always wave towards the parting and never wave in straight lines.
- Ensure that the underneath hair is waved. Lifting the hair into place when finger waving can distort the roots.

# Activity

This activity has been devised to help you to understand the effects of different roller sizes on the hair. Divide your tuition head into six sections. Wind a different size roller onto each section. Dry the hair and remove the rollers. Examine the result then write your findings in the form of a table:

|  | Size of roller | Result |
|---|---|---|
| Section 1 | | |
| Section 2 | | |
| Section 3 | | |
| Section 4 | | |
| Section 5 | | |
| Section 6 | | |

## Drying hair: tools and equipment

Hair is usually dried with a dryer. Hand-held dryers are used when blow-drying, blow-waving or finger-drying the hair whereas a stand dryer is used when the hair has been set. Infrared heat produced by an 'octopus', climazone or rollerball machine is normally used when the hair requires natural drying.

### Brushes

Natural bristle brushes are kindest to the hair. Both hair and bristle are composed of keratin, so neither wears against the other. Nylon brushes have a harsher effect on the hair and tend to increase static electricity and cause hair fly, but they are useful in hairdressing because they are easily cleaned and sterilised, thus cutting down the risk of infection between clients. The bristles of any brush should have even tufts or rows to allow loose, shed hair to collect in the grooves without interfering with the action of the bristles. Styling brushes are used when blow-drying the hair. They can be obtained in various sizes and shapes depending upon the result required. They are made from nylon, bristle or a combination of both.

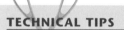

**TECHNICAL TIPS**

If the bristle tufts of brushes are spaced too close together, they will not penetrate the hair.

### Electrically heated styling irons

- **Hair tongs** – round and usually obtained in small, medium and large sizes; they are used to create curl or movement, e g. after blow-drying or between sets.
- **Crimping irons** – specifically designed to produce a crimped effect on the hair.
- **Straightening irons** – originally designed to temporarily straighten Afro-Caribbean hair but now also used on Caucasian (European) hair to produce straight or flattened results.

**POINTS TO REMEMBER**

Metal tools should not be left in a vapour-type sterilising cabinet for too long, as the chemicals used in these cabinets can cause corrosion.

## Hot brushes

Hot brushes work on the same principle and have the same use as round styling irons, but instead of just a smooth electrically heated barrel, the hot brush has vulcanite prongs that act as a brush. Thus, the hair can be combed and curled into position more easily.

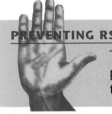

**PREVENTING RSI**

Take care when blow-drying as the wrist motion with the brush can result in painful inflammation of tendons at the elbows. Learn to alternate hands for the dryer and the brush.

## Pressing combs

There are two types of pressing comb: electrical and non-electrical. The comb has metal prongs (steel or brass) and a wooden or vulcanite handle. Pressing combs are used to temporarily straighten Afro-Caribbean hair and extremely curly hair. The comb is heated then combed through the hair.

## Combs

Combs are useful for drying short hair when a brush would give too much lift. A comb is often used when blow-waving men's hair as it allows more control, particularly in conjunction with the flattened nozzle attachment of the hand dryer.

## Diffusers

A diffuser is an attachment which fixes onto the end of the hand dryer in place of the nozzle. The diffuser disperses the air over a larger area instead of concentrating it in a stream onto the hair. The diffuser also makes it easier for the stylist to manipulate the hair with the fingers when either finger drying or scrunch drying.

## Drying techniques

### Blow-drying

Blow-drying is used to create a natural, soft effect and the finished result should be smooth and bouncy. There are many methods of blow-drying the hair and each stylist may use slight variations to achieve the same result. But all methods should include certain precautions to achieve a successful finish. See Unit 1.1 for how to blow-dry long, one-length hair.

## Before a blow-dry

1. Always talk to the client to find out their requirements before beginning the treatment.

2. The client must be well protected with gown and towel.

3. The client's hair must be clean and in good condition. It is often beneficial to use a conditioner after shampooing; use an oil-free conditioner if the hair tends to be greasy. A conditioner will give a healthier, shinier finish to the style.

4. Note the texture of the hair. Fine hair will need more body than thick hair; so the finer the hair, the smaller the diameter of the hairbrush.

5. Note the amount of curl present in the hair. Curly hair needs more control than straighter hair, especially at the roots. Taking smaller sections of hair when drying helps to overcome this problem.

6. Note the direction of the hair growth. Do not work against hair growth as the hair could stick up and become unmanageable and the style will not last.

7. A conditioning blow-styling lotion gives a more durable style and helps to reduce static electricity.

8. The sectioning of longer hair helps the stylist work more quickly, methodically and efficiently.

9. Combing hair in the direction of the desired style, particularly short hair, helps the operator to dry the hair in the correct direction.

## While blow-drying

1. The jet of the air should follow the direction of the brush and hair. Never blow against the cuticle of the hair as this can be damaging and give a rough finish to the style.

2. Never allow the jet of air to flow onto the client's scalp as it can cause burns to the skin.

3. Make sure that each section of hair is completely dry before starting on the next section. If the hair is still damp, the shape of the style will not last.

4. The size of the section depends on the size of the brush. The smaller the brush, the smaller the sections. Taking too large a section and dragging the hair can make the style flat.

5. More curl and body can be achieved by winding the hair around the brush, drying with a hot jet of air and then allowing the hair to cool still wrapped around the brush. For speed, the brush is left in the hair while cooling takes place and another brush of the same size is used on the next section of hair.

6. Make sure the points of the hair are dried evenly around the brush. Rotating the brush while drying helps to prevent kinking of the hair.

7. Finger drying is sometimes more effective for very short hair. It is often better to use finger drying for short hair at the nape, on the sides or on the fringe, as a brush gives too much lift.

8. Blow-drying long hair can be tedious and time-consuming. To save time it is often easier to dry off the roots of the hair by brushing it in the opposite direction than the finished style and allowing the jet of air to dry the root section in this position. When the hair is combed back into its original position there is then a good degree of lift at the roots. The points of the hair are then dried in the direction of the style.

### After a blow-dry

1. When blow-drying is completed, allow the hair to cool thoroughly then check that the hair is completely dry. Warm hair often gives the illusion of dryness while it is still damp.
2. Comb or brush the hair into the finished style. Check that the sides are blended into the back, pay particular attention to the nape area to make sure the shape is pleasing and check the balance of the finished dressing from the front, sides and back of the head, making full use of the mirror.
3. Apply a fine spray of lacquer or shine and smooth down any flyaway hairs with the back of the comb or palm of the hand.

## Finger drying

Drying the hair with the fingers creates a tousled, natural effect. The hair is combed in the direction of the finished style and the fingers are then used to create lift and movement where needed. A hand dryer with a diffuser attachment is often used and the air is directed to the roots of the hair as it is moulded by the fingers. The hair may also be squeezed between the fingers while it is dried to give more movement. This is known as scrunch drying the hair. This is particularly useful for clients who prefer a more natural look to their hair.

## Blow-waving

Blow-waving the hair is a method of waving the hair, producing soft natural movements with the aid of a comb or brush and heated air from a hand hairdryer. The hair is held in a wave position and a flattened nozzle dryer attachment directs and concentrates the flow of heated air. The control required to form wave shapes is determined by movements of the comb or brush and dryer, in relation to the hair position. It is mainly used in men's hairdressing.

**SAFETY TIPS**

Take care not to burn the fingers with the jet of air when finger drying the hair.

## Natural drying

Natural drying means leaving the hair to dry naturally. Comb the hair into the position of the finished dressing. It is sometimes easier to use a very wide-toothed comb to do this, particularly if the hair is curly. Putting the head upside down then letting it fall back is a way of achieving root lift. When the hair is in position the client is placed under an infrared heat machine to speed up the drying time.

Do not be tempted to recomb or brush the hair while it is drying; curly hair will frizz and the effect will be spoilt.

## Dressing hair

Dressing the hair is of equal importance to setting or blow-drying, for although good setting or blow-drying will make the style durable and easier to dress, the actual dressing of the hair will give the final image.

Dressing the hair requires plenty of practice to gain the confidence to work quickly and efficiently and to know when enough work has been carried out on the head. It is almost like putting the finishing touches to a painting. A good artist will know almost instinctively when the picture looks right and will stop working on it. By dabbling about too much after this stage, the image can be completely ruined.

## Dressing hair

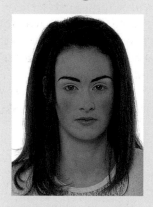 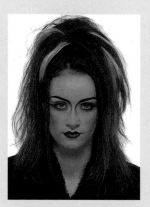 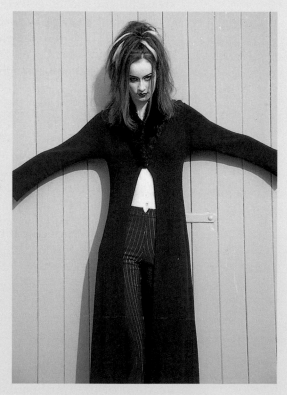

Before dressing, the hairstyle is smooth and flatter. The hair is then backcombed and false hair incorporated into the style to give volume and create an avant-garde look. The clothes and make-up complete the overall image.

*Source*: Hair by Plassey Hair Studio, Wrexham

## Dressing creams, shine enhancers and waxes

Dressing creams, shine enhancers and waxes are used to reduce static electricity and to replace any natural oil that may have been removed when shampooing. They will also add a shine or gloss to dull, dry hair. Most of these products are made from mineral oil with perfume added. Mineral oil is used in preference to vegetable oil because it does not go rancid and does not penetrate the hair shaft. It remains on the surface, giving a better shine than vegetable oil. This also helps to protect the hair from dampness.

### Dressing creams

Dressing creams do not need to be used on every head of hair but only if the hair is dry or very flyaway. Do not use them on hair which tends to be greasy as they will encourage this condition. After brushing the hair thoroughly, apply a small amount of the cream to the palm of the hand (about the size of a pea). Rub the hands together then gently stroke the hair with the hands, making sure the cream is also applied to the underneath layers. Take care to avoid applying too much as this will make the hair too greasy and lank. When the cream has been applied, rebrush the hair thoroughly to distribute the cream evenly throughout the whole head.

### Shine enhancers

Dressing oils or shine enhancers as opposed to creams can be obtained in sprays or aerosols and are known as spray-on shine or hair gloss. They are usually applied after completion of the dressing to add shine and lustre to the hair. Hold the can or spray about 30 cm (12 in) away from the scalp and direct the spray just above the head to prevent the oil being concentrated in one area. The oil will then drop onto the hair and will coat it more evenly if applied in this manner. It is very important to use this type of dressing oil sparingly; too much will make the hair appear greasy and lank.

### Waxes

Waxes are used to give texture to the hair (Fig. 2.3.12). A small amount is rubbed quickly between the hands. The friction of the rubbing movement creates heat which melts the wax. The wax is then quickly applied to the hair before it cools. Once cool it becomes more solid again which helps to hold the hair in position in addition to giving it a more textured look. Do not use waxes on fine, lank hair.

## Backcombing for extra volume

### Backcombing

Backcombing is pushing the hair back on itself at the root to give a lifted full effect using a comb. Backcombing is also sometimes used to temporarily

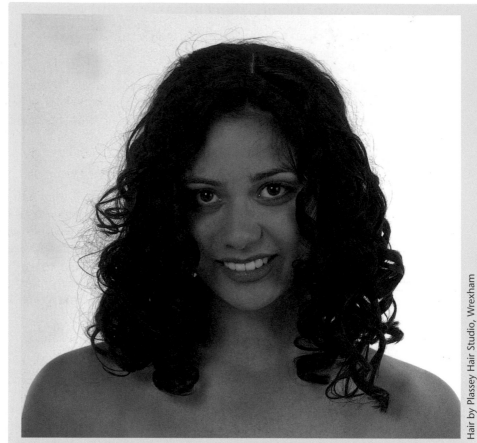

Hair by Plassey Hair Studio, Wrexham

**Fig. 2.3.12**    Below shoulder length hair has been dressed with the fingers then wax has been used to keep the textured curl

straighten overcurly hair. Backcombing the hair at the roots underneath the hair section will give volume. Backcombing on top of the section will help to blend the hair together and give an even spread of hair; this is often called **teasing**.

### Basic backcombing

1. Brush the hair into the shape and direction of the style then decide which area of the head needs extra volume; usually this is on top of the head and the crown area.

2. Start at the top or front of the head and take a narrow section of hair in the direction of the style.

3. Lift out from the scalp at right angles. Holding the hair section firmly in one hand and the comb in the other, insert the comb into the section approximately 2–3 cm ($\frac{3}{4}$ to $1\frac{1}{8}$ in) away from the scalp.

4. Push back the hair to the root repeatedly until enough hair has been pushed back to form a padding at the root. The more the hair is pushed back, the greater the lift.

5. Continue until the areas which need extra volume are completed.

6. Always remember to hold the hair firmly while backcombing. If you allow the hair section to sag while the comb is pushing back the hair to the roots, this will prevent the hair from being pushed back correctly and will make the style flop.

7. The size of the section depends upon the density and thickness of the hair and the amount of volume required, but the finished backcombing should not be visible at the front of the section as this creates difficulties when smoothing the hair over the backcombing.

8. If the backcombing does penetrate through to the front of the section then the section is too fine.

It is usually only necessary to backcomb the hair at the root area as this is where the lift is needed. Only if extreme height is required by the hairstyle is it usually necessary to backcomb the hair past the mid-lengths towards the points.

A common fault when backcombing is not pushing the hair right back to the scalp, creating a padded effect at the mid-lengths instead of at the roots. When the hair is smoothed over, the root area remains floppy, giving no lift whatsoever.

## Backcombing

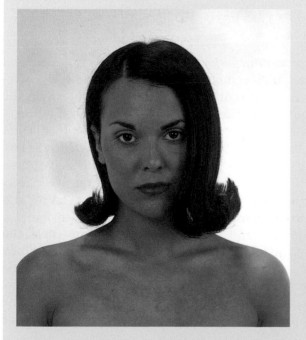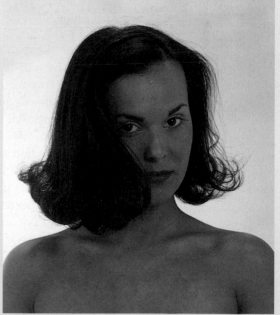

A smooth hairstyle can be backcombed to give fuller, more unstructured effect

*Source*: Hair by Plassey Hair Studio, Wrexham

### The teasing method

Teasing does not give the same lift to the hair but it is used to blend the hair together, giving an even spread of hair and a smoother finish to the dressing. It can be used with backcombing or on its own.

Larger sections of hair are taken where needed and held between the fingers and thumb. The hair is then pushed back on itself on top of the hair section while the hair between the fingers is pulled in the direction of the style. When smoothing the hair after teasing, take care to smooth the hair gently so as not to remove all the backcombing.

### Removing backcombing

Clients should always be advised how to remove backcombing from their hair. Incorrect removal can be very painful for the client and damaging to the hair. Start removal at the nape of the neck, with the wide-spaced teeth of a dressing comb. Always start at the points of the hair and work downwards towards the roots.

## Backbrushing for extra volume

This is pushing the hair back on itself either under or on top of the hair section to give a lifted effect using the brush.

Backbrushing gives a softer effect than backcombing and is useful for longer hair; backcombing long hair tends to create too much lift and there is the danger of the hair becoming too entangled.

## Line and balance

Balance refers to the shape of the dressing in relation to the client's face, head and neck. The lines of the hairstyle should complement the wearer, and each movement should complement or flow naturally into the next. Judging when the finished style is balanced requires practice and that indefinable something – instinct or flair perhaps – that tells the stylist the dressing looks right on the client.

The use of the mirror while dressing the hair helps to keep a check on the balance of the hairstyle by putting the style in perspective. Dressing the hair at close quarters limits the vision of the stylist to one area only; so by frequently checking the outline and shape of the dressing in the mirror, the stylist can see at a glance where the shape needs to be altered.

When the dressing is complete, stand away from the head and check the line and balance of the style at the front, sides and back of the head. First look at the silhouette of the hairstyle; this will help to show up any defects in the balance of the dressing. Then check that the movements and/or smoothness within the silhouette are correct. Next check that the edges along the hairline are even and that the lines blend into each other and complement the face and neck.

## Final image

It is the final image on which the client will largely judge the salon. It is worth a few extra seconds therefore to check that nothing mars the line of the hairstyle. Remove any stray, wispy neck hairs with the scissors. When you are completely satisfied with the result, show the client the finished style from all angles in a hand mirror. Do not apply any lacquer before making sure the client is pleased with the result; the style may have to be changed slightly and this is difficult after the lacquer has been applied.

### How to apply the lacquer

1. Protect the client's eyes and face with a face shield or with the free hand.
2. Aim the spray just above the dressing to allow the lacquer to drop onto the hair. While lacquering the hair, the spray should be moved in the direction of the hairstyle so that any movement of air does not disturb the dressing.
3. Spray the lacquer from a distance of 30 cm (12 in) so that a fine even spray coats the hair. Spraying the hair too near to the head will saturate only one area and this could wet the hair too much, causing it to drop. Alternatively, the lacquer may form blobs on the hair, which dry into white nodules.
4. When enough lacquer has been applied to the hair, recheck the dressing carefully and smooth any flyaway hairs with the flat of the hands or the back of the comb.

### Hair-fixing sprays

Hair-fixing sprays are developed from synthetic plastic polymers dissolved in alcohol; they coat the hair with a clear plastic film. A mixture of two plastic film formers is often used, e.g. polyvinyl pyrrolidone (PVP) and polyvinyl acetate (PVA):

- General use – 60%PVP, 40% PVA
- Hard holding – 70% PVP, 30% PVA

When lacquer is sprayed onto the hair the alcohol evaporates leaving the resin or plastic coating on the hair. This tends to stick or mildly glue the hair in place when the alcohol solvent evaporates. Hair lacquers can be sprayed onto the hair using either a hand-pumped spray or a pressurised aerosol spray can. Public concern for the environment has made manufacturers more aware of the need to produce aerosol spray cans which are ozone friendly, i.e. they do not contain **chlorofluorocarbons** which destroy the ozone layer.

**SAFETY TIPS**

Because lacquer sprays are often **flammable**, do not allow a client to smoke when lacquering their hair. As the contents are under pressure, heat will increase the pressure and may cause the can to burst. Do not store spray cans on heaters or in direct sunlight. Do not puncture or burn them, even when empty.

## How to dress a basic set

1. Gown the client to protect their clothing.

2. Check the hair is completely dry by removing one of the rollers (usually where the hair is thickest or longest) and test the ends of the hair. If the hair is damp, it will lose its springiness and will not comb out into shape.

3. Remove the rollers and clips from the hair gently without tugging, then allow the hair to cool for a few minutes.

4. Loosen the set and help eradicate any roller partings by double brushing or by using the brush and comb to brush the hair thoroughly from root to point in all directions over the head.

5. Apply a small amount of dressing cream if the hair appears dry or flyaway. If an aerosol or spray type is used, this may be applied when the dressing is complete.

6. Brush the hair into shape using one brush and following each stroke with the other hand to smooth and shape the hair. Stroke the brush in the planned direction of the set, taking into consideration any wave or curl movements.

7. Backcomb or backbrush any areas of the hairstyle that need extra volume or lift; remember that not all styles need backcombing.

8. Lightly comb the surface of the hair to shape and smooth it into position; the free hand can also be used to follow the comb, helping to smooth the hair. It may be necessary to tease certain areas at this stage so that the lines and movements blend into the shape.

9. Check the line and balance of the hairstyle from all angles making sure it is the correct shape and suits the client. Remove any wispy neck hairs.

10. Show the client the finished style in the hand mirror. If they are satisfied then apply a light spray of lacquer, remembering to use a face shield or the hand to protect the face and eyes.

## Precautions and considerations

1. Make sure the hair is completely dry before combing or dressing the hair. Straighter hair will drop if it is damp, whereas permed or naturally curly hair will frizz.

2. Use the correct tools. For example, do not use a tail comb for disentangling or smoothing the hair; the teeth are too fine and it can be painful for the client.

3. Fine hair should not be brushed as vigorously as normal or thick hair as it loses its springiness more easily.

4. Always work in the direction of the set when brushing, backcombing or smoothing the hair.

5. Use dressing creams and oils sparingly. Using too much may result in the hair having to be shampooed again to remove the excess grease.

6. Only backcomb or backbrush the hair where necessary. Putting too much backcombing into the hair is time-wasting and can damage the cuticle scales.

7. Take hair sections of the correct size when backcombing: too fine and the backcombing will be visible at the front of the section; too thick and the backcombing will not penetrate into the section far enough and it will be floppy.

8. Do not backcomb right to the points of the hair.

9. Make sure the backcombing is at the root of the hair to give the necessary lift; if it is only present at the mid-lengths, the hair will flop.

10. Do not let the comb penetrate too deeply through the section when smoothing, as this can remove too much backcombing.

11. Any areas that still need lifting even after backcombing can be lifted by the tail end of a tail comb.

12. Check regularly in the mirror when dressing the hair; this makes it easier to create the correct shape and balance.

13. Make sure the movements within the style complement each other and check the hair is blended.

14. The final dressing should be balanced from all angles, so check the style at the front, sides and back.

15. Asking the client to stand is sometimes a good idea; this helps to check the finished dressing in relation to the client's body proportions.

16. When the dressing is complete, remove any fallen hairs, etc., from the client's neck and shoulders with a neck brush.

17. Only use the lacquer after the client has been shown the finished style; if the style needs to be altered slightly, it can then be done with the minimum of fuss.

18. Do not spray the lacquer too close to the head as this concentrates it into one area and can wet the hair, causing it to drop.

19. Use only a fine spray of lacquer. Too much can cause beading of the lacquer and when dry it will look like white nodules on the hair.

20. Finally, do not overwork the hair. When the balance, shape and smoothness are correct, leave it alone.

## Dressing long hair

### Dressing long hair into a vertical roll pleat

1. Backcomb or backbrush the hair if necessary to give volume and hold the hair together (Fig. 2.3.13(a)). The backcombing or backbrushing is usually done underneath the hair section at the roots and possibly mid-lengths.

2. Leave out the top sections and take one side of the back section just past the centre back (Fig. 2.3.13(b)). Secure firmly with hairgrips positioned alternately up and down next to one another to prevent any hair from slipping through.

3. Brush the hair from the other side of the back section and brush towards the centre. Fold this hair under and secure with hairgrips making sure they do not show (Fig. 2.3.13(c)).

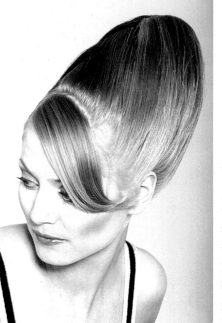

Goldwell/Michael Balfre Photography

4. Smooth the top hair and blend it in with the pleated back hair either by twisting it round into a curl, as shown in (Fig. 2.3.13(d)), or under like an envelope. Secure firmly with hairgrips.

### Dressing long hair into a horizontal roll

1. Backcomb or backbrush the hair, if necessary, to give volume and hold the hair together (Fig. 2.3.14(a)). The backbrushing should be placed underneath the direction in which the hair is to be dressed.

2. Smooth the top hair in the direction of the finished dressing, decide on the height at which to place the roll, then carefully place a row of hairgrips in an arc around the sides and back of the head. The hairgrips are usually placed approximately 2.5 cm (1 in) below the height of the finish roll to allow for the actual rolling of the hair (Fig. 2.3.14(b)).

3. Starting at one side of the head, the underneath hair is folded over into a roll in the direction indicated by the arrows in Fig. 2.3.14(c). Work in sections round the head, securing each rolled section with a hairgrip when it is thoroughly smoothed and in the correct position. Care should be taken to avoid showing any hairgrips in the final dressing.

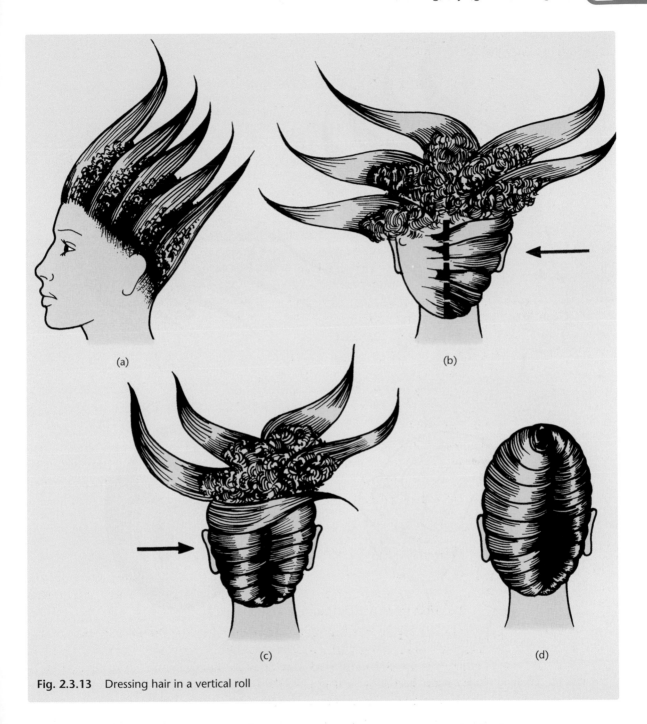

(a)

(b)

(c)

(d)

**Fig. 2.3.13**    Dressing hair in a vertical roll

4.  Figure 2.3.14(d) shows the finished dressing. Rolls can be varied by making them fuller or tighter, higher or lower. When dressing long, layered hair into a roll, it may be easier to brush the lower sections into a roll first, then smooth and blend in the top layers afterwards.

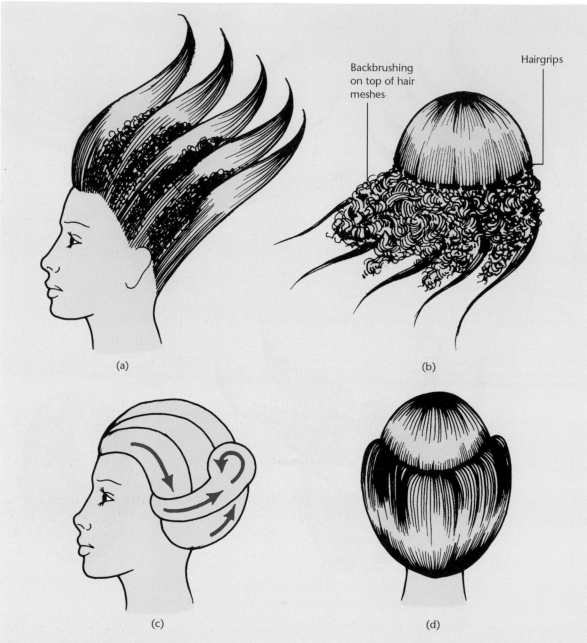

(a)

(b)

Backbrushing on top of hair meshes

Hairgrips

(c)

(d)

**Fig. 2.3.14**    Dressing hair in a horizontal roll

## Plaiting the hair

A plait is a method of weaving strands of hair together. The techniques are the same for both European and Afro-Caribbean hair. Any number of hair strands from two to sometimes more than seven may be used to create various effects. Plaits do not always have to be woven down towards the nape; they can be positioned across the head or plaited from the nape upwards. The way in which the hair is woven, under or over the hair strands, will also give variety.

When learning to plait, you first need to master how to manipulate your fingers for a three-stem plait. When you are used to weaving the hair strands over each other, experiment by bringing in extra strands, twisting the hair, weaving the hair under instead of over and placing the plait (or any number of plaits) in different positions on the head. Do not worry if your first attempts at plaiting are not very neat and your fingers feel too wooden to cope; remember that practice makes perfect and the more you experiment, the more confident and adept you will become.

### Plaiting a three-stem plait (English plait)

1. Divide the hair into three equal strands (Fig. 2.3.15(a)).
2. Take strand A to the right and wrap over strand B. Pull strand B in the opposite direction (left) to aid the wrapping (Fig. 2.3.15(b)).
3. Strand C is then taken to the left and wrapped over strand A (Fig. 2.3.15(c)).
4. Strand B is taken to the right over strand C in the same direction as strand A (Fig. 2.3.15(d).
5. Strand A is now taken back in the opposite direction and over the centre strand B (Fig. 2.3.15(e)).
6. Continue wrapping the strands over each other always taking the outside strands in towards the centre until all the hair has been plaited (Fig. 2.3.15(f)). Secure the ends of the hair with a covered band, or wrap a piece of the hair tightly round then tuck in the ends securely.

### Plaiting the hair to the scalp (French braid)

1. To plait the hair to the scalp, begin by gathering the top hair, from the temples to the crown, into a thin ponytail.
2. Divide this hair into the three equal sections and begin plaiting in the manner shown in Fig. 2.3.15(a) and (b). Hold the braid in the right hand, keeping the strands separate.

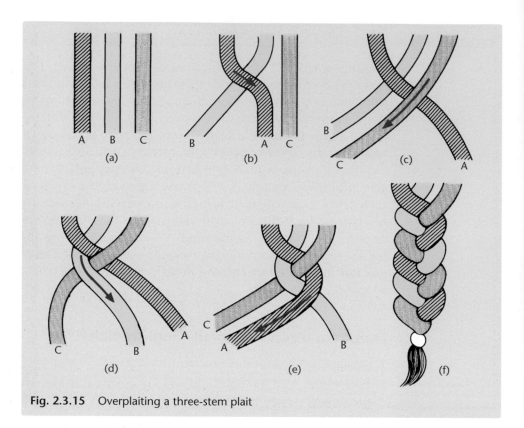

**Fig. 2.3.15**    Overplaiting a three-stem plait

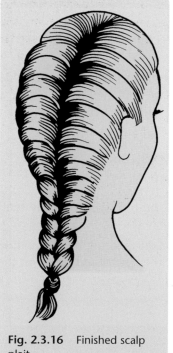

**Fig. 2.3.16**    Finished scalp plait

3. With the left hand, take a strand of hair from the front through to the back – about half the width of the originals – then draw it back towards the ponytail. Combine this new strand of hair with the left strand and cross over the centre.

4. Hold the plait in the left hand with the strands separated and take a section in the same way as before but on the opposite side of the head, making sure it is the same width as the previous strand and therefore equal on both sides of the head. Add this newly gathered hair to the right strand and cross over to the centre.

5. Continue taking fine, equal sections of hair from alternate sides of the head until the nape is reached and there is no more hair to section. Plait the remaining hair in an English braid as described previously (Fig. 2.3.16).

## Underplaiting the hair to the scalp

Underplaiting is carried out in almost the same way as a French braid. The hair is gathered into a fine ponytail from the temples through to the crown then divided into three equal sections. Commence plaiting as described previously, but wrap the hair **under** instead of over.

Fine strands of hair are then taken alternately from each side of the head and combined with the original strand of hair from that side, remembering to cross each strand under the centre instead of over. The finished result is a plait which rests on top of the hair instead of being incorporated into it. Underplaiting can also be done along the edge of the hair by including sections from only one side of the hair and combining them with the plait strands on that side.

1. Start the plaiting by wrapping strand A under strand B. strand B is taken to the left in the opposite direction (Fig. 2.3.17(a)).

2. Strand C is then taken to the left under strand A (Fig. 2.3.17(b)).

3. Strand B is taken to the left, in the opposite direction and then under strand C (Fig. 2.3.17(c)).

4. Figure 2.3.18(a) shows an underplait down the centre of the head. Note how the finished plait sits on top of the hair.

5. Underplaiting can be done along the edge of the hair on both sides of the head. The two plaits are held together with a covered band and the ends are then turned under and secured at the nape with hairgrips (Fig. 2.3.18(b)).

Usually known as **corn rowing**, the plaiting shown in Fig. 2.3.18(c) is extremely popular for Afro-Caribbean styling. Many small plaits are used throughout the head and the ends can be secured with cotton thread, or beads to give more decoration. The direction of the plaits creates the style, and an experienced plaiter can produce almost limitless variations.

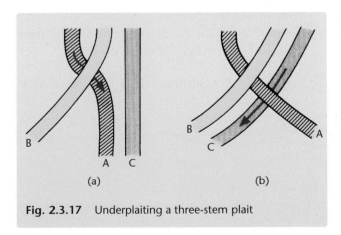

(a)                                    (b)

**Fig. 2.3.17**  Underplaiting a three-stem plait

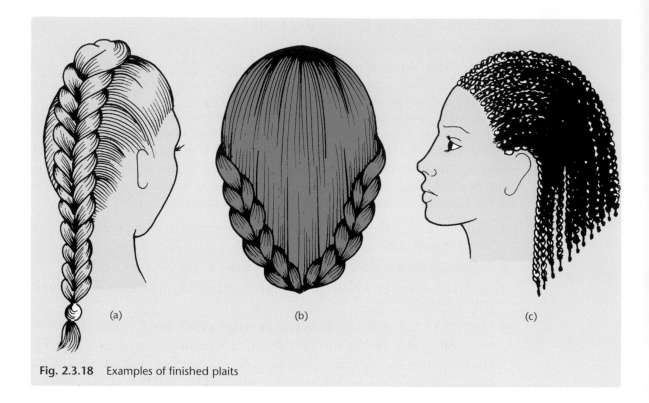

(a)                                        (b)                                        (c)

**Fig. 2.3.18    Examples of finished plaits**

## Using ornamentation

A client with very long hair is not usually able to achieve a change of style by having a new shape cut into the hair. Any new style must therefore be achieved by setting and blow-drying or dressing the hair in different ways. When used imaginatively ornamentation such as ribbons, ornamental grips, decorative combs, beads and embroidery thread, can alter the effect of a hairstyle and give the client more variety.

## Consultation checklist

Talking to clients can be a very daunting prospect for some trainees. To help you to overcome any initial shyness, fill in the following checklist for each client over a period of one week. At the end of this time you should then feel more comfortable when talking to the clients.

1. Is the client: New ☐
   Been once before ☐
   Regular ☐

2. What is the client's name?

3. Where does the client live?

4. What is the client's occupation?

5. Does the client have any hobbies? If yes, what?

6. Does the client have a family (including pets)? If yes, what?

7. Is the client going somewhere special? If yes, where?

8. Is the client going on holiday? If yes, where and when?

9. What products does the client normally use on their hair (mousse, gel, lacquer, etc.)?

10. Does the client's hairstyle usually stay in well? If no, what could be the cause?

11. Does the client's hair need a perm/conditioning treatment or colour?

12. If yes, what have you recommended?

13. What after-care advice have you given to the client?

14. Are there any retail sales suitable for the client's hair? If yes, what?

15. Has the client made another appointment?

## Practising plaits

Plaiting requires flexible fingers. This assignment has therefore been devised to help you to handle strands of hair more easily and with greater confidence. You will need:

- A4 size piece of card
- Large safety pin, scissors and stapler
- 19 strands of very thick wool about 25 cm (10 in) long
- Old cushion

1. Take three strands of the wool, knot the ends together and attach the safety pin 2.5 cm (1 in) to the ends of the wool.
2. Attach the safety pin and wool to the cushion and plait the wool into a three-stemmed plait. Secure the ends by twisting one strand of the wool around the others and knot. Remove the safety pin and place the plait to one side.
3. Repeat the procedure using four strands of wool, then five then seven until you have four completed plaits of different sizes.
4. Draw or collect an illustration of a hairstyle for each type of plait.
5. Attach the plaits to the card with the stapler (or adhesive tape); display them to their best advantage together with the relevant illustration. Ornaments or dried flowers, etc., may be used to emphasise the plaiting. Label each plait clearly using block letters.
6. Write a short report on how you carried out the task and any difficulties you encountered.

## What do you know?

- List **five** influencing factors which need to be considered before drying the hair.
- What type of style favours a **long** face?
- How can a style be designed to minimise a **heavy** jawline or chin?
- What type of **drying** makes hair appear fullest?
- **Contrast** the hair design for someone who regularly plays sport with the hair design for someone who regularly entertains.
- List the different hair **textures**.
- What are the reasons for considering the hair **growth direction** when drying hair?
- Explain what happens **inside** the hair when it is wet, moulded then dried.
- Explain what is meant by **hygroscopic**.
- List the drying techniques **currently** available to the stylist.
- What holds the **polypeptide** chains of hair keratin together?
- What is the effect of **moisture** on a set?
- Give **four** examples of dry sets and wet sets?
- What is meant by **hair direction**?
- Why should placing rollers in straight, ladder-like rows be **avoided**?
- What effect does using a hair section **too wide** for the roller produce?
- List the **main** types of pincurls.
- How does a **setting aid** produce a longer-lasting set?

- What type of **accident** is particularly associated with dry setting techniques?
- In wet sets, what causes the **cross-linkages** to reform?
- Why should a client **not smoke** when laquer is being applied?
- Why is it necessary to use dressing creams **sparingly**?
- Which teeth of the comb are used to **smooth out** backcombing?
- Where should the hair be **backcombed** to create lift?
- What is meant by **balance** in relation to hairstyling?
- Why is dressing **cream or oil** used when dressing the hair?
- How would you advise the client to look after **long** hair?
- When dressing the hair into a **pleat**, why may it be necessary to use some backcombing or brushing?
- What is a **plait**?
- What is the **difference** between a French brad and underplaiting?

# 4

In this unit you will learn about:

- Tools and equipment used when cutting hair.
- Methods used to sterilise cutting tools and equipment.
- Client preparation and consultation needed before cutting hair.
- Cutting techniques and their effects.
- Health and safety considerations when cutting hair.

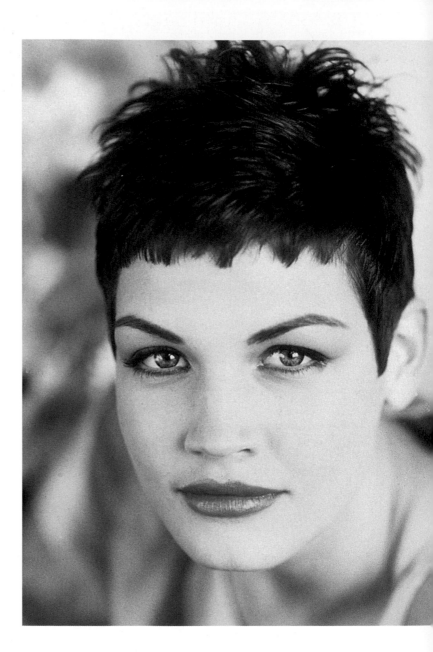

# Cutting hair

## Haircutting tools

Being able to cut hair well is a very important hairdressing skill. A good haircut can make even the worst head of hair look special. Each head of hair is different, so it is wise to spend some time analysing the client's hair (and their personality) and discussing their needs.

**POINTS TO REMEMBER**

A good haircut is the basis of all good hairdressing. When a blow-dry or set has dropped from the hair, all that is left is the shape of the haircut!

### Scissors

Scissors can be- bought in a variety of lengths and weights. The choice of length and weight is entirely up to you but it is important that the scissors feel comfortable. When buying a new pair of scissors, test them first by holding between the thumb and the third finger; they should feel like an extension of the fingers.

Hairdressing scissors should *only* be used for cutting hair. Using them for cutting string, paper, etc., will blunt the blades very quickly and then they will tear the hair.

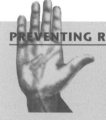

**PREVENTING RSI**

Choose your scissors carefully. Make sure they fit your hand; operate smoothly with the minimum of effort; are a proper size for the job; are as light as they can be while being sturdy enough for the amount of use they will get; are balanced for easy control; and can be sharpened easily. Get the best you can afford and replace them when you find a better pair.

#### Types of scissors

- **Plain straight edge** – used for most cutting techniques. Longer blade lengths are used in men's haircutting (Fig. 2.4.1).
- **Very fine serrated edge** – similar in appearance to straight-edged scissors, they are intended to be self-sharpening. They can be used for all cutting techniques except slide cutting. In slide cutting, the finely serrated edge of the scissors tends to drag on the hair and does not cut it as cleanly as the straight-edged scissors.
- **Wide-spaced serrated edge** – these are known as aesculap scissors. Either one blade or both blades are serrated to limit the amount of hair which can be cut. They are normally used to remove bulk or weight from the hair, i.e. thinning.

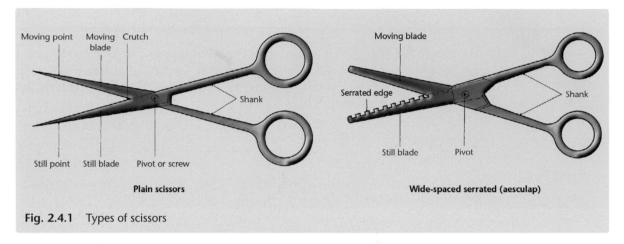

Fig. 2.4.1    Types of scissors

However, there are many different types of aesculap scissors, some designed to remove far more hair than others. The choice of aesculap depends upon the required result and also the stylist's own personal preference. They are normally used on dry hair; on wet hair they can remove too much hair as the wet hairs tend to stick together (Fig. 2.4.1).

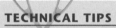

**TECHNICAL TIPS**

To maintain their balance, do not drop scissors on the floor. To maintain their sharpness, make sure each pair of scissors is used by one person only. Sharing scissors will blunt the blades very quickly.

### Cleaning and sterilising scissors

- After use on wet hair, dry them and wipe them carefully with spirit.
- Place them in the sterilising cabinet or autoclave for the correct length of time.
- Treat the pivot with oil to prevent stiffness.

To keep scissors in good working order:

- Keep them away from strong chemicals such as bleach or perm lotion.
- Never use them for anything except to cut hair.
- Have them sharpened by experts.
- Store them away from dust as it harbours bacteria.

## Razors

Razors are only used on wet hair. They tend to pull and tear dry hair, which is *very* painful for the client and not very good for the hair. The **safety razor** is mainly used in salons nowadays. It is called a safety razor because it has a

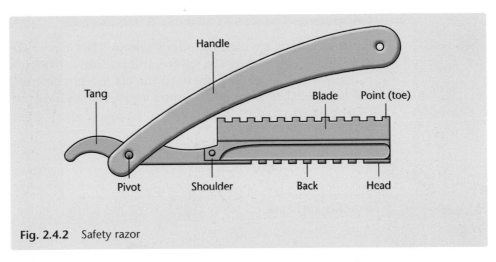

**Fig. 2.4.2**  Safety razor

replaceable blade which is protected by a metal guard. This means it is safer for the stylist to use as they are less likely to cut their fingers than with the old open razors, which did not have a guard. For hygiene and safety reasons, a new blade should be used on each client.

Safety razors come in various shapes. The 'shaper' razor has a straight, fixed handle; other razors have a movable handle and are the same shape as the old open razor but with a guard over the blade (Fig. 2.4.2). The type you choose will depend on which one you feel most comfortable with.

The old open razors are rarely used in salons today. They are far more dangerous to both the stylist and the client because of their very sharp, unguarded blade. Safely in the workplace is very important but if you should cut the client, wear rubber gloves when you stop the blood flow. Do not let the blood come into contact with any open wound because of the risk of AIDS, hepatitis B or other infections.

### Cleaning and sterilising razors

- Carefully remove the blade (sharp) and dispose of it in a special sharps bin or box.
- Dry the remaining razor parts then wipe them with surgical spirit.
- Place the razor in the sterilising cabinet or autoclave for the correct length of time.

**SAFETY TIPS**

Combs with broken or irregular teeth should not be used as they may scratch the scalp or tear the hair.

## Clippers

Electric clippers are used in today's salons. They have two blades with sharp-edged teeth. One blade stays fixed and the other blade moves across it. This cuts the hair. The distance between the blade teeth determines the closeness of the haircut. They are used for men's and women's haircutting to produce very short haircuts.

### Cleaning and sterilising clippers

- Remove loose hairs with a tissue.
- Remove any grease with surgical spirit.
- Apply antiseptic oil to the clipper head and joints (Fig. 2.4.3)

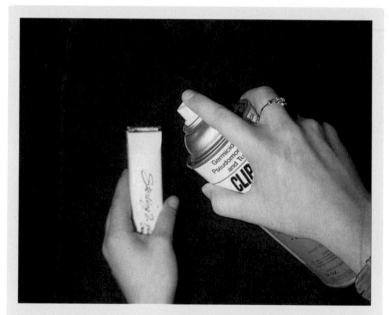

**Fig. 2.4.3**    Using an antiseptic oil spray on cordless clippers

### Combs

Cutting combs are smaller and thinner than other combs. They are also more pliable and allow the hair to be cut nearer to the scalp; in men's graduation or short back and sides.

**SAFETY TIPS**

Combs with broken or irregular teeth should not be used as they may scratch the scalp or tear the hair.

### Cleaning and sterilising combs

- Place the comb in warm, soapy water then gently scrub the teeth with a nail brush.
- Rinse in warm water.
- Place the comb in chemical sterilising fluid until needed, or in the sterilising cabinet or autoclave for the correct length of time.

**SAFETY TIPS**

When not in use and after use on each client, combs should be kept in the sterilising cabinet or completely submerged in an antiseptic solution of the correct strength.

### Neck brushes

Neck brushes are used to remove the loose hairs from the face and the neck after cutting the hair. They are made from bristle, nylon or a combination of both.

### Cleaning and sterilising neck brushes

- Swish the bristles of the brush in warm, soapy water; do not wet the handle if it is wooden.
- Rinse the bristles carefully in clean water.
- Pat the bristles dry on a towel then place the brush in the sterilising cabinet or autoclave for the correct length of time.

**POINTS TO REMEMBER**

Three main sterilisation methods are used in the salon (see Unit 2.9).
- Heat – dry and moist
- Chemical
- Ultraviolet rays

**Table 2.4.1  Summary of sterilization methods**

| Tool | Method |
| --- | --- |
| Scissors | Wipe with surgical spirit and keep in sterilising cabinet or use autoclave |
| Razors | Wipe with surgical spirit and keep in sterilising cabinet or use autoclave |
| Clippers | Wipe with surgical spirit; spray with antiseptic oil |
| Combs | Clean then place in sterilising fluid, sterilising cabinet or autoclave |
| Neck brush | Clean then place in sterilising cabinet or autoclave |

## Four basic techniques

### Club cutting

Club cutting is cutting the hair bluntly straight across, removing the length from the hair but retaining the weight. Because the weight is left on the points of the hair, it tends to discourage any natural hair curl.

Hair can be club cut wet or dry, either using the scissors or a razor. However, club cutting with a razor requires a lot of practice and should only be attempted when the stylist is fully proficient in razor cutting.

Club cutting allows the hair to be cut very precisely, but remember that the head is a curved object, and although the hair may be cut in a straight line, the angle at which the hair is held away from the scalp is very important to produce the correct shape for the finished haircut.

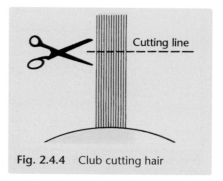

Fig. 2.4.4   Club cutting hair

#### Club cutting wet or dry hair

Vertical or horizontal sections of hair are held from the scalp at an angle and the points of the hair are cut straight across between the fingers or, if the hair is to be cut very close to the scalp, over a comb, using scissors (Fig. 2.4.4).

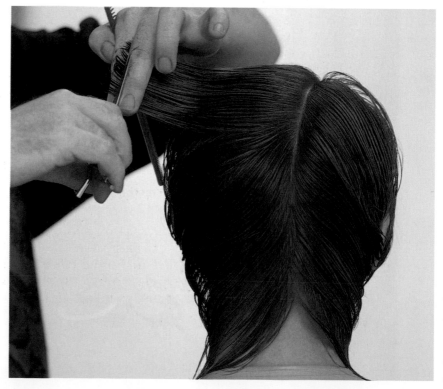

Joe Patterson for Clynol

**Uses and effects**

- To keep as much weight as possible with fine hair.
- To discourage curl on overcurly hair.
- To keep the weight of hair needed in fashion cutting.

## Scissors or clippers over comb

Cutting over a comb can produce extremely short haircuts and it was originally used in men's haircutting and the women's shingle of the 1920s.

A fine, pliable comb is used so that the hair can be cut as close to the scalp as possible. The hair is combed upwards from the nape and the hair which protrudes through the teeth of the comb is cut off. If scissors are being used, they should rest along the length of the comb and should open and close quickly while the comb is moving up the head. If the scissor movement is too slow then steps will occur in the haircut.

Clippers and comb may be used instead of scissors and comb. Make sure the clipper head is in the correct position to remove all the hair protruding through the comb.

The angle at which the comb is held will determine the length of the hair. If it is held next to the scalp, the hair will be very short. The further away the comb is held, the longer the hair.

Electric clippers can also be used without a comb. The clipper heads have attachments numbered according to their depth; the lower the number, the shorter the haircut.

**Uses and effects**

- To create very short graduation on men's and women's hairstyles.
- To blend in difficult growth patterns on the nape hairline.
- To create interesting shapes within the haircut, e.g. double baseline cut.

## Thinning

Thinning removes unwanted weight without altering length. It may be done with scissors, razor or aesculap scissors, but remember that the scissors and aesculap scissors should only be used to thin out dry hair and the razor to thin out wet hair.

Check the hair carefully to decide where on the head the weight needs to be reduced, as it is not always necessary to thin out the whole head. The following areas on the scalp should never be thinned; this is because of their growth direction patterns and the possibility of unwanted spiky effects or odd hairs sticking out from the scalp if the hair is cut too short:

- The hairline, particularly at the front
- Along a parting
- The crown area

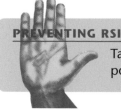

**PREVENTING RSI**

Take note of your hand and wrist positions and motions. Try to keep in neutral position and to alternate motions.

### Thinning dry hair using scissors

Divide off the areas that should not be thinned, then taking sections approximately 10 mm (½ in) wide, hold the hair out from the scalp at right angles. Using the points of the scissors, remove a few hairs from the root area and along the hair shaft. Continue in this way until the whole head, or the parts that need thinning, have been completed. Take care not to remove too much hair at the root area as these hairs will tend to spike out when they grow if too many have been removed.

### Thinning dry hair using aesculap scissors

Divide off the areas that should not be thinned. Now take sections approximately 2 cm (1 in) wide; these sections are wider than when thinning with ordinary scissors. Hold the hair out from the scalp at right angles. Insert the aesculap scissors into the sections at an angle. Cut the hair in a zigzag pattern along the length (Fig. 2.4.5). Continue until all the selected parts have been thinned.

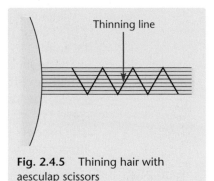

**Fig. 2.4.5** Thining hair with aesculap scissors

### Thinning wet hair using a razor

Divide off the areas which should not be thinned, then taking approximately 1 cm (½ in) sections hold the hair out from the scalp at right angles. With the tip of the razor, remove a few hairs at the root and along the hair shaft. The hair can also be thinned by using shorter and extra slicing movements on each hair section while actually razor cutting the hair (removing length at the same time); in this case you should begin the slicing movements closer to the scalp (see Fig. 2.4.6).

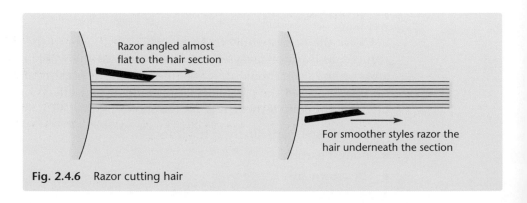

**Fig. 2.4.6** Razor cutting hair

**Uses and effects**

● To remove excess weight from the hair.

● To give a finer, feathered effect to certain areas of a hairstyle.

● To remove the weight from overclubbed hair.

## Razor cutting

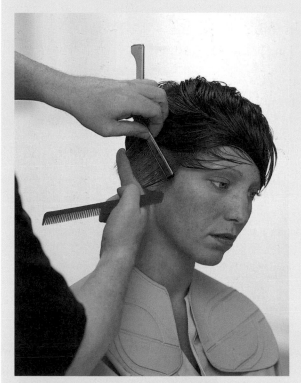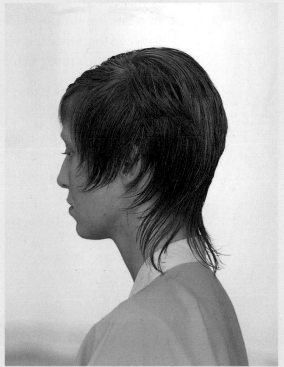

Using razor cutting techniques on wet hair creates a fine feathered effect.

*Source*: Joe Patterson for Clynol

## Freehand Cutting

Cutting hair freehand needs skill and confidence; it means cutting the hair without holding the hair in place. Many of the more advanced cutting techniques such as slither cutting or chipping into the hair are done freehand plus most clipper cutting and work on Afro-Caribbean hair.

It is absolutely essential that you have an understanding of shape and balance before attempting freehand cutting. It is very easy to hit problems and get carried away when not cutting to guidelines.

**POINTS TO REMEMBER**

No matter what type of haircut is being carried out, it is very important to keep the client's head in the correct position. If it is held to one side during cutting, then the finished haircut will be lopsided.

### Uses and effects

- To create less structured effects within the haircut.
- To blend short hair and very long hair (slide cutting).
- To add texture to the hair.

**Table 2.4.2** Summary of cutting techniques

| Technique | Description | Effect |
|---|---|---|
| Thinning | Aesculap scissors or scissors on dry hair Razor on wet hair | Removes bulk and weight Encourages curl |
| Club cutting | Cutting straight across the hair section | Removes length only. Retains weight Discourages curl |
| Scissor or clipper over comb | Cutting the hair through the teeth of the comb: using clippers or scissors | Can create very short haircuts on both men and women |
| Freehand cutting | Cutting the hair without holding it in place | Creates less structured effects Can blend short and very long hair |

## Haircutting shapes

### Solid form

Commonly known as the bob, the solid form is where all the hair is cut to the same perimeter or baseline. There is no graduation or layering in this haircut.

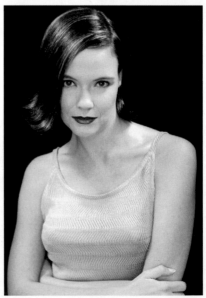

Hair by Russell Hyde for VeroColour; Sabre Corporation Australia

#### Effects

- Keeps weight on ends of the hair.
- Produces a squarer, chunky effect on the hair.
- Makes finer hair appear as thick and dense as possible.

### Uniform layering

Uniform layering is when all the layers in the haircut contain hair of the same

## Cutting a solid form style

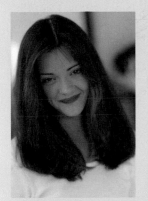 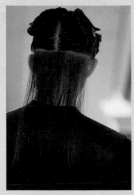 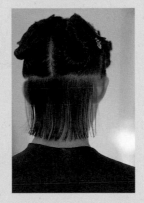 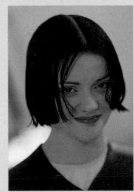

Below shoulder length hair is shampooed and sectioned down the centre from the forehead to nape then from the top of the ears across the back, occipital area of the head. The hair is cut flat to the skin, beginning at the centre nape and working forward to the top of the head. The front section is cut starting at the bottom of the side. Sections are combed flat onto the face and cut close to the skin, angling the cutting line on a slight diagonal to connect with the nape outline To allow for ear protrusion, remember not to use too much tension on side hair.

*Source*: Hair by Sharon Peake of Francesco Group Hanley for Clynol

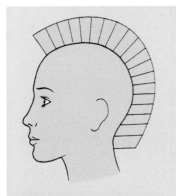

**Fig. 2.4.7** Cut hair lengths for uniform layering

length. If the hair is cut to 75 mm on the crown then it is cut to 75 mm at the nape and front, etc. (Fig. 2.4.7). This is done by lifting the hair out from the head at a 90° angle all over the head.

**Effects**

- Produces a rounded silhouette which mirrors the shape of the head.
- Can make thicker hair appear less thick.
- Can look stunning if the hair is cut very short, but the client needs good bone structure for this.

### Low layering

Low layering is when the top layer contains much longer hair than the layers beneath (Fig. 2.4.8). A wedge cut is an example of low layering.

**Effects**

- Creates a triangular silhouette.
- Because the top hair is left longer, much of the weight remains.
- Makes finer hair appear thicker.

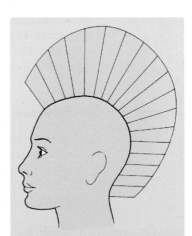

**Fig. 2.4.8** Cut hair lengths for low layering

# Cutting a uniform layering

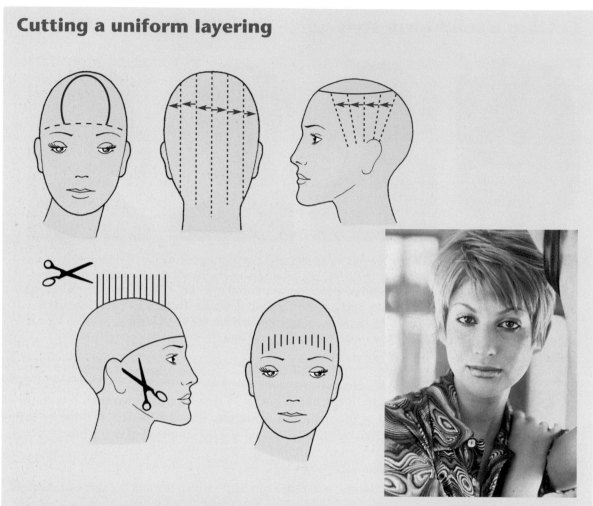

Hair is sectioned off on top of the head from the crown area to each temple. Hold the hair out at a 90° angle and cut a guideline at the crown. Work down the head to the nape until all the back hair has been cut. Work through to the sides then cut the fringe guideline. Cut the top hair by working from the crown towards the front and blending in with the back and sides. Overdirect the front two sections and blend with the fringe. Dry the hair with a Denman brush for a soft finish.

*Source*: Sabre Europe Ltd

## Reverse graduation

Reverse graduation is when the top layers contain longer hair that falls *below* the underneath layers and perimeter line (Fig. 2.4.9). Used when the top hair needs to be moulded over the underneath layers; a pageboy style is an example.

### Effects

- Creates a smooth effect on a bob shape.
- Can make finer hair appear thicker.

# Cutting a low layered for low layering

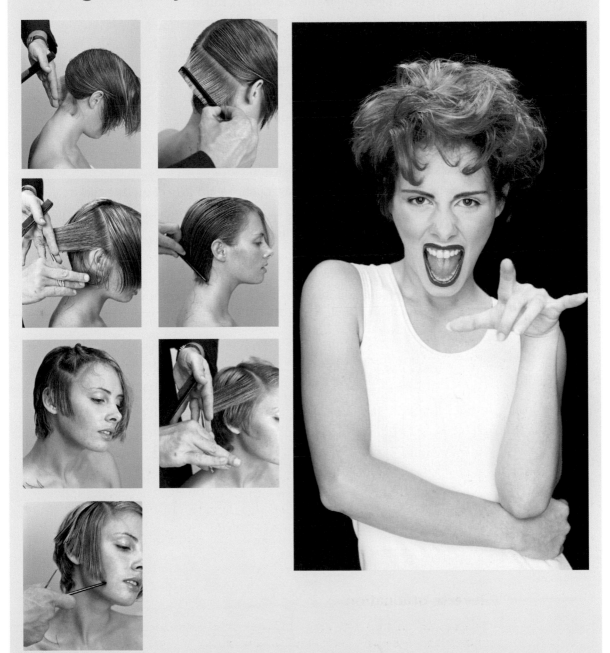

The guideline is cut at the centre back with fingers pointing towards the nape. All hair is cut to the guide, creating longer lengths at the occipital area and above. Work through to the front of the head, pulling the front hair back to create length and weight in this area. Recut a guideline at the side to blend with the back guide. Bring the hair down, holding it out from the head to graduate it but still leaving weight through the front.

*Source*: Hair by Russell Hyde for VeroColour; Sabre Corporation Australia

## Increased layering

Increased layering is when the top hair is much shorter than the underneath layers, creating very steep angles (Fig. 2.4.10). A guideline is cut at the shortest point (usually the top of the head) then all the hair is combed up to this guideline and cut straight across at this point. This is a simple way of achieving the very steep graduation. When the head is held upside down the haircut resembles a bob.

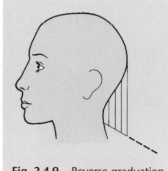

**Fig. 2.4.9**    Reverse graduation

### Effects

- Makes thick hair appear less thick and dense.
- Encourages curl as there is not as much weight to pull out the curl.
- Allows long hair to remain long but without the weight of a solid form.
- Allows greater variety when styling the hair.

## Layering and graduation: a summary

Increasing the graduation increases the amount of layering in the hair. The more the hair sections are lifted, the greater the graduation. A bob effect is produced

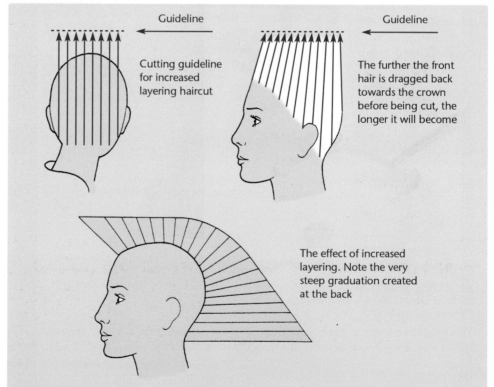

Guideline

Cutting guideline for increased layering haircut

Guideline

The further the front hair is dragged back towards the crown before being cut, the longer it will become

The effect of increased layering. Note the very steep graduation created at the back

**Fig. 2.4.10**    Increased layering. Usually a box shape is cut on top of the head then all hair is cut to this guide.

Graduation is often called **layering**. Increased layering is when the hair is steeply graduated and low layering is when there is little graduation. Graduation is achieved when the top layers of the hair lie above the lower layers. The top layers may lie well above the lower layers in which case there would be a lot of graduation, but if all the top layers lie just above the lower layers then there is little graduation.

when the hair is held down close to the head at a 0° angle; this contains no graduation. For each degree the hair is lifted away from the head, more graduation is achieved. To help understand the degrees of lift, it is useful to remember that a 90° lift means the hair is held straight out from the head at right angles. Thus, a 45° lift is half this amount and a 180° lift is double (Fig. 2.4.11).

- **45° lift** – this will create slight graduation, usually used for wedges, etc.
- **90° lift** – this will create twice as much graduation, usually used for short, uniform layered shapes.
- **90 – 180° lift** – this will create a great deal of graduation, usually used for long, high layered styles.

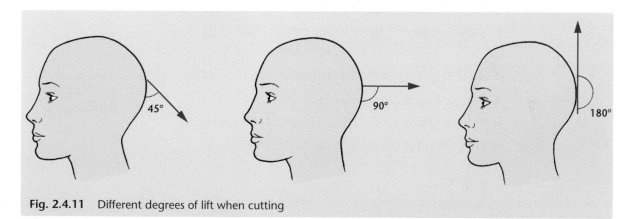

**Fig. 2.4.11**　Different degrees of lift when cutting

Before you start the haircut, consult the client and do a hair analysis. If you do not carry out a thorough discussion with the client, you may not cut the hair correctly or how they want it. If they do not like their haircut when it is finished, they will tell their friends and perhaps they won't return to the salon. Very bad for business!

## Health and safety points

Health and safety is important at all times. Make sure you know and understand your salon's procedures and any local by-laws in connection with the safe disposal of sharp objects. In particular, you need to be aware of working safely in the following areas.

### Storing and handling cutting tools

- Use scissors only for cutting hair.
- Close scissor blades when not actually cutting the hair.
- Carry scissors in a safe manner – potentially they are a lethal weapon.
- Clean and sterilise scissors after use then store them safely.

### Storing and handling electrical equipment

- Check for loose or frayed wires before use.
- Switch off equipment at the socket after use.
- Clean equipment after use.
- Store equipment safely in the correct place.

### Disposing of waste materials

- Put cut hair in the correct bin.
- Put any sharps in the correct disposal bin or box.
- Observe any local by-laws on waste disposal.

**POINTS TO REMEMBER**

Minimise risk of harm to yourself and others, maintain a professional salon image and minimise the risk of cross-infection or infestation. Follow this checklist:
- Make sure the client is well protected before you begin cutting.
- Protect yourself by wearing shoes without open toes.
- Make sure the client is comfortable and in the correct position at all times.
- Close scissor blades when not cutting hair.
- Take extra care when cutting near to the eyes or skin.
- Keep tools and equipment clean and sterile.
- Keep the work area clean and tidy.
- Remove any cut hair from the client's neck and protective clothing.
- Sweep up all hair as soon as you have finished the haircut.
- Dispose of all waste materials safely.

# Factors that influence a haircut

It cannot be stressed too often that before placing a pair of scissors near to a head of hair, the stylist must know exactly what the client wants and how best to achieve it. It is too late when the hair has been cut to realise that the client's requirements have been misunderstood, or even ignored.

Client's are often nervous when they visit a salon for the first time, particularly for a haircut. Talking to the client and discussing what they want helps the stylist to find out exactly what the client expects from the haircut. It also helps to build up a relationship of trust and confidence between the client and the stylist. To provide a good service, you should assess the client and assess the client's hair.

## Assessing the client

Assessing the client is a two-way process. It is not just about asking the client questions. It is about getting a holistic view of the client and then offering advice if what they want seems unrealistic. Clients sometimes have difficulty describing a haircut or style. It is useful to have books or magazines with up-to-date hairstyles so the client can *show* you what they want. This can also help you to explain why the client's hair is unsuitable for the chosen haircut and offer more suitable suggestions. When you assess a client, think about the following aspects.:

### Face shape

Take a good look at the client's face by drawing the hair away from the face to decide whether it is round, square, long, oval, etc.; this can affect the amount of hair that needs to be cut and will also help you decide the shape of the finished haircut. Next check whether there are any prominent features or blemishes that need to be camouflaged, e.g. a receding chin. Some prominent features can be attractive and therefore need to be emphasised, e.g. the eyes can be emphasised by a fringe.

### Neck length

If the client has a very long neck the hair needs to be left longer in the nape. However, a very short neck looks less obvious if the hair is kept shorter in the nape or is swept up towards the top of the head to make the neck appear longer.

### Body size

The finished haircut should be part of a total look, not just a separate item that happens to be attached to the client's head. For example, a very tall, slim client with a small head would look ridiculous with a short, scalp-hugging haircut.

### Age

The age of the client is a very important consideration. A middle-aged person cannot always wear the same style as a teenager, although a current fashion trend can often be adapted to meet the needs of both, as long as it is not too extreme.

## Assessing the hair

Assessing the hair will help you to decide on the type and method of cutting to use. Remember that you will sometimes have to combine a variety of haircutting techniques on one head to get the result that you and the client want.

Whenever possible, use the type of hair to its best advantage – it is very difficult, if not impossible, to create a long, smooth bob style on very thick, wiry, naturally curly hair. It is far better to use the curl and thickness of the hair to create a style that needs these features. Here are some things to consider:

### Hair texture

Texture refers to the **diameter** of the hair. it can be fine, medium or coarse:

- **Fine hair** – needs to keep as much weight as possible to make it seem thicker; this is helped by club cutting the hair and choosing solid forms or styles with low layering.
- **Medium hair** – not usually a problem and adapts to most haircutting techniques.
- **Coarse hair** – may need to have some of its volume and weight removed or reduced; thinning and layering help to do this.

### Hair volume

Hair volume is the number of hairs on the scalp, or how densely they grow. A client may have fine textured hair but with plenty of hairs on the scalp, making it quite abundant; or they may have thick, coarse hair which is very sparse. The density of hair can vary throughout the head, e.g. hair may be denser at the nape than the crown. There are many combinations and each head is slightly different.

### Hair length

Clients do not always realise that some haircuts need a lot of length in certain areas and often do not appreciate how much time it takes to grow to that length. Often you will have to compromise with a hairstyle, and it may take a few months and quite a few haircuts to achieve the final effect. A good example of this is when a client has had a layered or steeply graduated haircut and wants to grow out the top layers until the hair is all one length. This can take up to 12 months, depending upon how short the hair was originally. Advise your client on the types of style and haircut they can have to keep the hair well shaped without loss of length from the areas which need to grow longer.

### Hair curl and movement

Always try to use any natural curl or movement in the hair. Ignoring or fighting against the curl can often ruin a haircut. By using any natural curl or movement the haircut will stay in shape longer and will be easier for the client to manage.

### Hair growth patterns

Strong growth direction patterns can cause difficulties. Cutting the hair when wet without tension allows extra length in these problem areas and prevents an uneven line when the haircut is finished. Strong patterns include:

- Double crown
- Nape whorls
- Widow's peak
- Cow's lick

## Preparing for a haircut

- Always be aware of the safety aspects.
- Carry out a client consultation.
- Protect the client with gown and towels according to your salon's procedure.
- Disentangle the hair by combing or brushing through.
- Carry out a hair and scalp analysis; remember to look for any infectious or contagious conditions.
- If the hair is to be cut wet, shampoo the hair and towel-dry. You have no need to do this if the hair is to be cut dry, unless it is very greasy, dirty or sticky with dressing aids such as lacquer.
- Comb through the hair to disentangle it.
- Section the hair if necessary.

## Cutting angles around the hairline

The hair may be cut at many angles around the hairline to create different shapes and styles. But always remember to take into consideration any strong hair growth direction patterns.

The areas to consider when cutting angles around the hairline are:

- The forehead or fringe (Fig. 2.4.12)
- The sides of the head (Fig. 2.4.13)
- The nape of the neck (Fig. 2.4.14)

### TECHNICAL TIPS

When using the features of the face or ears, etc., as a guide to form the cutting angles; always check they are even on either side.

You will need to know the technical names for various parts of the head. The main ones are listed here and illustrated in Fig. 2.4.15:

- Temple
- Forehead
- Crown
- Occipital area
- Nape

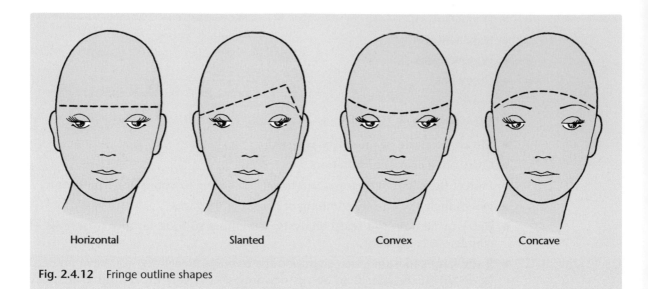

Horizontal          Slanted          Convex          Concave

**Fig. 2.4.12**   Fringe outline shapes

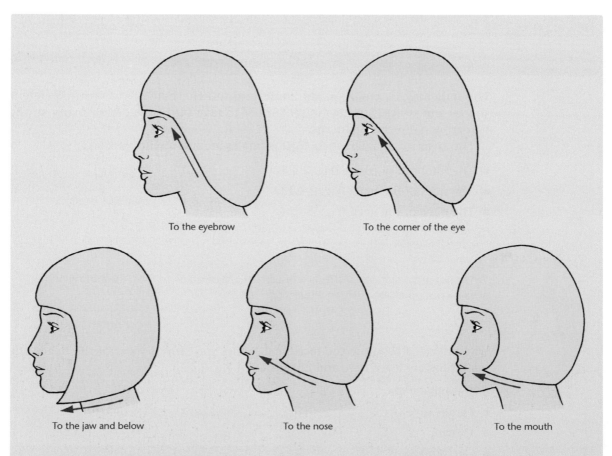

To the eyebrow          To the corner of the eye

To the jaw and below          To the nose          To the mouth

**Fig. 2.4.13**   Cutting shapes around the face

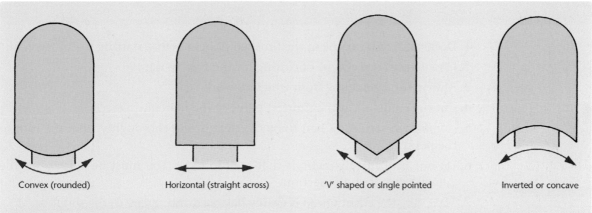

Fig. 2.4.14    Neckline (nape) shapes

| Convex (rounded) | Horizontal (straight across) | 'V' shaped or single pointed | Inverted or concave |

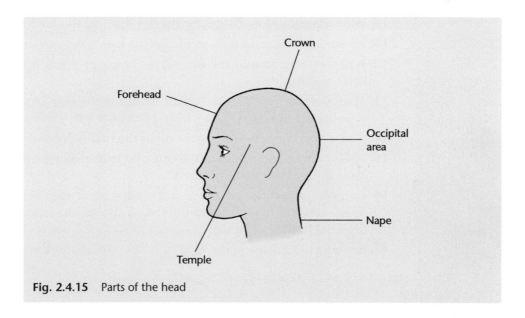

Fig. 2.4.15    Parts of the head

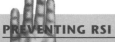

**PREVENTING RSI**

Try not to bend or twist your neck. Adjust and turn the chair so you can be exactly centred at the section you are cutting. This also gives you the best results. Try to face straight ahead and look down slightly. If you bend your neck forward, you can easily put a 60° slant on it and this leads to headaches and backaches. After 20° of slant, the weight of your head (4–6 kg) is transferred from your skeleton to your muscles and that is a great strain. Imagine carrying 4 kg of sugar around and you will get the idea. Let your bones carry the weight – they don't strain.

## Basic guidelines when cutting hair

1. Decide the exact shape of the finished haircut before starting to cut the hair.
2. Choose the correct type of cutting for the type of hair.
3. Always cut a guideline from which to work.
4. Cut the guideline at the shortest point of the haircut.
5. Comb each section of hair to be cut cleanly and thoroughly from the root to the point.
6. Do not take cutting sections that are too large. You must be able to see the guideline through the section.
7. Make sure the client's head is evenly balanced and square to the shoulder.
8. Cut with the hair growth pattern and use any natural curl or movement.
9. Never cut the hair too short. It is easy to cut off more hair but impossible to put it back on again.
10. When cutting wet hair, allow for the fact that hair will lift 5 mm ($\frac{1}{4}$ in) when dry.
11. When precision cutting, do not allow the hair to dry out – always keep it wet.
12. When cutting around the ear, allow for ear protrusion and do not cut the hair too short.
13. Always cross-check a basic haircut by lifting the hair away from the head in the opposite direction from which it has been cut.
14. Give a final check to the haircut when the hair is dry and dressed.
15. Always advise the client on the care and maintenance of their haircut, especially if they have had a new style.
16. For beginners: if the guideline at the nape is cut with the client's head bent forward, it will help to avoid the risk of cutting the hairline too short when the head is lifted upright.
17. Be aware of health and safety at all times – yours and the client's.

**SAFETY TIPS**

If the hair is cut short around the ears, take particular care to protect the ears with the fingers.

## Cross checking the hair

Every haircut should be checked very thoroughly across the sections to make sure it is level and even from all angles. This is known as **cross-checking**. However, when cross-checking a fashion cut remember not to get too enthusiastic and alter the line or shape of the style, particularly if the angles already cut are very steep.

Check carefully around the hairline at the sides, front and nape. If the hair has been held and cut away from the head, the underneath hair will be slightly longer, leaving wisps of hair which can make the finished line untidy. Unless intended as part of the style, these wisps should be removed.

## Things to do

This assignment should help you get used to diagnosing the hair growth patterns of your clients and give you practice in selecting suitable haircuts.

1. Look carefully at the hair growth of **two** of your friends or family members then draw the position of the hair growth pattern at the front, nape, sides and crown area.

2. Compare the different growth patterns for each person and write a brief summary of each.

3. Describe a suitable haircut for each and give reasons for your choice.

4. Draw or cut out from magazines haircuts which would be suitable for someone with a:
   (a) double crown
   (b) strong upward-growing napeline
   (c) cow's lick at the front of the head
   Give reasons for your choice.

## What do you know?

List **six** things that help to keep scissors in good working order.

- Name the **three** main methods of sterilisation used in salons.

- Describe how you would clean and sterilise **combs**.

- List **four** haircutting techniques and give the use and effect of each.

- What is the effect of a **solid form** haircut?

- Briefly describe how would you cut a **uniform** layer.

- What is **increased** layering?

- Why should consultation and hair analysis be carried out **before** cutting hair?

- How would you store and handle **electrical** equipment?

- How should you **dispose** of waste materials?

- Give **eight** health and safety considerations when cutting hair.

- List **four** areas that you need to think about when assessing the client.

- Why is it important to take note of any **strong** hair growth patterns when cutting hair?

- Describe how you would **prepare** a client for a wet cut.

- How would you **cross-check** a basic, uniform layer haircut?

# 5a

In this unit you will learn about:

- What happens to hair when it is permed.
- Types of basic winding techniques and the perming and neutralising process.
- Testing hair to make sure that it is suitable and safe to perm.
- Contra-indications and health and safety aspects when perming hair.

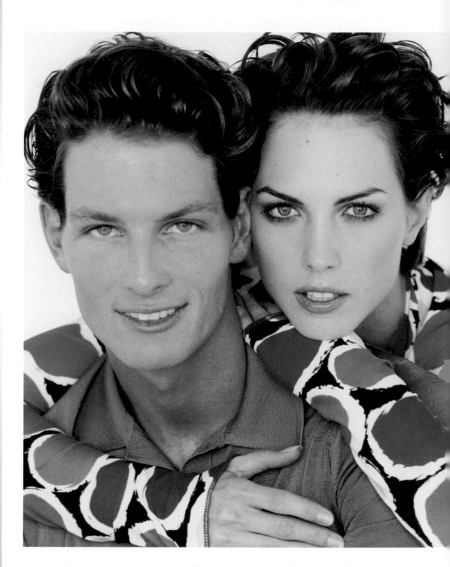

# Perming hair

# Perming – what happens in the hair

Perming and setting both involve the breaking of the cross-linkages between the polypeptide chains of hair keratin. The type of cross-linkage broken in setting is different from that broken in perming:

- In setting, some of the weak water-breakable cross-linkages between the polypeptide chains are broken and reformed. So hair that is dried or set into a style quickly drops or washes out.
- In perming, some of the stronger linkages are broken and reformed.

Perming can be used then to permanently curl, wave or straighten hair.

Much practical expertise is needed in perming but the basic operation can be thought of as three stages:

- **Softening** – by using the **perm lotion**.
- **Moulding** – rolling or combing the hair to give the required amount of curling or straightening.
- **Fixing** – this permanently 'fixes' the hair in the styled position. This last stage is often called **neutralisation** and the chemical used, a **neutraliser**.

## Stage 1 – Softening

Traditional cold perm lotion has a pH value of 9 to 9.5 (it is alkaline on the pH scale). This dissolves some of the cement-like keratin which usually holds down the hair cuticle scales. The alkaline factor in turn allows the lotion to get into the hair cortex and to then work on the cross-linkages between the polypeptide chains in the cortex. First, the water in the perm lotion breaks some of the water-breakable cross-linkages (in the same way as wet setting) and second, and more importantly, a chemical called **ammonium thioglycollate** attacks and breaks the water-unbreakable cross-linkages made up of sulphur bonds (about 60–70 per cent of them).

In 'acid' perms, another chemical is used, called **glycerol thioglycollate**, which has a pH value of about 4, but the hair is made alkaline first to cause the outside scales to open and the lotion to penetrate the hair cortex. Another point about 'acid' perms is that only about 10 per cent of the sulphur bonds are broken, because these bonds are stronger in acid conditions.

In both cases, the sulphur bonds are broken by the perm lotion forcing some of the sulphur atoms making up the cross-linkages to take hydrogen atoms instead of linking together between the polypeptide chains.

Sulphur atoms can only form two links or bonds with other chemicals, i.e. one is used up holding the sulphur atom on to the polypeptide chain and the other is used to link to a sulphur atom of a neighbouring chain (i.e. from a cross-linkage). Accepting the hydrogen from the perm lotion means the bond that is used to form the cross-linkage is taken up by the hydrogen atom and the cross-linkage is broken. This is shown in Fig 2.5.1.

In chemistry, the adding of hydrogen atoms like this is called a **reduction**, with the chemical giving the hydrogen called a **reducing agent** (in this case the perm lotion) and the substance accepting the hydrogen being said to be reduced (in this case the hair keratin).

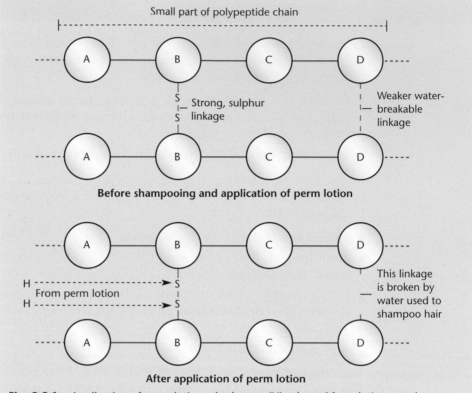

**Fig. 2.5.1**   Application of perm lotion – hydrogen (H) released from lotion attacks sulphur atoms (S) of sulphur linkage

## Stage 2 – Moulding

Most often, this involves winding hair around rollers. The hair is stretched slightly and **tension** is applied. Since some of the water-breakable and non-water-breakable sulphur cross-linkages are broken in stage 1, the stretching causes the polypeptide chains to slip past each other very slightly. This very tiny movement on the minute scale of polypeptide chains adds up, by slightly moving millions of chains,

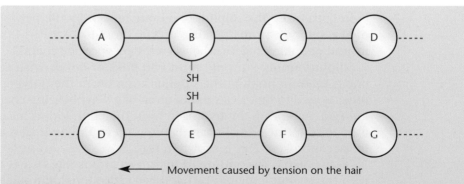

**Fig. 2.5.2**   Winding hair causes the polypeptide chains to change positions slightly (A, B and C of lower chain have moved off to the left)

and allows the individual hairs, and therefore the hair in general, to be styled. How much the chains are caused to slide determines just how much curl will be in the hair when the perm is finished. This sliding of the polypeptide chains is shown in Fig. 2.5.2. The hair is then rinsed thoroughly to remove the perm lotion.

## Stage 3 – Fixing

This stage uses a neutraliser. In order to fix the perm, the polypeptide chains must be locked into the positions they are in after stage 2. To do this, the hydrogen atoms added by the perm lotion in stage 1 have to be removed to allow the sulphur atoms to reform cross-linkages between the polypeptide chains. As keratin, being a protein, contains a high proportion of sulphur-containing amino acids, there is a good chance that even after moving the polypeptide chains, the sulphur atoms of one chain will still be near other sulphur atoms of other chains.

The hydrogen atoms are removed by using a chemical that can pull hydrogen away from the sulphur. In practice this is done by one of two reagents:

- Hydrogen peroxide (often 6 per cent).
- Sodium perborate (often 5 per cent).

Both these chemicals when applied to hair release highly reactive single atoms of oxygen (called nascent oxygen) which pull the hydrogen off the sulphur, allowing the cross-linkages to reform. In fact, each atom of nascent oxygen pulls two hydrogen atoms off and combines with them to form water. (See Fig. 2.5.3.)

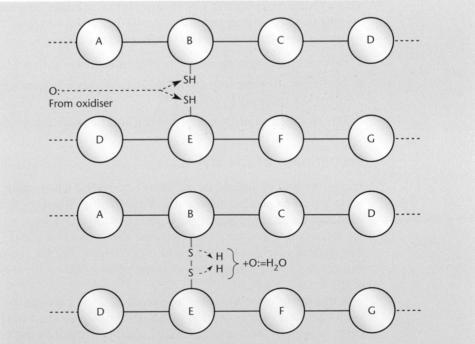

**Fig. 2.5.3** Nascent oxygen removes hydrogen from the sulphur atoms and combines to form water ($H_2O$)

In chemistry, the removal of hydrogen atoms in this way is called **oxidation**, with the chemical doing the removal called an **oxidising agent**, and the substance the hydrogen is removed from being described as **oxidised**.

## The perming and neutralising process

### Hair and scalp analysis

Consultation with the client *before* starting the perming process is essential to allow the client's requirements to be thoroughly discussed and understood.

Examine the hair carefully to make sure that it is really suitable for perming and question the client on any previous treatments, referring to record cards if the client has attended the salon previously. If in any doubt carry out a pre-perm test to support the analysis.

The client's scalp must also be checked for the presence of any inflammation, excessive dryness, cuts or abrasions (this can be done when disentangling the hair prior to shampooing). If these conditions are minor they can be protected with barrier cream but if they are major then the treatment must be postponed. Remember, if in doubt postpone the treatment.

### Preparation for perming

Preparation involves making sure all the equipment, reagents and sundries (sundries are things like towels, cotton wool and endpapers) are ready to hand. It is also about preparing the client and stylist in order to protect them from the chemicals used in the perming and neutralising process. These chemicals are hazardous and come under the COSHH Regulations:

● Personal protective equipment (PPE) in this case gowns and overalls.
● Reduction of exposure by taking care to avoid chemicals getting onto the client's or the stylist's skin.
● Safe storage and disposal of perming and neutralising products.

### Preparation of the stylist

Protective gloves should be worn by the stylist while applying the permanent wave lotion to prevent dermatitis of the hands. However, if the rods are wound with water and the lotion applied after the rods have been wound (post-damping technique) it is not necessary to wear the protective gloves when winding the hair. In this case it is often a good idea to apply barrier cream to the hands as it will protect them if they should come into contact with the lotion at any stage of the perming process.

A tinting apron worn over the overall helps to prevent the lotion from splashing and drying on the overall. Although it does not stain in the same way as tint, perm lotion can leave an unpleasant smell if allowed to dry on any clothing.

## Preparation of the client

The client's clothing should be protected at all times during the perming process. A gown should be placed around the client to cover all the clothing and a towel should be securely tucked in at the nape to prevent it from slipping on to the floor. A neck strip or strip of cotton wool may also be placed at the nape to prevent any lotion or water from seeping down the neck.

Barrier cream applied to the skin around the hairline protects it from any lotion that may accidentally run on to this area and prevents burning or sensitising of the skin by the lotion. This is particularly important if the client already happens to have a sensitive skin. But remember that the barrier cream must be applied to the skin only. Any cream that accidentally coats the hair will prevent lotion penetration of that hair and will therefore affect the curl.

## Preparation of the hair

Most perms are wound on wet hair but the hair should not be oversaturated with water as this could dilute the perm lotion and makes it less effective. Towel-drying the hair after shampooing removes the excess water but leaves the hair damp enough to give better absorption of the lotion.

The hair should be shampooed with a soapless shampoo as this not only cleans the hair and scalp but also removes any natural sebum that may be coating the hair. If the sebum remained, it could create a barrier between the lotion and the hair which would prevent the lotion from entering the cortex and the perm would not produce a satisfactory curl.

## Routine hygiene

Make sure that the rollers to be used are clean and have been sterilised. Use fresh, clean gowns, cotton wool, towels and neck strips for each client.

## Testing the hair

If the hair is structurally damaged or porous it may be necessary to apply a restructurant or special pre-perm treatment after shampooing to even out the porosity of the hair and to strengthen the cortex. Always take a test curl if the hair is very porous or damaged to make sure that it can withstand the perming process. If in any doubt at all, do not perm until the hair is strong enough. A full list of the tests to use on hair is given later in this unit.

## Preparation of the tools and equipment

All the equipment and tools that you will need should be assembled before beginning the permanent wave. A lot of time and energy can be saved if everything is to hand when it is needed.

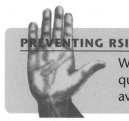

**PREVENTING RSI**

Winding perm rods or rollers uses small muscles of the hands that tire quickly, as well as putting a strain on the tendon at your elbow, so try to avoid several winding tasks one after the other.

## Contra-indications for permanent waving

The stylist should not go ahead with permanent waving if:

- Incompatible chemicals are present on the hair.
- Hair is excessively porous or weakened, e.g. overbleached.
- The elasticity of the hair has been impaired.
- A previous permanent wave is present – remember that a perm will stay in the hair until it is cut off. However, specialised techniques like 'blocking out' with conditioner or specially designed restructurants may be used over the old curl in some cases.
- Hair or scalp suffers from contagious or infectious disease, e.g. tinea, pediculosis capitis, etc.
- Perming after childbirth. The nutrients in the blood which are usually given to the hair to feed it are required to return the body to normal, leaving the hair in poor condition. It is usually more successful to perm the client's hair before the birth of the baby, during pregnancy.
- When the client is taking drugs (after/during illness). Perming hair during this time is often unsuccessful. If in doubt, always take a test curl.

## Sectioning for a basic perm

### Reasons for sectioning

- Ease of working.
- Minimum of wasted time.
- Cuts down the risk of overprocessing.
- Divides the hair into neat, controllable divisions.
- Helps rod selection.
- Keeps the size of the rods balanced by dividing the head into smaller areas.

### Method of sectioning

1. After shampooing with soapless shampoo, towel-dry and disentangle the hair.
2. Divide the hair into nine sections as shown in Fig. 2.5.4. The numbers refer to the order in

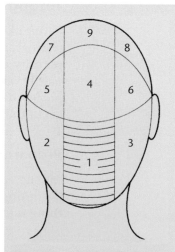

**Fig. 2.5.4    Basic nine sections**

which the sections are wound, Section 1 being divided into subsections. Note how the sections curve to the shape of the head. Each section should be the same width and slightly longer than the perm rod.

**POINTS TO REMEMBER**

Always work to the shape of the head. If the hair is extremely short, thick or abundant it may be necessary to add extra sections to hold the hair securely. The sections can be altered slightly as sectioning progresses but remember that the sections should always be the same width as the rods used otherwise problems are created when placing the rods during winding.

## Winding a perm

Before starting to wind a perm the following points must be taken into consideration as they will determine the size of rod to be used and the amount of curl to be achieved.

- **Texture of hair** – thick hair will need a larger rod than fine hair to achieve the same effect.
- **Type of curl required** – a tight curl needs small rods, a loose curl needs large rods.
- **Type of hair** – i.e. bleached, tinted, porous, resistant, or normal. Bleached, tinted and porous hair will need a special weaker lotion while resistant hair will need a stronger lotion. If in doubt, take a test curl of the hair. Remember that the condition of the hair after perming is very important. Using too strong a lotion for the type of hair will leave the hair in poor condition and could even cause hair breakage.
- **Finished result** – this will also determine the amount of curl needed.

### Method of winding a basic nine-section perm

1. The hair is ready for winding when it has been shampooed with soapless shampoo, towel-dried and sectioned into nine sections.
2. Start winding at the centre nape. Using a tail comb divide the hair to produce a subsection which is exactly the same depth as the rod.
3. Apply the lotion approximately 1 cm ($\frac{1}{2}$ in) from the scalp to prevent the lotion from running onto the skin. This is known as **presaturation**.
4. Comb the hair out from the head at right angles making sure that the hair is thoroughly combed from the roots to the points. Then comb the hair upwards towards the crown to allow for the width of the rod when wound.
5. Make sure that the tension is even on both sides of the section, otherwise the hair will 'loop' at one end producing an uneven finished curl.

   - When looking down the section (Fig. 2.5.5), the points of the hair should be directly in the centre, giving even tension to the hair on both sides.
   - If the hair is pulled slightly to one side the tension becomes uneven.

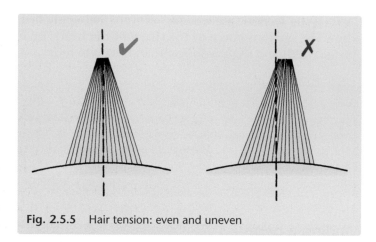

**Fig. 2.5.5** Hair tension: even and uneven

6. Place the endpaper over the ends of the hair past the hair points which helps to avoid 'fish-hook' ends (Fig. 2.5.6).

7. Carefully wind the endpaper and ends of hair around the rod and wind down to the root. Winding the hair from the points down to the root is known as **croquignole** winding. Do not pull the hair too tightly when winding as this creates undue tension on the hair and could cause hair breakage, or 'pull-burns' on the skin.

   The hair should be spread evenly along the length of the rod. 'Bunching' all the hair in the centre will give an uneven curl.

8. Secure with the rubber band across the top of the rod, making sure that it is not twisted or cutting into the hair, otherwise breakage may occur.

9. Proceed down the first major section. Keep each section the same size as the rod.

10. Continue winding each major section, checking for development at frequent intervals during the wind.

11. When the whole head is completed, post-damp with lotion, taking care that the lotion does not run onto the skin.

12. Check the first and last rod wound for development.

13. To use the body heat from the scalp, place a disposable polythene cap over the head and await development. Check every three to five minutes.

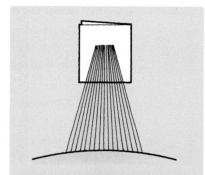

**Fig. 2.5.6** Make sure the endpaper is past the ends of the hair

## TECHNICAL TIPS

Plastic pins can be inserted to lift the rubber band off the hair and to prevent marking the hair.

## Neutralising the hair

1. Before fixing the curl, a development test curl should be carried out to make sure that enough disulphide bonds have been broken to obtain the amount of curl required.

2. Rinse the hair thoroughly in warm water. Check the temperature and pressure of the water used. If a front wash is used, take particular care to avoid water running into the client's eyes and to rinse front rods thoroughly. If a back wash is used (preferred as this reduces the chances of anything washing into the client's eyes) pay particular attention to the rods at the nape.

3. Remove excess water by blotting thoroughly with cotton wool. Leaving the hair too wet will dilute the neutraliser and make it less effective. To check that enough moisture has been removed from the hair, press the palm of the hand onto the rods – if the palm is wet when it is pulled away from the head, the hair requires reblotting.

4. Apply a strip of cotton wool around the hairline to protect the face and neck.

5. Apply the neutraliser to the wound rods, making sure that each one is completely covered. Neutralisers are designed by the manufacturer to work with a particular perm lotion; keep them matched. There are a variety of ways of applying the neutraliser, including cream, foam or liquid. These may be used straight from the container or by using a sponge or brush. It is important to

## Basic perm wind

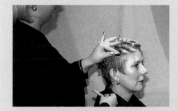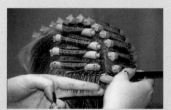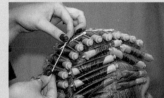

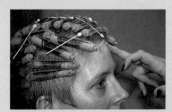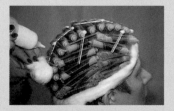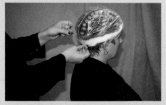

Winding a partial perm wind in a basic nine-section pattern. If needed, weaving the hair instead of taking straight sections will prevent 'tramlines' on the finished result. When the wind is finished, plastic pins are placed under the rubbers to prevent marking and breakage. Barrier cream is applied around the hairline to protect the skin, then damp cotton wool is placed around the hairline for added protection. The stylist uses cotton wool to stop any spillage of the perm lotion. Once the lotion has been applied thoroughly to each rod, a plastic cap is placed over the head to retain body heat and decrease the development time.

*Source*: Plassey Hair Studio, Wrexham

use the neutraliser quickly once it has been mixed or poured otherwise it will lose oxygen as it is released into the atmosphere.

6. Leave for the time recommended by the manufacturer, usually about five minutes. Cotton wool around the hairline prevents the neutraliser from dripping onto the client's face and neck.

7. Carefully remove the cotton wool and the rods. The hair should not be pulled or stretched at this stage as the curl is not yet fully 'fixed'.

8. Apply neutraliser gently to the points of the hair as each rod is removed. Do not drag the hair or massage the neutraliser into the hair as this could alter the curl. Check that all the hair has been treated with the neutraliser then leave for a further five minutes.

9. Rinse the hair thoroughly and apply a pH balance conditioner if necessary to remove any traces of alkali that may be left in the hair, and to make sure the perming process has stopped.

10. Always advise the client on the after-care needed for a permanent wave. Clients do not always realise that a perm will dry the hair and make it more porous, therefore the hair will usually need to be conditioned regularly. Other further chemical processes (e.g. bleaching, tinting) should be approached with caution, again because the hair will be more porous and also because the scalp will be more sensitive for a few days after the perm. The hair should be protected from dampness (such as rain or bathing) after a perm as it will revert back to its new alpha stage when wet – that is, it will become curly.

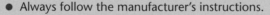

**SAFETY TIPS**

- Always follow the manufacturer's instructions.
- Cotton wool around the hairline prevents chemicals from dripping on face and neck.

**POINTS TO REMEMBER**

- The sulphur bonds are not completely fixed until the hair is dry. This means that care should be taken when setting or blow-drying after the permanent wave. Stretching or pulling the hair at this point can loosen the curl so if the hair is to be blow-dried after the perm (which does involve stretching and moulding the hair) it is often better to allow slightly more curl than required during development to counteract the loosening effect of the blow-dry.
- The hair should be thoroughly rinsed in warm water before the neutraliser is applied.
- All excess moisture must be removed after rinsing and before the neutraliser is applied to prevent dilution of the neutraliser.
- The neutraliser must be left in contact with the hair for the correct length of time to ensure adequate fixing of the curl.
- When permanent waving above a graduated neckline, the curl should be large enough to blend into the straight hair at the neckline.

## Other basic winding techniques

### Directional winding

Directional winding is used mainly on shorter hair. The hair is wound in the direction of the style, therefore it would be impossible to give any definite method of winding as the variations are limitless. By alternating or mixing the size of the rods a mixed curl strength can also be achieved.

### Brickwinding

As the name suggests, this type of wind resembles a brickwork pattern (Fig 2.5.7) and is used to prevent 'tramlines' that may be caused by conventional winding. It is important to start the wind on the top crown area and work outwards and down the head to the nape to allow all the rods to be placed correctly.

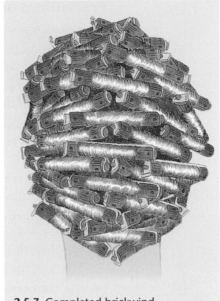

**2.5.7** Completed brickwind

**TECHNICAL TIPS**

When brickwinding, the sides may be wound directionally, either forwards or backwards, according to the finished style.

## Record cards and computer records

Always complete and update the client's record when the process is completed. This should contain the following information:

- Date.
- Hair condition.
- Product used, including the strength of the lotion.
- Size of rod used.
- Development time.
- Any precautions necessary.
- Finished result and any comments necessary.
- Recommended after-care treatment.

Remember that if the records are put onto a computer there is a duty under the Data Protection Act to:

- Protect the client's confidentiality.
- Allow the clients to see the information stored about them if they ask for it. Make sure any remarks about the client are professional.

## Precautions and considerations

1. Always carry out an elasticity, porosity and pre-perm test curl on bleached hair. Bleached hair is in a very porous condition; therefore too strong a lotion can cause irreparable damage.

2. Always use a special or weaker lotion on tinted hair. Tinted hair is also in a porous condition.

3. Test unknown hair for any incompatible chemicals on the hair shaft, e.g. hair colour restorers, with an incompatibility test.

4. Before starting a perm check the scalp for cuts and abrasions. If these are minor, cover and protect with petroleum jelly or barrier cream; if major, postpone the treatment.

5. The porosity of the hair must be taken into consideration when selecting the correct strength of lotion. The porosity can, in some instances, vary along the shaft of the hair, in which case a pre-perm treatment may be needed to even out the porosity.

6. Use the correct size rods for the result you want. Hair sections should be the same size as the rod, as too large a section will result in too great a difference between the root and point curl.

7. Partings should be clean and straight, unless 'weave winding' the hair to prevent rod partings on some types of hair.

8. Each section should be combed thoroughly from root to point.

9. The points of the hair should be wound completely round the rod to prevent fish-hook ends.

10. The tension on the wound hair must be even and the hair evenly distributed along the length of the rod. Do not 'bunch' the hair in the middle of the rod.

11. The rubber of the rod should lie flat and untwisted along the top of the wound hair.

12. The perm lotion should not be allowed to come into contact with the skin as it could cause dermatitis.

13. Barrier cream may be used round the hairline to prevent burning of sensitive skin.

### TECHNICAL TIPS

When leaving hair to develop, remember that heat will speed up the processing time but excessive heat can damage the hair. Therefore always follow the manufacturer's advice regarding development times.

14. Hair should be checked for development every five minutes unless otherwise stated by the manufacturer.

15. Perm lotion should not be allowed to come into contact with anything metallic as this could discolour the hair.

16. If there are any difficulties before, during or after the perming process *always* seek advice from a senior staff member.

## Testing hair for perming

Perm lotion can sometimes damage the hair and it is therefore extremely important to test the hair both before and during perming to make sure that the hair is strong enough to withstand the process and also that the condition of the hair is maintained. Some permanent waving faults, causes and remedies are listed in Table 2.5.1.

### Elasticity test

Carried out before perming to determine the general condition and strength of the hair. A few hairs are removed from the front of the head and they are then pulled between the fingers. If the hair is in a weakened, fragile state then it will break. Hair with good elasticity should be capable of stretching up to half its own length when wet and a third of its own length when dry. If the hair breaks or appears weakened, do not proceed with the perm.

### Porosity test

This test is used to check the hair cuticle for damage. The cuticle is the protective layer of the hair and, if it is damaged in any way, it will absorb the perm lotion very quickly. If this is the case, it will be necessary to even out the porosity with a pre-perm lotion or restructurant and then use a weaker or specially formulated perm lotion.

To determine the hair's porosity, gently slide the fingers down the length of the hair shaft from root to points. Healthy hair feels smooth; the more porous the hair, the rougher it will feel.

Previously treated hair such as tinted or highlighted hair is often damaged (porous) and will therefore need extra care when perming.

### Incompatibility test

This test determines whether there are any chemicals on the hair which will react with the perm lotion.

Take small cuttings from various parts of the head and place them in a simple bleach (a mixture of hydrogen peroxide and ammonia). If there are incompatible chemicals on the hair, the mixture will foam, get hot and the hair will finally disintegrate. It is therefore important not to carry out the perm if this test is positive.

**Table 2.5.1** Permanent waving faults, causes and remedies

| Fault | Possible cause | Action required |
| --- | --- | --- |
| Development time excessively long | Rods too large<br>Use of too few rods<br>Hair sections too large<br>Wrong strength of lotion<br>Cold salon | Change rods if necessary<br>Redamp with correct strength of lotion and leave until fully developed |
| Hairline and scalp irritation | Cuts and abrasions on the scalp<br>Reagent running onto scalp<br>Too much reagent applied<br>Cotton wool placed around hairline or between rods has not been damped | Apply a soothing lotion to the affected areas<br>Use cool water for rinsing and do not massage the scalp |
| Pull-burn | Rods wound too tightly allowing lotion to penetrate hair follicle | Apply soothing lotion to affected area<br>Refer client to doctor if serious |
| Hair breakage (within a week or two) | Rods wound too tightly<br>Rubbers too tight or twisted<br>Overprocessing<br>Reagent too strong<br>Incompatible reaction | Condition the hair using restructurants and deep penetrating conditioner |
| Straight finished result (no curl) | Rods too large<br>Insufficient processing<br>Reagent too weak<br>Insufficient neutralising<br>Too few rods used<br>Poor shampooing | Take test curls, if hair is in a good condition, reperm<br>If hair is in poor condition, treat with conditioning treatments and reperm with weaker lotion |
| Discoloration of the hair | Use of metal tools<br>Use of containers used for other purposes<br>Presence of incompatible chemicals on the hair | If incompatible chemicals are present on the hair, rinse off reagent immediately<br>If the hair remains discoloured after rinsing, apply toning or semi-permanent or temporary rinse |
| Curl weakening | Use of wrong or too weak neutraliser<br>Incorrect timing of neutraliser<br>Insufficient blotting of hair after rinsing<br>Faulty neutraliser<br>Hair pulled excessively when not completely 'fixed' | Take test curls; hair in good condition can be repermed; hair in poor condition should be treated with deep penetrating conditioners before reperming |
| Frizz (curl may appear straight when dry, excessively curly when wet) | Reagent too strong<br>Rod size too small<br>Overprocessing<br>Overheating during development | Condition the hair thoroughly using penetrating conditioner and restructurant<br>Cut the hair if possible |
| Fish-hooks on hair points | Points of the hair doubled back while winding | Remove by cutting |
| Hair too curly | Rod size too small | Hair in good condition can be relaxed by combing through perm lotion then neutralising<br>Hair in poor condition should be treated with deep penetrating conditioners and restructurants and not subjected to further chemical treatments |
| Good curl result when wet, poor result when dry | Hair overstretched when drying<br>Overprocessing | Condition the hair thoroughly and cut if possible |

**Table 2.5.1** continued

| Fault | Possible cause | Correction |
|---|---|---|
| Uneven curl along the hair length | Section too large for rod size<br>Uneven tension along length of the rod<br>Incorrect use of endpapers<br>Hair not combed smoothly from roots to points<br>Hair 'drag'<br>Uneven application of reagent/neutraliser | When hair is in good condition, relax with perm lotion. If curl strength is too great; reperm if curl strength is too weak<br>If hair is in poor condition treat with conditioning agents first |
| Uneven curl throughout the head | *See* section above<br>Section too short for rod length, causing drag at the sides of the section<br>Wind started at the more porous area instead of the most resistant<br>Lotion insufficient or unevenly applied<br>Lack of control when winding causing 'looping' | When hair is in good condition, relax with perm lotion if curl strength is too great; reperm if curl strength is too weak<br>If hair is in poor condition treat with conditioning agent first |
| Straight hair at sides and nape | Incorrect angling or placing of rods<br>Rods too large for length of hair<br>Section too large for rod size<br>Wispy hair around the head left out of the rod | If hair is in good condition reperm the straight hair, making sure that the perm lotion does not come into contact with the curled areas |

## Pre-perm test curl

Winding a couple of rods with the chosen perm lotion at the back of the head will tell the stylist whether the hair is suitable for perming or not. A pre-perm test curl will also show the strength of lotion to use and how long it should be left in contact with the hair.

## Development test curl

This test is carried out during the perming process, once the perm lotion has been applied, to decide how much processing has occurred.

Gently unwind a rod, without removing it completely, then push the hair back gently towards the roots. If the perm is ready the hair will form an S-shaped movement the size of which depends upon the amount of curl needed. A large S-movement gives a loose curl while a small S-movement will give a tight curl. Check different rods at various parts of the head to make sure there is an even development throughout the whole head. Keep hair points round the rod by holding with the thumbs while pushing the hair towards the roots.

# Activity

Discuss with your supervisor at what point, and for what type of problems, should you alert them either before, during or after perming or neutralising.

## Other types of perm

### Acid perms

These are believed to be less damaging to the hair than alkaline perms. They are usually supplied with an activator and their own neutraliser. When the hair has been wound, the lotion is mixed with the activator and applied to the hair making sure, as with all post-damping, that each rod is thoroughly dampened with the lotion.

Most acid perms need heat to speed up their development and even then they tend to be slow-acting. When checking the development of an acid perm, look at the 'stranding' of the hair section as well as the S-shape formed. The hair should separate into about seven strands when it has developed.

### Foam perm

This needs a special machine which is powered by electricity and has two separate guns, one to pump air into the perm lotion and the other for the neutraliser, making a foam of each. Because of its aerated nature, this perm is applied after the rods are wound and is very comfortable for the client as the lotions do not drip.

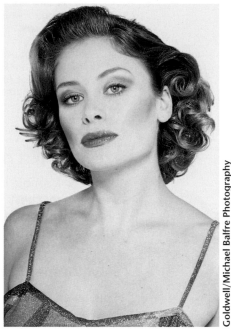

Goldwell/Michael Balfre Photography

### Uni perm

This perm is processed by heat from a machine similar to the old heat perm machine. The machine has heated bars which then heat up the clamps attached to it. The hair is wound taking large sections to accommodate the size of the clamps which are placed over the wound rods and then left to cool. The hair must be pushed to the centre of the rod and the rubber band placed along its top to allow the hair to be properly heated and prevent the rubber band from melting.

### Exothermic perming

This type of perm is wound in exactly the same as a cold perm way except that the lotion is always applied after, instead of during, winding. It is therefore important not to allow the hair to dry out during winding – if it does, redamp with water. When the wind has been completed, mix the two chemicals together according to the manufacturer's instructions. The mixture will become warm. Apply this warm mixture evenly over the wound rods and await development. When the required amount of curl is achieved, rinse and neutralise according to the manufacturer's instructions.

## Things to do

**You will need:**

- Tuition head and clamp.
- Sectioning clips.
- Tail comb.
- Rods of uniform size and endpapers.
- Permanent waving lotion and neutraliser for normal hair with applicator bottles.
- Permanent waving lotion and neutraliser for treated hair with applicator bottles.
- Cotton wool and towel.
- Water spray.

1. Wet the tuition head thoroughly with water, remove excess moisture with the towel.
2. Divide the hair into three sections, forehead to crown (the width of a rod), then from ear to ear at either side. Pin the remaining hair out of the way.
3. Wind both the front two sections using the same size rods. When they are wound, place cotton wool around them to protect the other hair.
4. Apply the perm lotion for normal hair to the left side section and apply the lotion for treated hair to the right side section.
5. Leave to develop until an S-shaped curl is formed.
6. Rinse thoroughly in tepid water, then blot dry and place cotton wool around the rods.
7. Apply the neutraliser and leave for five minutes (or according to the manufacturer's instructions).
8. Remove the rods and apply more neutraliser to the hair ends. Leave for a further five minutes then remove by rinsing the hair thoroughly in warm water.
9. Towel-dry the hair and comb through.

Compare the results of both sides of the tuition head. How does the curl strength differ? How does the hair feel on each side?

## What do you know?

- Name the chemical process occurring during the **first**, softening stage in perming.
- What is the **main** ingredient in alkaline perms?
- What happens in the hair during neutralisation?
- What is meant by presaturation?
- What is meant by post-damping?
- What can happen if the rod rubbers are **twisted** on the hair?
- How often and how should perming **development** be checked?
- When neutralising, why must the hair be thoroughly **blotted** after rinsing to remove the excess moisture?
- What factors can cause an excessively **long** processing time?
- List **three** important pieces of advice which can be given on the after-care of permed hair.

# 5b

In this unit you will learn about:

- How to safely perm, relax, and neutralise curly hair, particularly African Caribbean hair.
- How to consult with the client, carry out diagnostic tests, prepare tools and equipment, and organise methods of work.
- Basic perming techniques.
- Relaxing techniques using a range of products.
- Neutralising techniques.

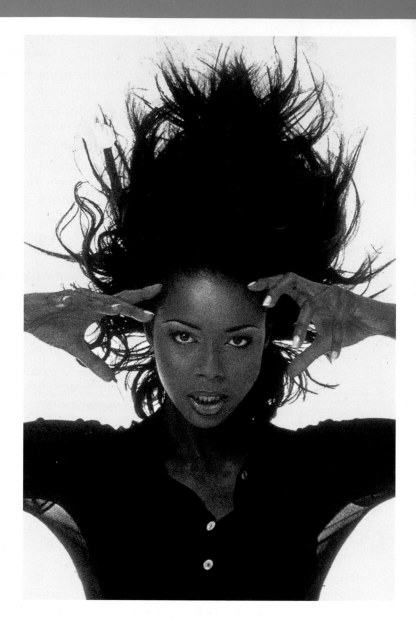

# Perming and relaxing hair

This unit is about relaxing African Caribbean hair but the techniques can also be used on Caucasian tight curly hair. Much of this material is covered in Unit 2.5a and here is an activity to help you find the information from Unit 2.5a that is relevant to this unit.

# Activity

Use Unit 2.5a to find answers to the following questions:

1. How should the client be gowned and positioned?
2. How should their hair be prepared?
3. What personal protective equipment should be used by the stylist?
4. What are the following tests and when are they used?
   (a) elasticity
   (b) porosity
   (c) incompatibility
   (d) pre-perm test curl
   (e) development test curl
   (f) strand
5. How are the following products used?
   (a) barrier cream
   (b) pre-perm treatment
   (c) acid perm lotion
   (d) alkaline perm lotion
   (e) neutralising agents
6. List the sundries used in the perming and neutralising process.

There are several key differences between the structure of African Caribbean, and non-curly Mongoloid or Caucasian hair which influence the products and procedures used when carrying out a perming or straightening process.

## Structure of African Caribbean hair

### Medulla

The medulla is the centre layer of the hair and, unlike Caucasian hair, it often has colour pigment present. Therefore it is often difficult to detect the medulla in African Caribbean hair.

## Cuticle

The cuticle of African Caribbean hair has seven to eleven layers, which is more than the four to seven layers of Caucasian hair but less than the eleven plus layers of Mongoloid hair. However, the continual everyday brushing and dressing of the tight curl of African Caribbean hair tends to damage and remove some of the cuticle layers towards the ends of the hair, making them more porous than the root area. The better the hair condition then the more resistant it is to chemical products. However, because of the uneven porosity along the length of the hair shaft, the stylist must be very thorough when analysing the hair to determine the strength of chemicals to use.

The twisting, bending nature of African Caribbean hair also prevents the cuticle layers lying as flat as they do for Caucasian or Mongoloid, preventing light from reflecting as easily and making the hair appear duller. Spray gloss is often used to counteract this and to make the hair more supple and less likely to break.

## Cortex

African Caribbean hair is flattened in shape, which means that it has a smaller amount of cortex than the round-shaped Caucasian or Mongoloid hair. Therefore, once chemicals have penetrated into the cortex they react more quickly and great care has to be taken to prevent the hair becoming over-processed or destroyed.

The tight curl of most African Caribbean hair gives two different cortex types within each hair. These types are known as **orthocortex** and **paracortex**. The orthocortex contains less sulphur and is on the **outside** of the curl or wave curve; the paracortex is on the **inside** of the curve. This means that the orthocortex is stretched more than the paracortex, making it less dense than the compact paracortex.

The hair's natural colour pigment is deposited mainly in the cortex but, unlike Caucasian hair, a small percentage is also present in both the cuticle and the medulla. The colour pigment (melanin) granules of African Caribbean hair are larger than those in Caucasian hair. The cortex also gives the hair 75 per cent of its strength and the cuticle gives it 25 per cent.

The cortex contains the following bonds (Fig. 2.5.8):

- **Disulphide bonds** are strong bonds between the sulphur atoms. These are the bonds which are broken during perming and relaxing processes.
- **Hydrogen bonds** are weaker bonds between the hydrogen and oxygen atoms. These bonds are broken by heat and stretching during setting and pressing.
- **Salt linkages** are formed between the negative and positive ions in amino acids. These bonds are found between and within the polypeptide chains, and are easily broken by weak acids and alkalis.

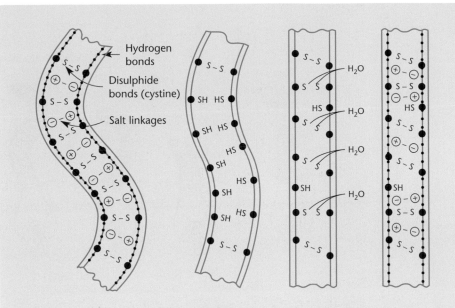

**Fig. 2.5.8** African Caribbean hair contains disulphide bonds (cystine), hydrogen bonds and salt linkages. When an ammonium thioglycollate straightener is applied, it produces hydrogen (H) which reacts with the cystine to produce two cysteines (SH). The hydrogen bonds and salt linkages are also broken and the hair's natural curl then relaxes. The straightener is then rinsed from the hair and a neutraliser applied. The neutraliser contains oxygen atoms. One oxygen atom combines with two hydrogen atoms to form water ($H_2O$). When the neutraliser is rinsed from hair, all three bonds (disulphide, hydrogen and salt) reform in a new, straightened position.

## How the natural curl of African Caribbean hair is formed

There are several theories regarding the formation of the distinctive tight curl of African Caribbean hair. The curl formation is believed to be due to the way cell division takes place at the base of the hair in the germinal matrix of the papilla. The cell division here is uneven in that one side divides more quickly than the other. However, to further complicate matters, this additional cell division is not constant on one side but shifts from side to side. The hair bends away from where the cell division is greatest and it is therefore made to bend from side to side which causes it to curl. The process of cell division is known as **mitosis**; therefore the curliness of African Caribbean hair, and some other types of hair, is often said to be caused by uneven rates of mitosis (Fig. 2.5.9).

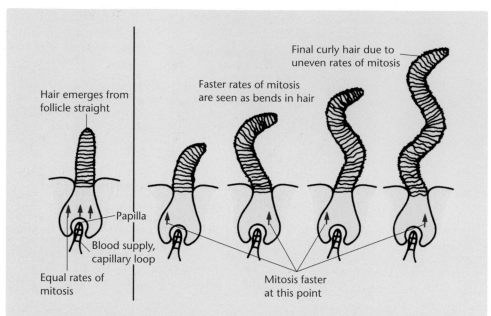

**Fig. 2.5.9** The cyclical theory of hair growth. The first hair on the left has emerged from the follicle as a straight hair because the rates of cell division (mitosis) in the papilla are equal. However, the second hair has emerged curly because the rate of cell division has not been even; the arrows on the diagram show where the cell division is fastest.

## Perming African Caribbean or tight curly hair

### Specially formulated products

Although perming products are similar for Caucasian, Mongoloid and African Caribbean hair, it is always better to use products which have been formulated for the specific type. Always make sure that the correct neutraliser is used in conjunction with the perming lotion to ensure a successful result and avoid hair breakage. Here are some of them:

- **Curl rearranger** – ammonium thioglycollate is the active ingredient in these products and it is used in cream or gel form. It is available in three to four strengths, from mild to super or maximum, depending on the manufacturer. Curl rearrangers are used before perming to soften and straighten the hair.

- **Curl booster (perm lotion)** – this is often the name given to the perm solution. Ammonium thioglycollate is also the active ingredient in curl boosters although it is in a weaker form than in curl rearrangers. They are used in exactly the same way as a cold perm on Caucasian or Mongoloid hair.

- **Neutraliser** – the main ingredient is either hydrogen peroxide or sodium bromate. Both act as oxidising agents although sodium bromate does not lighten the hair as much as hydrogen peroxide and tends to be less likely to cause irritation to the scalp.

- **Pre-perm lotion** – this coats the hair with a protective polymer film to even out the porosity. It is left in the hair prior to perming but should be used sparingly otherwise it will prevent penetration of the curl rearranger.

- **Moisturiser** – glycerine is often used as the base for moisturisers. They help to prevent moisture loss from the cortex by coating the hair with oils. Hair needs to be sprayed with moisturisers at least every other day after curly perming to keep the hair and scalp supple. Moisturisers also prolong the life of the perm as they prevent it becoming dry and brittle but use them sparingly or they can be difficult to remove when shampooing.

- **Hydrolysed keratin conditioner** – used after a curly perm to minimise chemical damage by helping to replace some of the lost amino acids and maintain the moisture level within the cortex.

The active chemical ingredients in many of these products can be hazardous and may be covered by the COSHH Regulations:

- Always follow the manufacturer's instructions.
- Avoid spillage.
- Avoid skin contact.
- Dispose of the containers with care.
- Protect the client.
- Protect yourself as the stylist.
- Keep careful records.
- Look out for any contra-indications.

## Perming African Caribbean hair

### How perming works

An African Caribbean perm is usually called a curly perm, or sometimes a curl redirector or wet-look perm. Ammonium thioglycollate is the active ingredient in the perm lotion, and it is also used for **curl rearranging**, carried out before the perming process to soften and straighten the hair.

The hair structure is altered in exactly the same way as when perming Caucasian hair. The alkalinity of the ammonium thioglycollate swells the hair, causing the cuticle scales to lift and open, this allows the perm lotion to penetrate into the cortex more easily. A reducing action takes place, breaking the disulphide bonds. When enough bonds have been broken, the action is stopped by rinsing the hair thoroughly in warm water. The hair is then permanently 'fixed' in a new position by reforming the disulphide bonds in this new position through the addition of oxygen in the form of a 'neutraliser'. The hydrogen and salt bonds are also reformed in the new position. This chemical process was explained in greater detail in Unit 2.5a.

## Testing the hair before perming

Tests which can be carried out include the porosity test, elasticity test, incompatibility test and pre-perm test curl. The choice of test will depend on the hair condition and what information the stylist requires. See Unit 2.5a for details of how these tests are carried out.

## Test curl for a curly perm

This is carried out before the perm, using different strengths of lotion to decide the most suitable strength to use and to make sure that the hair can withstand the process.

### Method

1. Shampoo the hair and apply pre-perm treatment if necessary (according to the manufacturer's instructions).
2. Section off a small section of hair, enough to hold two or three perm rods, at the nape of the neck. If there are any problems, the hair in this area can be more easily covered.
3. Clip the remaining hair out of the way and coat with conditioner to protect.
4. Apply the **curl rearranger** to the nape hair. Straighten the hair with the back of the comb then cover with a cap to retain body heat. When ready, rinse from the hair and blot out excess moisture.
5. Apply **perm lotion** (**curl booster**) then comb the hair with a wide-toothed comb. Wind one or two rods, protect surrounding hair from the lotion by placing a strip of damp cotton wool around the wound rods. Cover with a cap then leave to develop, checking every two to three minutes.
6. When developed rinse in warm water. Blot out excess moisture then neutralise.
7. Rinse out neutraliser and apply conditioner. Assess condition, porosity and elasticity of the hair.
8. Record the results.

Full and detailed records are very important. If kept on computer, the Data Protection Act gives the client a right to confidentiality and a right to see the records.

## Curly perming African Caribbean hair

This involves using two lotions, in two stages to alter the hair structure. In the first stage (unless the hair is extremely porous), a curl rearranger is used to soften and break down some of the disulphide bonds. This is then followed by the second, curl booster, stage which moulds the hair into a new curled shape which is softer and less curly than the hair's original state (Fig. 2.5.10).

### How to curly perm

1. Carry out any necessary tests. If they are satisfactory, protect the client with towels and gown and self with tinting apron and gloves.

2. Do not shampoo the hair unless it is heavily coated with oils or gloss. Indeed, it is preferable not to shampoo the hair for at least three days beforehand. However, always follow manufacturer's instructions as this will give specific guidance for their product.

3. Apply pretreatment to the hair if necessary. Blot to remove any excess then place the client under a hairdryer to harden and dry the treatment into the hair.

4. Apply protective cream around the hairline and ears then section the hair into four major sections: forehead to nape then ear to ear across the crown.

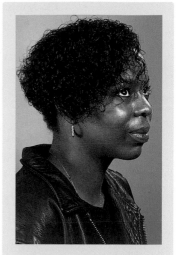

**Fig. 2.5.10** African Caribbean curly perm

5. Starting at the nape, as this is usually the most resistant area, take small subsections of hair approximately 0.6 cm ($\frac{1}{4}$ in) wide. Apply the correct strength curl rearranger 0.6 cm ($\frac{1}{4}$ in) from the scalp and along the length of the hair section. Work as quickly as possible, from side to side, up towards the front of the head making sure that the hair is thoroughly coated with the curl rearranger.

6. When application is complete, smooth the hair with the back of the comb or the fingers then cover with a plastic cap to retain the body heat and prevent dry-out. Leave to develop following manufacturer's instructions.

7. When the hair is sufficiently softened and straightened, remove the rearranger by rinsing the hair thoroughly in warm water for five minutes.

8. Blot the hair to remove excess moisture. Do not rub the hair as it is now in a fragile state.

9. Resection the head into nine basic sections, or in accordance with the salon's normal practice.

10. Start winding the hair as for a normal cold perm. The perm lotion (curl booster) may be applied either as each rod is wound (predamping) or when the winding is complete (post-damping). Always follow manufacturer's instructions for the best results.

11. Leave to develop. Heat may be applied to quicken the process but, if a dryer is used, make sure the head is covered with a plastic cap to prevent the hair drying out. Check for development at the front, nape and sides of the head.

12. When development is complete, rinse the hair thoroughly in warm water for five to ten minutes. Blot carefully to remove excess moisture then place a strip of cotton wool around the hairline to protect the skin.

13. Apply the neutraliser to the rods, pushing it well into the hair. Leave for the time stated by the manufacturer, usually five minutes.

**TECHNICAL TIPS**

The larger the perm rod, the looser the curl.

14. Gently unwind the rods then apply additional neutraliser to the ends of the hair where the endpapers have been. Leave for a further five minutes then rinse thoroughly from the hair.

15. Apply a keratin conditioner to the hair, taking care not to disturb the curl, and leave for three to five minutes. Rinse from the hair and apply an oil-rich 'curl activator' to prevent further moisture loss from the hair. Complete a record of work carried out and advise the client on the after-care of the curly perm.

**SAFETY TIPS**

Always use the correct neutraliser for the perm lotion. Do not mix different manufacturers' perming and neutralising products. At best the perm may not take; at worst there could be an adverse reaction on the hair.

## Regrowth application of a curly perm

In this case it is important to apply the curl rearranger to the regrowth area only, but again apply the lotion 0.6 cm away from the scalp. The remaining hair may be coated with conditioner or a protective polymer to help prevent overlapping and possible breakage. When the hair is sufficiently softened and straightened, proceed as for the second stage of a full head curly perm.

If the hair is porous the curl rearranger stage is omitted and the hair is permed using the post-damping technique to prevent overprocessing.

## Precautions and considerations

The same considerations and precautions are necessary for perming African Caribbean hair as for perming Caucasian hair. These have been previously covered in detail in Unit 2.5a. However, there are also the following additional factors to take into account when carrying out perming processes on this hair type:

1. Do not use curl rearranger or perming products on highly porous or bleached African Caribbean hair.

2. Always carry out the necessary tests before the treatment to make sure that the hair is strong enough to withstand the double application of perm lotion.

3. Use a conditioner or pre-perm lotion on porous hair.

4. Do not curly perm over previously relaxed hair.

5. Do not overlap the curl rearranger onto any previously treated hair.

6. Rinse off any of the lotions immediately if irritation occurs.

7. Always use the correct neutralisers for the perm lotion being used.

8. Condition and moisturise the hair before and after the treatment. Always advise the client on the after-care of their hair.

## Relaxing hair

Relaxing hair permanently alters its internal structure, reducing any wave or curl movement that the hair may have. For this reason, it is usually better to cut the hair after the relaxing process as it is then more manageable and easier to judge the overall hair length.

Calcium hydroxide, potassium hydroxide and sodium hydroxide are chemicals used to relax the hair. All are extremely alkaline with a pH of between 10 and 14 and if used incorrectly can cause irreparable damage to the hair. Sodium hydroxide, known as caustic soda or lye, is the most commonly used base for relaxers and, under the 1989 Cosmetic Products (Safety) Regulations, relaxing products in Britain are only allowed to contain 4–5 per cent sodium hydroxide. Relaxers also contain skin coolers and conditioning agents to help lessen skin irritation, replace lost oils and maintain the hair's moisture content. Relaxers can usually be obtained in three strengths: mild, regular and super.

### Sodium hydroxide relaxers

#### Advantages

● They are very quick acting.

● They straighten the hair more effectively than any other straightening agents.

● The hair is less likely to revert back to its previous curly shape after neutralising.

#### Disadvantages

● The hair may become brittle and break off.

● If left longer than ten minutes, the hair may dissolve.

● They can cause severe burning of the skin.

● If sodium hydroxide is left too long the hair may turn red.

### How a relaxer works

The process of relaxing differs from perming or straightening the hair with ammonium thioglycollate in that the disulphide bonds, hydrogen bonds and salt bonds (these are the bonds within the cortex which hold the hair in its natural shape) are broken and rearranged by a chemical reaction known as **hydrolysis**.

This is a very complex process but, put simply, the relaxer (sodium hydroxide) adds water and hydrogen to the disulphide bonds (cystine) forming cysteine and sulphenic acid. As the hair straightens, the newly formed cysteine and sulphenic acid react together to form the amino acid lathionine. Lathionine has only one sulphur atom instead of the two of cystine, therefore the spare sulphur atom attaches itself to the water to form hydrosulphide.

The above process is continuous. The newly formed lathionine is able to hold the hair in a new straightened shape, therefore it is not necessary to reform the sulphur bonds by neutralising as in conventional perming. Instead, the action of the alkaline sodium hydroxide is stopped by rinsing it from the hair and then applying a special **acid** shampoo to neutralise the alkalinity of the relaxer. When the hair is dried, the hydrogen bonds and the salt bonds are reformed in the hair's new position, helping to hold it permanently in its new straightened shape.

A test cutting should be taken before any relaxing process because of the high alkalinity of the relaxer cream.

## Testing the hair before using the relaxer

Incorrectly used relaxers can seriously damage the hair. Pre-testing the hair before starting the treatment enables the stylist to select the correct strength of relaxer and will also give an indication of how long the development should be. The relaxer can be tested either on test cuttings of hair or while still on the head.

### Method 1

Take a few strands of hair from various parts of the head and apply a small amount of the relaxer cream evenly along the lengths. Do not leave the relaxer in contact with the hair longer than recommended by the manufacturer and observe constantly. Shampoo with neutralising shampoo then assess the relaxation of the hair or any damage that may have been sustained. If the test shows any sign of breakage or excessive elasticity, postpone the treatment until the hair has been conditioned and retested at a later date. Record the results of the test.

### Method 2

Take a section of hair from the nape area of the head, pull through a piece of aluminium foil with a slit in it, alternatively use an easi-meche packet to hold the hair section. Apply relaxer and allow to process checking frequently. Rinse, then shampoo with neutralising shampoo. Check hair porosity and elasticity. Record findings including the processing time.

## Application of sodium hydroxide relaxers

1. Check the client's records for any previous treatments.
2. Examine the scalp for any cuts, abrasions or inflammation – if any disorders are present then postpone the treatment.
3. Examine the hair for:

- tightness of curl
- elasticity and tensile strength
- texture and porosity
- any breakage

4. Examine and assess the results of the preliminary pre-perm test.

5. Make sure the client is adequately protected by a gown and towel. Apply protective cream (petroleum cream or jelly usually) evenly in order to cover the scalp and around the hairline (known as basing) to prevent burning or irritation of the skin by the product. Do not shampoo the hair or rub/brush the scalp. Some products only require basing around the hairline and ears.

6. The stylist must wear protective gloves.

7. Read the manufacturer's instructions carefully before the treatment starts.

8. Section the hair into four: forehead to nape then ear to ear across the crown.

**SAFETY TIPS**

Use specialist African Caribbean products for best results.

9. Start application by taking small sections, applying enough relaxer cream to the hair 0.6 cm ($\frac{1}{4}$ in) away from the scalp. Do not allow the relaxer to touch the scalp.

10. With previously relaxed hair, apply to the regrowth only.

11. When application is complete use a gentle smoothing technique to straighten the hair, starting where the cream was first applied. It is important that the hair should not be pulled or stretched during the application.

12. The approximate times for relaxing hair are as follows:
    - Fine hair takes two to three minutes.
    - Medium hair takes three to five minutes.
    - Coarse hair takes five to seven minutes.

    The maximum time for even the most resistant hair should not exceed eight minutes.

13. Rinse at a back wash with a strong force of warm water. Start at the hairline and hold the hose 10–12.5 cm (4–5 in) from the head. Do not use hands to remove the cream from the hairline; let the force of the water remove it.

14. Use a neutralising acid shampoo to thoroughly shampoo the hair. On the second shampoo, gently but firmly comb the hair straight and leave for five minutes, then rinse. All relaxers have their own specialist neutralising shampoos. Always follow the manufacturer's instructions.

15. Remove excess moisture from the hair by blotting; do not rub the hair. Apply a pH moisturising conditioner as a treatment and leave for at least ten minutes before rinsing thoroughly.

16. Complete a record of work.

## Curly perming African Caribbean hair

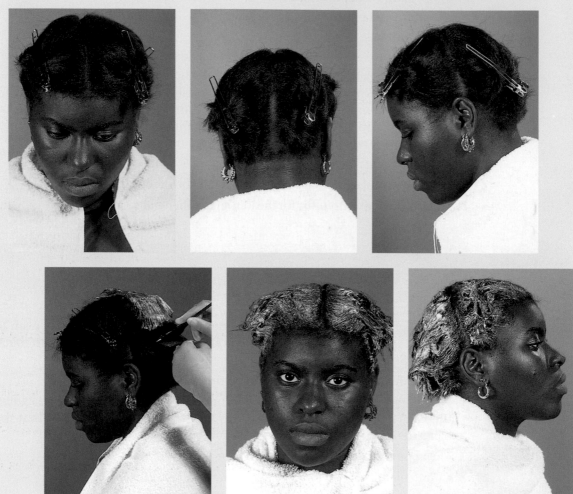

Hair is sectioned into four: forehead to nape then ear to ear across the crown. Relaxer cream is applied to the hair at least 0.6 cm ($\frac{1}{4}$in) away from the scalp. The sylist must always remember to wear protective gloves while working through each section, towards the front.

**Note:** When styling the hair after relaxing do not use high heated equipment, e.g. hot brushes, etc.

### Contra-indications when relaxing hair

Do not start a relaxing process in any of the following cases:

- Cuts, abrasions or inflammation on the scalp.
- The hair is coated with incompatible chemicals.
- Fragile or broken hair.

- Hair has been chemically damaged, particularly bleached.
- Hair or scalp with an infectious or contagious disease.
- On children under ten years of age.

## Health and safety

1. Always carry out a preliminary pre-perm test.
2. Carry out an incompatibility test if necessary.
3. Read the manufacturer's instructions very carefully and use only as directed.

**SAFETY TIPS**

Apply protective cream to the scalp and skin around the hairline to protect them from the chemicals.

4. Examine the hair and scalp carefully to decide the correct strength of relaxer. If in doubt, choose a weaker type.
5. Protect the skin and scalp with a protective cream.
6. The stylist must always wear protective gloves.
7. Do not allow the relaxer cream to come into contact with the scalp or any part of the skin.
8. Do not pull or stretch the hair during the application; it could break.
9. Do not use hot brushes, heated curling tongs or any other heated implements on the hair either during or after relaxing.
10. If the cream relaxer enters the eyes, rinse immediately with water and seek medical aid. Sodium hydroxide could cause blindness.
11. If the cream relaxer causes skin irritation, rinse off immediately and shampoo the hair with a non-alkaline shampoo. If irritation persists, seek medical aid.
12. Use a timer when processing to prevent the relaxer being left in contact with the hair too long.
13. Test frequently for development. Do not exceed the maximum time permitted by the manufacturer.
14. When rinsing the relaxer cream from the hair, great care must be taken to see that the chemical does not run into the eyes or ears by careless directing of the water.
15. Use the force of the water to remove the cream. Keep hands protected.
16. Always complete a record of the treatment carried out.
17. Advise client on after-care and the importance of conditioning and moisturising treatments after relaxing.
18. Pay attention to health, safety and hygiene at all times.
19. In the event of any unforeseen problems, refer to a senior staff member in charge.

## Things to do

Collect information on the products and techniques for African Caribbean hair. Present this as a report on African Caribbean hairdressing.

## What do you know?

- Name the **two** different cortex types of African Caribbean hair.
- What is mitosis?
- What is the **main** active ingredient in curl rearrangers and curl boosters?
- Describe how to carry out a **test curl** for a curly perm.
- Name the **main** ingredient in hair relaxers.
- List the contra-indications to relaxing hair.

- Explain what happens to the **internal** structure of the hair when relaxing it.
- What is the purpose of using a neutraliser **after** curly perming the hair?
- What is the purpose of the neutralising shampoo **when** relaxing the hair?
- List the **disadvantages** of using a sodium hydroxide relaxer.

# 6

In this unit you will learn about:

- The types of products used to colour and highlight hair.
- How temporary, semi-permanent, quasi and permanent colours work.
- How bleach works.
- The tests needed before colouring and highlighting hair.
- Preparation of the client and yourself for colouring hair.
- Methods of applying the different types of colour.
- How to solve any problems that might happen when colouring hair.
- How to work safely and efficiently when colouring hair.

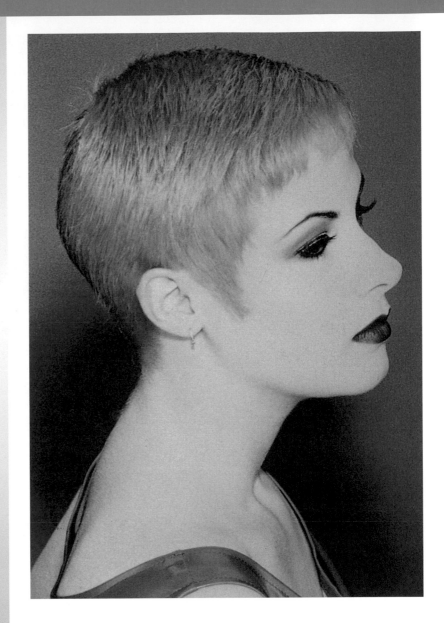

# Colouring hair

## Non-permanent hair colouring

Colouring the hair is often called **tinting** and there are a range of products for safe and effective tinting (Fig. 2.6.1). Permanent colours have to be cut out of the hair; non-permanent colours may last up to about 12 weeks and are usually classified into three types: temporary, semi-permanent and quasi (Table 2.6.1).

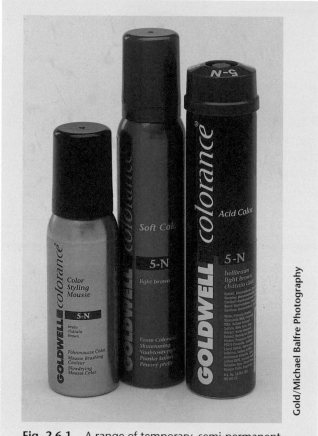

Gold/Michael Balfre Photography

**Fig. 2.6.1**    A range of temporary, semi-permanent and permanent coluring products in the same colour

**Table 2.6.1**  The four main types of tinting product

| Type | Approximate lasting time |
| --- | --- |
| Temporary | Washes out at the first shampoo |
| Semi-permanent | Lasts for 6 to 8 shampoos |
| Quasi | Fades over about 12 weeks |
| Permanent | Has to be cut out |

## Temporary colours

### Temporary rinses

Temporary rinses are applied to wet hair. They have large, coloured molecules which coat the outside cuticle of the hair (Fig. 2.6.2), and are therefore easily washed out.

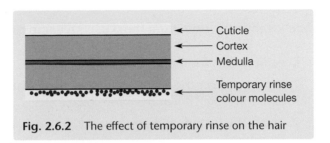

Cuticle
Cortex
Medulla
Temporary rinse colour molecules

**Fig. 2.6.2** The effect of temporary rinse on the hair

**POINTS TO REMEMBER**

A common acid dye used in temporary rinses is an azo dye (e.g. parahyroxazobenzene). The acid used is an organic acid (citric or tartaric) and has a pH of between 2.5 and 4.0. These acids are soluble in water and this makes them easier to remove by shampooing. Temporary rinses can be found in the following forms:

- **Coloured setting lotion** – contains synthetic resin, polyvinyl pyrrolidone (a plastic) and alcohol in addition to the acid dye. On drying, the alcohol evaporates leaving a coloured plastic film on the hair.
- **Coloured mousse and gel** – normal mousse or gel with a suitable acid dye added.
- **Temporary toners** – ready mixed for use on bleached hair to get rid of unwanted gold tones. They often contain a mild conditioner in addition to the acid dye.

### When to use temporary rinses

1. As an introduction to colour, particularly useful for younger clients.
2. To brighten dull or faded hair. May also be used between permanent dye retouches if the colour has faded.
3. To tone bleached hair or to temporarily rectify a colour fault.
4. To mingle in grey hair. But remember that these rinses will not completely cover the grey hairs.
5. To darken natural coloured hair.
6. To add multi or partial colouring to the hair.

### How to apply a temporary rinse

Temporary rinses are easy to use as most can be applied straight from the bottle. Coloured mousse and gel can be applied as normal but read the manufacturer's instructions.

1. Shampoo hair, towel-dry and comb through.

2. Protect client with dark gown and towel and protect yourself with apron and rubber gloves.

3. Apply rinse straight from the bottle by sprinkling onto the roots (these are less porous) then rubbing through to the ends of the hair.

4. Comb hair through to make sure the rinse is evenly distributed throughout the head.

5. Remove any rinse from the skin with damp cotton wool.

### Considerations for temporary rinses

1. Always protect the client's clothing, particularly at the neck area, by tucking a dark towel well down over any collars, etc.

2. Assess the texture and porosity of the hair before starting to apply the temporary rinse.

3. Pre-towel-dry the hair thoroughly to stop the rinse being diluted.

4. Never choose a temporary colour a shade lighter than the natural colour of the hair – it will not show.

**SAFETY TIPS**

Make sure the client is adequately protected from splashes or spillage.

5. Do not apply strong red shades to hair that contains any white hair, particularly on the front hairline.

6. When applying temporary rinses to freshly bleached hair, make sure that an antioxidant cream rinse is applied beforehand. Any hydrogen peroxide left in the hair could cause a bleach-out of the colour rinse.

7. For hair with an uneven or high degree of porosity, either apply a good hair conditioner or restructurant, or leave the hair wet by not towel-drying thoroughly before applying the rinse.

8. Use only a fine hairspray when dressing out after a temporary rinse. Heavy lacquering could redissolve the colour and give a patchy effect.

9. Do not display temporary coloured setting lotions near sunlight or heat, as either can cause deterioration and colour distortion.

**POINTS TO REMEMBER**    Porous hair needs extra care as it will absorb the rinse very quickly, making the final colour too dark or uneven. Applying the rinse with a tinting brush instead of straight from the bottle gives greater control and allows the rinse to be applied evenly and where necessary, this reduces the likelihood of a patchy result.

**Temporary colour sprays, paints and hair mascara**

These are all applied to dry hair and are good for special effects. The colours are limited and they are usually very bright. There are four types of this temporary colour:

- **Aerosol can form** – has a lacquer type base and is sprayed onto the hair, usually after it has been dressed.
- **Puff on powder** – this is a coloured powder that is just puffed onto dry hair where it is needed.
- **Coloured mascara** – vibrant colours in a mascara type applicator. The colour is stroked on where needed using the applicator brush.
- **Hair paints** – small pots of thick, water-soluble hair paint that is stroked on the hair in streaks where needed.

**SAFETY TIPS**

Metallic gold or silver temporary sprays or powder must be completely removed from the hair before perming, tinting or bleaching as they will react with the hydrogen peroxide used in these processes, causing rapid decomposition of the peroxide and, consequently, hair damage. In other words, they are incompatible with the peroxide used in other processes.

## Semi-permanent colours

Semi-permanent dyes are applied to wet hair. They have smaller coloured molecules than temporary rinses and are able to go deeper into the cuticle of the hair to just inside the cortex. This means they last longer, between six to eight shampoos (Fig. 2.6.3).

Semi-permanent dyes have a limited colour range with not many brown shades to choose from. They do not lighten the hair and if a shade is chosen that is lighter than the base shade (existing hair colour) of the client then it will not show.

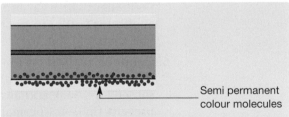

Semi permanent colour molecules

**Fig. 2.6.3** The effect of semi-permanent on the hair

**When to use semi-permanent colours**

1. To brighten dull or faded hair.
2. To tone bleached hair.
3. To mingle in grey hair.
4. For use on clients who are allergic to para dyes.
5. To rectify colour faults, e.g. a green discoloration can be rectified by red.
6. For preliminary pigmentation when returning bleached hair to its natural colour.

7. In conjunction with bleach to give subtle or striking effects to the hair (depending upon the colour of the semi-permanent used). For example, streaking or scrunch bleaching the hair, then applying a semi-permanent over the whole head will give lighter and darker tones of the semi-permanent colour.

**POINTS TO REMEMBER**

Semi-permanent dyes are made from synthetic, organic dyes known as nitro dyes. Nitro dyes are small coloured molecules which can pass through the cuticle into the cortex, but because they are small they pass out again too. This means they are gradually washed from the hair. Semi-permanents also usually contain:

- **Benzol alcohol** – this is added as a solvent because nitro dyes do not dissolve easily in water. Adding benzol alcohol lets the dye penetrate deeper into the cortex.
- **Sodium lauryl sulphate** – this is a detergent which produces a foam and helps to improve contact between the hair and the dye.

### How to apply a semi-permanent dye

1. Shampoo the hair and towel-dry unless instructed otherwise by the manufacturer — some semi-permanents are shampooed into the hair.

2. Protect the client with a tinting gown, dark towel and preferably a disposable plastic cape to cover the whole of the client and the chair. Protect yourself with apron and rubber gloves.

3. Section the head into four main sections (Fig. 2.6.4).

4. Apply barrier cream around the hairline to prevent skin from staining. Take care to apply it to the skin only.

5. Start application at the nape and apply semi-permanent with a brush (or sponge or applicator bottle) to the roots and along the hair shaft (Fig. 2.6.3).

6. Continue application towards the front hairline with the front two sections. Take the subsections back and away from the face to prevent the semi-permanent running onto the face.

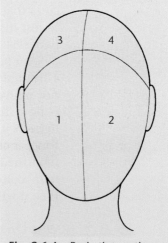

**Fig. 2.6.4    Basic tint sections**

7. Apply the semi-permanent carefully to the last 1 cm ($\frac{1}{2}$ in) of the hairline. This is best done with a brush, even when using a sponge or applicator bottle on the remainder of the hair. A brush gives more control and helps to avoid skin staining on the face and neck.

8. Cross-check the application by taking sections across the subsections. Make sure that the application is thorough and that the semi-permanent dye is even along the hair shaft.

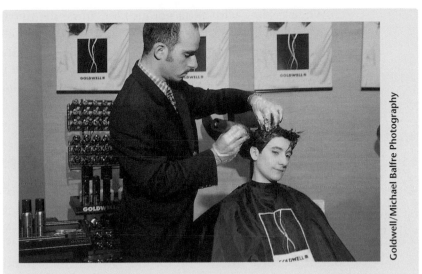

**Fig. 2.6.5**   Semi-permanent application using an applicator bottle

9. Comb the hair thoroughly up towards the crown.

10. Remove any staining to the skin with cotton wool.

11. Leave to develop for about 10–20 minutes, or according to the manufacturer's instructions.

12. When developed, add warm water and massage the head. Rinse thoroughly until the water runs clear.

13. Complete a record of work carried out and advise client of any after-care needs.

### Considerations for semi-permanent tinting

1. Read manufacturer's instructions carefully *before* application.

**SAFETY TIPS**

Always give a skin test when unsure of the client's skin sensitivity, or when the semi-permanent tint contains a para dye.

2. Some semi-permanent tints will cover up to 50 per cent of white hair but they cannot cover white hair where it is concentrated in one area.

3. Do not use bleach to remove an unwanted semi-permanent – it could cause complications. Try using an alkaline soap shampoo (or toilet soap) which will open the cuticle scales. Apply a second, soapless, shampoo to remove any soap scum deposit then apply a conditioner.

4. Poor shampooing, or lacquer left on the hair before the application, prevents the colour penetrating the hair and gives unsatisfactory result.

5. When dealing with extra porous hair, dilute the tint with water or reduce the development time or apply a pretreatment restructurant.

6. If a regrowth appears on very porous hair, apply semi-permanent to the roots. Leave ten minutes, then apply to the lengths of the hair and comb through, leave for a further five to ten minutes. This will produce an even result.

## TECHNICAL TIPS

Any stubborn skin stains can be removed by industrial strength methylated spirit (semi-permanent colours are soluble in alcohol).

7. A client wanting a natural brown shade may be better advised to have a permanent tint as the semi-permanent range of browns is limited.

8. Do not leave the tint on for longer than the recommended time, otherwise the resulting colour will be too harsh and deep.

9. Perm lotion will remove some of the colour and could cause patchiness. Therefore, when perming and colouring, the perm should be carried out before the semi-permanent tinting.

## Quasi colours

Quasi colours are sometimes called tone on tone. They come somewhere between a semi-permanent dye and a permanent dye but they will not lighten the hair. Quasi colours last longer than semi-permanent colours; they fade over a period of twelve weeks.

## POINTS TO REMEMBER

Quasi colours usually have a *para* base like the permanent dyes. It is mixed with a colour releaser (oxidiser), usually in the ratio 1:2. Some clients may be allergic to para, so you must carry out a skin test on the client 24–48 hours before the quasi tint is applied.

### How to apply a quasi colour

Manufacturers may differ slightly, so always read their instructions carefully. However, the usual method of application is as follows:

1. Protect the client and yourself as for other tinting processes.

2. Mix the quasi colour as directed by the manufacturer's instructions.

3. Apply to dry, unwashed hair like a shampoo (Fig. 2.6.6).

4. Leave to develop for approximately fifteen minutes or according to the instructions.

5. Rinse off thoroughly and apply a conditioner if necessary.

6. Towel-dry the hair, comb through and complete a client record card.

7. Advise the client on the after-care of the tint.

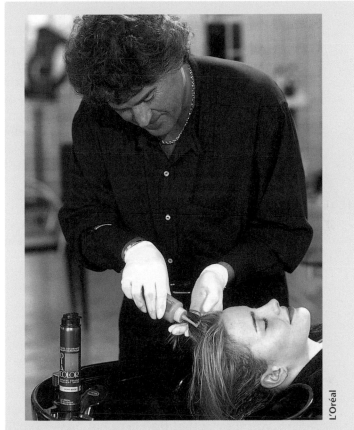

**Fig. 2.6.6**    Application of quasi colour (tone on tone)

**When to use quasi colours**

- To give shine to the hair.
- To add sheen to newly permed hair.
- To pre-pigment highlighted hair returning to natural colour.
- To correct colour.
- To refresh new and old highlights.
- For men's coloration.

**TECHNICAL TIPS**

When using fashion colour shades on 30–40 per cent white hair, mix with the corresponding natural shade for a natural coverage.

## Permanent hair colouring

### Natural vegetable dyes

Originally, all products for colouring hair came from plants, the main one being henna.

Henna is a natural vegetable dye, also known as Lawsone. It is produced from the crushed, dried leaves of the Egyptian privet plant which grows in Iran, Egypt and along the Mediterranean coast. It is a non-toxic dye which is mixed with water and does not need a skin test before application.

Pure henna stains the hair red and the shade of red varies slightly according to where it was grown. The depth of red depends on the length of time that it is left in contact with the hair, i.e. the longer the development time, the deeper the red. Henna will not lighten the hair therefore the shade of red will depend on the base shade of the client. The lighter the base shade, the lighter the red produced.

**TECHNICAL TIPS**

Henna should never be used on hair with over 10 per cent of scattered white hair, nor should it be used on highly bleached hair, as in both these cases the result would be too bright and harsh.

### Metallic dyes

Metallic dyes work by depositing **metal salts** in the hair cortex and on the hair cuticle. They are no longer used in salons but unfortunately clients can still buy hair colouring products that contain metallic salts for their own home use. The metals used in these dyes react badly with hydrogen peroxide. Unfortunately, hydrogen peroxide is used when we tint, bleach or perm the hair, so if a client has used a metallic dye on their hair they will not be able to have any of these services.

If you suspect that the client has used a product containing metallic salts on their hair, look carefully to see if it is a dull, flat colour with a slight greeny tinge – this is often a clue. If you have any suspicions at all, you must carry out an **incompatibility test**.

**POINTS TO REMEMBER**

Clients do not realise that a colouring product they have used on their hair may contain metallic salts. Hair grows at the rate of 1 cm ($\frac{1}{2}$ in) per month so it could still be on the ends of the hair six months later. Always carry out an **incompatibility test** if you are unsure what has been used on the hair by the client.

### How to carry out an incompatibility test

1. Take a small cutting of the hair from the crown area or the front. If the client has been tinting their own hair, this will have the highest concentration of tint.

2. Mix a simple bleach, which is a mixture of hydrogen peroxide and ammonia (or just use hydrogen peroxide).

3. Put the cutting in the simple bleach.

4. If incompatible chemicals are present on the hair there will be a reaction.

5. Bubbles of gas (oxygen) are given off. Steam rises and the mixture will get hot. The hair elasticity is increased and breakage occurs until the hair is completely destroyed.

## Para dyes

Para dyes are the permanent dyes that are used in salons today. They have a vast colour range from natural shades right through to exoctic greens, reds, blues and purples. They are manufactured in three forms: cream, liquid and gel. All para dyes need to be mixed with hydrogen peroxide.

Para dyes are water soluble and have small molecules (at this point they are often colourless) which will penetrate the cuticle and enter the cortex. When mixed with hydrogen peroxide, the oxygen released makes the small colourless molecules join together to form larger, coloured, insoluble molecules, which are then trapped in the cortex (Fig. 2.6.7). They are too large to pass through the cuticle and therefore do not wash out easily. In this way they mimic the hair's natural colour pigments. Para dyes are used in two ways: for darkening or changing tone and for lightening.

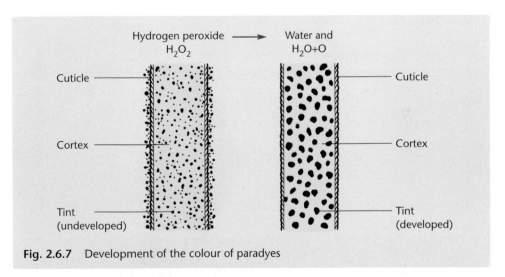

**Fig. 2.6.7** Development of the colour of paradyes

**POINTS TO REMEMBER**

Para dyes are synthetic organic dyes containing solutions of paraphenylendiamine, or similar 'para' compounds. Para compounds come from coal tar and are somtimes called synthetic aniline dyes. The tints that we use in the salon have other substances added to the para compounds:

- **Conditioners and antioxidants** – to help maintain the condition of the hair and keep it shiny. They also help to prolong shelf life.

- **Ammonia solution** – to speed up the breakdown of hydrogen peroxide, making it release its oxygen more efficiently.

### Darkening or changing tone

This is tinting the hair darker or a similar shade to the client's natural base colour, or matching white hair to the natural base colour.

The para dye is mixed with 20 vol. (6%) hydrogen peroxide as this releases enough oxygen to react with the para compounds.

Where maximum depth of colour is required, e.g. very dark or black hair or toning after bleaching, 10 vol. (3%) hydrogen peroxide may be used.

### Lightening

This is tinting the hair lighter than the base shade of the client (Fig. 2.6.8). To do this, the para dye has been mixed with hydrogen peroxide of a higher strength than is needed to react with the para compounds. This is important because the oxygen from the hydrogen peroxide combines with the para molecules to convert them to large coloured molecules; any additional oxygen attaches itself to the hair's natural colour pigment, making it lighter. The strength of hydrogen peroxide is usually 30 vol. (9%) unless a higher volume is recommended by the manufacturer.

It is useful to note that a higher volume strength of hydrogen peroxide sometimes throws up a golden tone. Therefore, when tinting the hair to pale ash

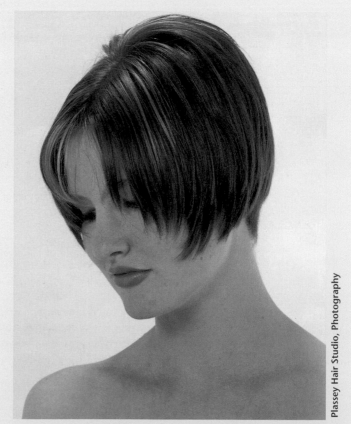

Plassey Hair Studio, Photography

**Fig. 2.6.8**   Highlights on front of hair emphasise the style and add interest and texture

shade (where no gold is required) some manufacturers recommend using 20 vol. (6%) hydrogen peroxide but in a greater proportion when mixing. In other words, the additional oxygen is obtained by adding more hydrogen peroxide. However, these proportions are only for certain tints and all manufacturers' instructions should be followed very carefully. Correct mixing of the tint in relation to the hydrogen peroxide is extremely important to get the shade you need.

**POINTS TO REMEMBER**

The base colour of the hair decides the volume strength of the hydrogen peroxide to be used. The lighter the colour required, the stronger the strength (or higher the volume) of hydrogen peroxide. The darker the colour required, the weaker the strength (or lower the volume) of hydrogen peroxide (Table 2.6.1).

**Table 2.6.1** Choosing the strength of the peroxide solution

| Volume strength of hydrogen peroxide | Purpose |
| --- | --- |
| 10 vol. (3%) | Gives maximum depth of colour |
| 20 vol. (6%) | For normal tinting |
| 30 vol. (9%) | Lifting peroxides for lightening |
| 40 vol. (12%) | |

## Hydrogen peroxide

Hydrogen peroxide is colourless and odourless and looks very much like its close relative, water. The difference is that hydrogen peroxide ($H_2O_2$) has an extra atom of oxygen compared with water ($H_2O$). Because of this extra atom of oxygen, the hydrogen peroxide molecule is unstable and will easily break down or decompose and release the extra oxygen atom as follows:

Hydrogen peroxide → Water + Oxygen
$H_2O_2$ → $H_2O$ + O

### Strength or concentration of hydrogen peroxide

**Volume (vol.) strength**

This refers to the amount, or volume, of oxygen that is released: 20 volume will release 20 times its own volume of oxygen, 30 volume will release 30 times, and so on. This means that the **higher** the volume, the more oxygen it releases and the faster it will work.

**Percentage (%) strength**

This is the **quantity** of hydrogen peroxide in the solution. In its pure form hydrogen peroxide is pale blue and very dangerous – explosive in fact. Therefore it can only be bought in a diluted form and this is what is meant by percentage (%) strength.

### Coversion

Volume stregth can be easily converted to percentage strength if you remember that 10 vol. = 3%, then the others can be calculated from this reference. For example, 60 vol. is six times stronger than 10 vol. 10 vol. = 3% therefore 60 vol. = $6 \times 3 = 18\%$.

**Table 2.6.2** Converting volume strength to percentage strength

| Volume strength (vol.) | Percentage strength (%) |
| --- | --- |
| 100 | 30 |
| 60 | 18 |
| 40 | 12 |
| 20 | 6 |
| 10 | 3 |

### SAFETY TIPS

Never use a higher volume of peroxide than necessary, as this causes hair damage and incorrect colour. As a general rule, 30 vol. (9%) hydrogen peroxide is the highest strength that can be safely used on the scalp and 40 vol. (12%) hydrogen peroxide is the highest strength that can be safely used on the hair; 60 vol. (18%) hydrogen peroxide should only be used with specially designed tints and the manufacturer's instructions should be strictly followed.

## Health and safety for hydrogen peroxide

Always follow the manufacturer's instructions on the safe storage of hydrogen peroxide. Here are some other guidelines for safe storage and handling:

- Do not store in direct sunlight or near heat.
- Always replace cap after use.
- Do not use at too high a volume or percentage strength.
- Do not splash onto the client's skin or your own skin.
- Mop up any spillage immediately.

## Preparation for para tinting

### Skin test

Para dyes are toxic dyes that can produce para poisoning in some clients. This para poisoning is known as **allergic dermatitis**. The symptoms are unpleasant, with itching and a blotchy appearance on the skin of the face and neck. In severe cases the face becomes so grotesquely swollen that the eyes cannot be opened and the mouth and lips swell to such an extent that swallowing and speaking become difficult. The skin may erupt and weep over the whole of the body. These symptoms are often accompanied by a violent headache, shivering and a high temperature and it may be many months before a full recovery is made.

It is important, therefore, to carry out a skin test before each application of para dye. Even a client who has had regular para dyes can still develop an allergic reaction (often called becoming sensitised). The skin test should be carried out 24–48 hours before the tint application and although this may often be inconvenient it is very much a case of better safe than sorry.

#### How to carry out a skin test

1. Clean a small area, either behind the ear or in the crook of the arm, with surgical spirit.
2. Mix a small amount of a dark shade of the tint to be used (the darker shades contain more para compound and are therefore more likely to produce a reaction) with hydrogen peroxide.
3. Apply the tint to the clean area, about the size of a one pence piece, and leave it to dry.
4. To protect the area, cover with collodion and leave to dry.
5. Leave for 24–48 hours without disturbing.
6. If no irritation occurs, the test is negative and it is safe to carry out the tint.
7. If irritation does occur, the test is positive and it is dangerous to carry out the tint.

### Elasticity test

This test is used to make sure the hair is strong enough to withstand the chemicals the stylist wants to use on it. It is quick and simple to perform.

1. Take a few strands of the client's most porous hair. This will usually be at the front.
2. Pull the strands between your fingers.
3. If the hair breaks or feels very elastic, postpone the tint and recommend conditioning treatments.
4. If you are unsure, carry out a strand test – this will show whether the hair is strong enough to be tinted.

## Porosity test

A porosity test will give you some idea of any precautions you need to take when you are tinting the hair. Porous hair will absorb more of the tint than hair that is in good condition. This will affect how you apply the tint and how long it is left to develop.

1. Take a few strands of hair at the front of the head.
2. Lift them out from the head at right angles then rub your fingers down the hair shaft.
3. If the hair is porous it will feel very rough.

## Strand test

These are taken before a full head tint, complete change of colour or whenever you are unsure of the outcome of the tint through hair porosity, base shade, etc. It is easiest to take a small cutting of the client's hair when they book an appointment, so that the hair can be tested before the actual tint application is carried out. A test cutting will tell you five things:

- Final shade of colour.
- Strength of hydrogen peroxide to use.
- Approximate development time.
- Breakage strength of the hair (stretching or elasticity).
- Whether pre-bleaching or softening of the hair is necessary.

### How to carry out a strand test

1. Take a small cutting of the hair from the front or nape area. (If the hair is white in one area in particular, take a cutting from there too.)
2. Mix a small amount of the tint and peroxide to be used in a bowl.
3. Place the cutting in the tint. To keep the cutting together, bind the ends with a small piece of Sellotape.
4. Await development.
5. When the tint has developed, rinse the hair and test for its strength by pulling between the fingers.
6. Dry and assess the results.
7. Record the results, together with the test cutting, on the client's record card as follows:
   - tint and shade used
   - strength of peroxide
   - strength of the hair
   - development time
8. Discuss the effect and final result with the client.

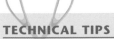

## TECHNICAL TIPS

The development time of the strand test should only be used as a rough guide, as warmth or heat will make the tint act more quickly. Therefore, even the temperature in the salon can have an effect on the length of the development time when actually carrying out the tint application.

## Client consultation and analysis

Consultation is the receiving and giving of information. A thorough consultation will help you to make sensible decisions about the client's hair and to offer them good advice. Make use of the shade chart, magazines and photographs to give you and the client visual ideas. For every consultation:

- **Look** at the hair and scalp.
- **Listen** to what the client has to say.
- **Feel** the hair to see what the condition is.

### Things to discuss

- What colour would they like? Warm, ash, lighter, darker, etc.?
- Have they had any chemicals on their hair in the past twelve months?
- Do they want an all-over colour, retouch or highlights/lowlights?
- Do they want a drastic change, subtle change or no change?

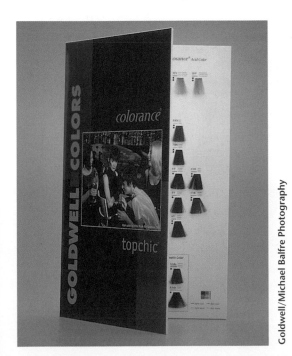

Goldwell/Michael Balfre Photography

### Choosing the colour

Use a shade chart when choosing a colour. A certain shade of colour may be difficult to describe and using the shade chart lets the client show you exactly what colour they want. All manufacturers use the International Colour Code (ICC) for their shade charts. This is a system that helps you to identify the **depth** and **tone** of colouring products.

*Depth of colour*  This means how light or how dark a colour is. A numbering system from 1 to 10 is used for this with 1 as the darkest colour (black) and 10 the lightest colour (blonde); see Table 2.6.3.

*Tone of colour*  Tone is the 'character' of the colour – how red, golden, ash or matt it is. There are three **primary** (first) colours from which all other colours are made. These primary colours can then be mixed

**Table 2.6.3**  The ten-point scale for depth of colour

| ICC number | Depth of colour |
|------------|-----------------|
| 1 | Black |
| 2 | Darkest brown |
| 3 | Dark brown |
| 4 | Brown |
| 5 | Light brown |
| 6 | Dark blonde |
| 7 | Blonde |
| 8 | Light blonde |
| 9 | Very light blonde |
| 10 | Lightest blonde |

to form three **secondary** (second) colours and it is the primary and secondary colours that make up the colour's *tone*. The primary colours are red, blue and yellow. The secondary colours are orange (red + yellow), purple (red + blue) and green (blue + yellow).

The colour star (Fig. 2.6.9)  shows the primary and secondary colours. Red, orange and yellow tones are know as **warm** colours and purple, blue (ash) and green (matt) tones are known as **cold** colours. Warm shades give the illusion of being lighter than cold colours – look at your salon's shade chart to see this. A red tone of depth 6 will look lighter than an ash tone of depth 6 even though they are both the same depth of colour.

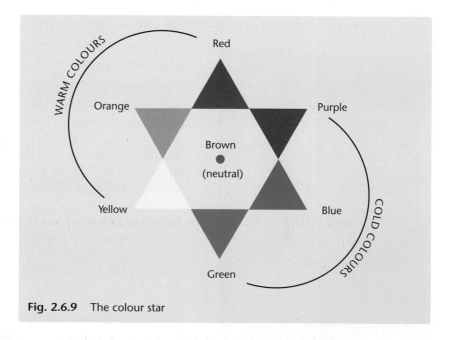

**Fig. 2.6.9**    The colour star

**POINTS TO REMEMBER**

Hair has two groups of pigment (colour) which are found in the cortex: melanin (brown or black) and pheomelanin (reddish yellow). Each head of hair has a different distribution of these pigments and depending on the reflection of light and the density of the hair, the base shade of the hair will be different on each head.

If the hair is in good condition it will reflect more light and will therefore appear lighter. If the hair is thick and dense, the colour will appear darker. This phenomenon can be easily seen by the black lines in Fig. 2.6.10, where the top diagram appears darker than the bottom diagram. The colour of the hair also reflects onto the face of the client and this too should be taken into consideration when choosing a colour.

### Other considerations

- Check the **porosity** and condition of the hair. Very porous hair will absorb or 'grab' the colour, and this could affect the outcome or give an uneven result.
- Look at the **texture** of the hair. Fine hair may need less product but could give a more intense result. Coarse hair may need a longer development time and more product.
- Always check the **scalp condition**. Do not proceed with the treatment if there are cuts, scratches or an excessively dry scalp – the tint could cause irritation.

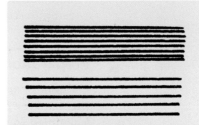

Fig. 2.6.10 The denser the hair, the darker it appears

- Look at the client's **skin tone**. Is it cool or warm? A warm skin tone suits warm colours such as gold, copper or red tones.
- Ask the client about any **previous treatments**. Always make sure that you know what has already been used on the hair. Has the client had any perms, bleaches or home colour treatments? If in doubt, test the hair.
- Decide on the **base shade** of the client's hair.
- Decide on the percentage of **white hair**. Fashion shades may be too intense if the hair has more than 25 per cent white in it.
- Find out whether you are **darkening or lifting** the colour of the hair and, if so, by how many shades.

After taking all these points into consideration, you can then select the shade and depth of colour tint that you need and mix it with the correct strength of hydrogen peroxide.

## Protecting the client and yourself

Personal Protective Equipment at Work Regulations 1992 state that you should be well protected for the task you are to carry out. A tinting apron to protect your clothing and rubber gloves to help prevent contact dermatitis and skin staining will meet these safety requirements.

It is important to protect the client's clothing at all times when tinting. Any stains to the clothing can be difficult to remove and you will have to replace any stained clothing.

- Place a tinting gown around the client to cover all their clothing and, preferably, it should be large enough to cover the chair also. This will prevent any tint from splashing onto the chair and perhaps staining another client's clothing later.
- Tuck dark towels firmly at the nape to prevent them from slipping.
- A neck strip or strip of cotton wool placed around the neck is also a safety measure. Special plastic, disposable capes can also be placed at the back, over the gown and the towel, to help protect the towels and the chair.
- Apply barrier cream around the hairline to prevent staining of the skin, but take care not to let the cream coat the hair. If the tint application is carried out carefully, there should not be any risk of skin staining.

## Preparation of products and equipment

Equipment and products should be assembled before you start to prevent rushing backwards and forwards across the salon. The equipment should be assembled so that it does not obstruct other staff, and on the flat top of a trolley for ease of working. It can also be easily wiped clean afterwards.

### Para dye

Para dyes are usually mixed with an equal amount of hydrogen peroxide, in the ratio 1:1. The manufacturers always state the amount of hydrogen peroxide to be used. There are one or two exceptions to the 1:1 ratio, but again, these are clearly stated in the manufacturer's instructions. To mix the tint:

1. Squeeze the tube (from the bottom and roll up to prevent oxidation, by the air, of the remaining tint if only using part of the tube) or empty the contents of the bottle into a non-metallic bowl.
2. If more than one colour is to be used they should be thoroughly mixed together in the bowl before adding the peroxide.
3. Mix the correct amount of hydrogen peroxide with the tint, adding it very slowly to form a thick, creamy mixture.

**TECHNICAL TIPS**

Add the peroxide slowly when mixing the tint, else it will become lumpy and the finished colour could be uneven.

## How to apply a para dye

Para dyes should always be applied methodically, carefully and as quickly as possible. How you apply the para dye can vary depending on the porosity of the hair and the degree of white hair present. Generally, the nape area is the most resistant as it does not get the same weathering as the front area and is therefore not usually as porous.

**POINTS TO REMEMBER**

The more resistant the hair, the longer it will take for the colour molecules to penetrate into the cortex. Resistant areas should therefore be treated first.

### Tint retouch

1. Assemble equipment and products; check that the client's skin test is negative.
2. Protect the client's clothing and skin.
3. Comb through the hair and check the scalp for cuts and scratches. If minor, protect with petroleum jelly, if major, postpone the treatment.
4. Divide the head into six sections: forehead to nape, ear to ear across the top of the head and ear to ear across the back.

**TECHNICAL TIPS**

If the hair is very greasy, wash with a mild, soapless shampoo, then thoroughly dry before sectioning. This is to prevent the hair's grease (sebum) from forming a barrier on the hair shaft.

5. Apply barrier cream around the hairline, making sure that it is applied to the skin only.
6. Mix the tint according to the manufacturer's instructions, then start application at the nape, unless more resistant elsewhere. Apply the tint evenly with the tinting brush to the regrowth area around the outline of the section.
7. Continue up the section. The tint should penetrate through to the next subsection, but try not to overlap onto the previously tinted hair. The brush is stroked in the direction of the hair.
8. Continue to apply the tint until the front sections are reached. Tint around the outline of the front section making sure that all wispy hairline hairs are covered.
9. Tint the roots of the front subsections.
10. Check your application by checking across the subsections to make sure that the application is even and thorough.
11. Remove any stains to the skin carefully with cotton wool.

12. Lift the hair away from the scalp with the tail end of the tinting brush to allow the air (and oxygen in the air) to circulate freely.

13. Cotton wool may be placed behind and above the ears to prevent the tinted hair from falling back and staining them.

14. Await tint development. Heat may be applied to quicken the process either with the aid of a steamer or an accelerator.

15. Check the development frequently by removing the tint from a small section of hair with a piece of damp cotton wool. Dry the section with another, dry, piece of cotton wool. The development is complete when there is no line of demarcation between the regrowth and the previously tinted hair.

16. When developed, add a small amount of water to loosen colour and massage the head. Rinse off the tint thoroughly with warm water until the water runs clear. Apply a cream or acid balance shampoo, massage gently, then rinse. Apply a second shampoo if necessary.

17. Apply an acid or pH balance conditioner, rinse, then towel-dry.

18. Complete a record of work carried out.

## Combing through

It is not necessary to comb through the lengths of the hair for every tint retouch. Tints tend to fade and lighten slightly because of the ultraviolet rays in sunlight. However, if the undiluted tint is always combed through the hair it will damage the cuticle scales, making it even more porous. A vicious circle is produced, whereby the more porous the hair becomes, the more quickly it fades. Acid balance shampoos and conditioners help to counteract fading by tightening the cuticle layers. If fading does occur, the tint should be diluted with water or a liquid shampoo before applying it to the hair.

**POINTS TO REMEMBER**   It is important when combing through either undiluted or diluted tint to make sure that the tint is applied to each strand of hair, otherwise the result will be very patchy. When the tint has been applied to the lengths of the hair, rub the hair gently between the fingers to distribute the tint evenly.

## How to apply a full-head para dye

### Darkening or same colour tone

1. Section the head as for a retouch and start the application at the most resistant area.

2. Apply the tint carefully to the roots and lengths of the hair shaft. The application must be thorough so that every hair is evenly coated throughout its entire length.

3. If the points of the hair are very porous, apply the tint to the roots and mid-lengths first and the points of the hair last.

**Lightening**

This is far more difficult than a darkening or same tone application. When you are lightening or using strong reds or purples for a full head application, you need to think about the effect of the body heat.

We lose almost 90 per cent of our body heat through the head, so it gets quite warm there. This heat from the scalp makes the tint at the root area develop more quickly than on the rest of the hair's length. To get an even colour result, you need to apply the tint to the roots last, when the rest of the hair is almost developed.

1. Prepare client, self and equipment as for a tint retouch until the actual application.

2. Apply tint to mid-lengths and ends of hair.

3. Place cotton wool strips along the root area to protect them from tint.

4. Leave to develop until just past the halfway stage.

5. Mix fresh tint and apply quickly to the roots.

6. Leave to develop until colour is even from the roots to the ends of the hair.

**POINTS TO REMEMBER**

When tinting long hair, allow for the effect of body heat, and also for the varying degree of porosity throughout the hair length. The hair points are the most porous due to wear and weather; the mid-lengths are usually the most resistant and will absorb the tint more slowly. Application should therefore be made first to the mid-lengths, then the points and finally to the roots.

## Keeping records

Always complete a record of the work you have done for each client after every application of tint. You may have to mix any number of colours to produce a certain shade of colour and it is very difficult, if not impossible, to remember exactly what has been used on every head. Any record should record the colours used and in what quantity, the strength of hydrogen peroxide, the date of each skin test and the result, the development time and any comments about the finished colour result. Any faults should also be recorded for further reference. Figure 2.6.11 shows a typical record card.

### Keeping client records on computer

If your salon keeps the client records on a computerised system, it must be registered with the Data Protection Register to comply with the Data Protection Act 1984. Other relevant points:

- All client information must be accurate.
- The information is confidential and must not be passed on to others without permission.
- The information must not be misused.
- The client has a right of access to any information you have about them on file.

| Name: ................................. | Base shade: ......................... |
| Address: ............................. | Percent white: ..................... |
| ............................. | Hair texture: ......................... |
| Tel No: ................................. | Hair condition: ..................... |

| Date | Skin test | Tint and peroxide used | Development time | Comments |
|------|-----------|------------------------|-----------------|----------|
|      |           |                        |                 |          |

**Fig. 2.6.11**    A tinting record

## Health and safety for para tinting

1. Take a skin test before each application.

2. If in doubt, always take tests of the hair to make sure that it can be tinted safely.

3. Products and equipment should not cause a hazard to other staff and clients.

4. Make sure that both you and the client are well protected.

5. Check that the correct shade of tint is mixed with the correct volume strength of hydrogen peroxide. In a busy salon it is easy to make a mistake by putting the tube of tint back in the wrong box.

6. Mix the correct amount of hydrogen peroxide with the tint, usually a 1:1 ratio.

7. Never use a higher strength of hydrogen peroxide than you need.

8. Be aware of your responsibilities under the COSHH and Personal Protective Equipment at Work Regulations.

**TECHNICAL TIPS**

Grease or heavy lacquer on the hair can form a barrier and prevent satisfactory penetration of the tint. If this is the case, shampoo then dry under a warm dryer before starting the application.

### Contra-indications for para tinting

- The client has a contagious or infectious disease of the hair and/or scalp, e.g. ringworm.

- Incompatible chemicals are present on the hair.

- You get a positive reaction to a skin test.

- Hair is very weak and fragile. This type of hair should always have a strand test, particularly before a full-head tint lightener.

## TECHNICAL TIPS

- A lighter shade of tint should not be applied over a dark dye. The previous dye must first be removed or lightened, otherwise the new lighter shade will not show.
- Work as quickly as possible. Remember that the colour molecules are being oxidised as soon as the tint is mixed.
- When a regrowth is too wide, in excess of 1 cm ($\frac{1}{2}$ in), and the hair is being lightened, it may be necessary to pre-soften the middle band of untreated hair with 20 or 30 vol. hydrogen peroxide, then dry under a warm hairdryer. Proceed with the root application as normal, overlapping the middle band. This will counteract the effect of body heat on the 1 cm ($\frac{1}{2}$ in) nearest to the scalp. Be careful: this is difficult and should only be attempted by experienced operators.
- Always check your application by cross-checking to make sure that the application is even throughout the whole of the head.
- Remove any stains to the skin after the application and before development. They are much easier to remove at this stage.
- Lift the hair away from the scalp when the application is complete. This allows the air to circulate more freely.
- Do not remove the tint before it is fully developed. All the colour molecules should be completely oxidised to give a satisfactory result.
- Never repeatedly comb through undiluted tint, it can make the ends of the hair very porous and cause colour fade.
- Always advise the client on the after-care of tinted hair. Explain the importance of regular retouching of the regrowth and the use of conditioning treatments.

## SAFETY TIPS

Always check the scalp for cuts and abrasions. If minor, protect with pertroleum jelly. If major, postpone treatment.

## Highlighting and lowlighting hair

Highlighting and lowlighting are methods of colouring or bleaching strands of hair to give a natural effect. They are kinder to the hair than a full-head permanent dye or bleach and there is not the same regrowth problems.

- **Highlighting** – lightens the hair. This can be done by using either a tint lightener or bleach. The bleach that is usually used is powder bleach but sometimes a salon will prefer emulsion bleach. (Unit 3.4 gives more information on these bleaches.)
- **Lowlighting** – keeps the same colour depth or slightly darker. Only colouring products are used for this method as bleach would lighten the hair.

**POINTS TO REMEMBER**

Bleaching lightens the hair. The two main colour pigments of the hair are melanin and pheomelanin. They are found as tiny granules, mostly in the hair cortex, but some occur in the outer hair cuticle. The bleaching process is a permanent lightening of these natural pigments and cannot be removed by shampooing.

In bleaches of all types the oxidising agent is the active ingredient in the bleach and it is the hair pigments which are oxidised. The main oxidising agent used in bleaches is hydrogen peroxide, which breaks down to release oxygen (Fig. 2.6.12). The bleaching process can be summarised as follows:

1. The oxidising agent in the bleach breaks down, releasing oxygen.
2. This oxygen penetrates the hair shaft and decolorises the hair's natural colour pigments.

This decolorisation can be seen, when bleaching black hair, as a series of colour changes as the pigment is increasingly oxidised:

black → brown → red → orange → yellow → pale yellow → white

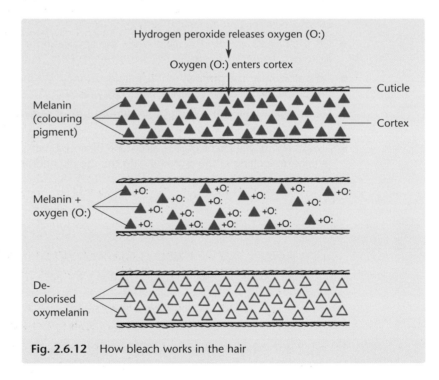

Fig. 2.6.12    How bleach works in the hair

# Highlighting and lowlighting techniques

## Traditional cap method

Although the traditional cap method does not have the accuracy of foil or plastic packets, it is much quicker and therefore popular with many salons. However, it is not recommended for use on long hair.

### How to highlight using the cap

1. Assemble equipment and products.
2. Comb hair into the position it is normally worn (if the hair is very greasy or heavily lacquered, shampoo it then dry thoroughly).
3. Place the highlighting cap firmly over the head by pulling it over the head from the front (Fig 2.6.13(a)).
4. Pull fine strands of hair through the holes in the cap with a crochet hook, starting at the nape and working through to the front hairline (Fig. 2.6.13(b)).

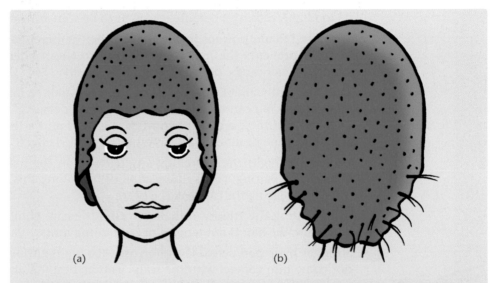

(a)          (b)

**Fig. 2.6.13**   A streaking cap is placed on the head and then strands of hair are pulled through the holes, beginning at the nape

5. When enough strands of hair have been pulled through, comb the strands gently with a wide-toothed comb to make sure that no hair is tangled or overlaps another.
6. Mix the bleach with the hydrogen peroxide to form a stiff paste to prevent the bleach from running down through the holes and causing 'spotting' at the roots.
7. Apply generously and evenly to the hair, but do not press the  bleach onto the cap – it could be forced through the holes.
8. Cover with a plastic, disposable cap to keep in the body heat and leave to develop. Apply heat if necessary to decrease the development time.
9. When the hair has lightened enough, rinse thoroughly. Apply a small amount of conditioner to the highlights as this will allow the highlighting cap to be removed more easily.
10. Take off the highlighting cap. Shampoo the hair, rinse thoroughly and apply a mild acid balance conditioner.
11. Complete a record of the work carried out. Leave the workstation clean and tidy.

## TECHNICAL TIPS

Always discard any highlighting cap that has become perished, or when the holes become too large, otherwise the bleach will seep through the holes.

### Precautions when using the cap

1. It is usual to pull only fine strands of hair through the cap. If the strands are too thick, it can give a striped effect, or alternatively the finished result can be too light, causing a definite regrowth to be seen within a few weeks.

2. Sprinkle talcum powder inside the cap before placing it over the client's head. It prevents the hair from sticking to the rubber of the cap so the strands of hair can be pulled through more easily.

3. Think carefully about how light you want the hair to be before starting the application. You can use bleach with tint lighteners, e.g. strands of hair may be treated with bleach at the front of the head and a tint lightener used at the back of the head to give a more subtle, shaded effect.

4. Do not highlight the hair along any partings in the hairstyle. If the client does have a parting, take a fine section of hair along this parting and section off before placing the cap over the head.

5. After pulling the strands of hair through the cap, comb them carefully to make sure the hair is not tangled or bent at the roots.

6. Stronger hydrogen peroxide can be used for highlighting as the bleach does not come into contact with the scalp. The highest volume that can be safely used on the hair is 40 vol. (12%), unless otherwise stated by the manufacturer.

7. Do not use a 'runny' bleach for highlighting as it can seep through the holes in the cap and cause 'spotting' at the roots.

8. Stroke the bleach onto the strands of hair. Do not dab or force the bleach down onto the cap – the bleach could be forced through the holes.

9. Always make sure that all the bleach is removed from the hair to prevent creeping oxidation. An acid balance conditioner used after rinsing helps to neutralise any traces of alkali that may be left on the hair.

10. Advise the client on the after-care of the highlights. The bleached strands of hair will be drier and more porous than the untreated hair; this must be allowed for if the client wants a perm or colour in the future.

### POINTS TO REMEMBER

- Comb the hair in the direction of the finished hairstyle before placing the cap on the head.
- Take only fine strands of hair, otherwise the final result could be striped.
- Check that there is no seepage of bleach (or tint) through the holes of the cap onto the scalp, otherwise the result will be patchy.

Be aware of the health and safety of yourself and your client at all times.

## Foil technique

The foil method needs more time and effort, but the finished result is far more subtle than using the cap. The whole head can be woven, or just certain areas (partial weaving) to add depth or lighten specific parts of the head.

Work as quickly as possible to prevent the first sections woven from becoming lighter than the other sections. If this happens, remove the foil from the developed sections and remove the bleach with water. The use of tint lighteners in place of bleach often gives a more subtle result – they do not lighten as quickly, nor do they make the hair as light as bleach.

**How to carry out full-head highlights with foil**

1. Prepare the client, self and equipment.
2. Section the hair as required, making sure the partings are clean and accurate.
3. Mix the hydrogen peroxide with the bleach to form a stiff paste or mix the tint.
4. Starting at the nape, weave in and out of a fine section of hair with a tail or pintail comb.
5. Place a strip of aluminium foil, non-shiny side next to and beneath the woven hair.
6. Brush the bleach evenly onto the woven hair, making sure that all the strands are completely covered.
7. Using the tail end of the comb, crease the foil to fold into a packet shape.
8. If necessary, fold another piece of foil into a long strip and wrap around the base of the parcel to prevent it slipping.
9. Continue weaving and wrapping up from the nape to the front of the hair, frequently checking the first wrapped parcel for development.
10. The number of parcels depends on the thickness of the hair and the effect you want to create. For subtle results, the woven strands of hair should be very fine; if they are thick they give a striped effect.
11. When weaving the front sections take a fine section of hair at the hairline, then weave the hair *behind* this section. If the actual hairline is woven the effect could be striped and there will be an obvious growth to be seen almost immediately.
12. When the weaving and wrapping are complete, check the first parcel wrapped, and depending upon the length of time taken to wrap the rest of the head, this should have lightened enough.
13. Remove the parcels in the same order as they were placed on the head.
14. Rinse the hair thoroughly, removing every trace of the bleach or tint.
15. Shampoo with a mild acid balance shampoo and apply a mild acid balance conditioner.
16. Complete a record of work carried out. Tidy and clean the workstation and equipment.

# Partial highlighting of the front hair

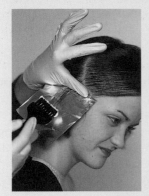
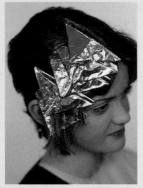
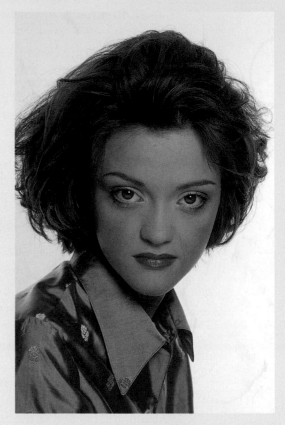
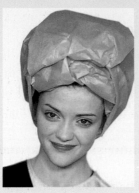

Bleach is used on finely woven sections of hair which is then wrapped in foil to form a triangular shape (instead of rectangular). The hair is then wrapped in brown paper to retain body heat. The finished result gives a subtle glint to the hair

**POINTS TO REMEMBER**

- Lowlights can be used to give a number of lighter and/or darker colours on fine streaks of hair for natural colour movement.

- Lowlights are very useful on grey hair as an alternative to a full-head permanent tint. Lowlights blend the white hairs with the natural coloured hair, so there is no need to retouch the roots every four weeks as with permanent tints. It is also much easier to return the client to their natural colour if they wish.

- Lowlighting can produce good results on bleached or very light hair using toning colours to put darker toning lights in the hair. One to three colours can be used and they are applied using either a streaking cap, plastic packets, spatula, or tinfoil.

## Plastic packet technique

Plastic packets are much easier to use than foil as they do not have to be folded. They also have an added advantage because the top layer of the packet is clear so that you can see the tint or bleach developing. Plastic packets have a sticky strip at the base – you must be careful not to let the tint go over this or it could seep onto the roots of the hair and cause spotting. The method of application for these materials is the same as for foil highlights/lowlights – just use the packets instead of the foil.

**TECHNICAL TIPS**

- The tint should be at least two shades lighter than the natural base shade when a lighter result is needed.

- Two shades of tint may be used instead of one, in which case the colours are alternated up the sections.

- For subtle effects, the colours should tone and complement each other.

- Faded red hair is given new vibrancy if gold and bright red shades (mixed as tint lighteners) are used. The colours may appear extremely bright on the shade chart, but as they are only applied to fine strands of hair they blend with the natural hair colour to give a brighter but subtle effect.

- The foil/plastic packet method of highlighting/lowlighting is more time-consuming but it gives a far superior result on long hair.

- Introduce a client to colour with subtle coloration. Once they have gained confidence they will become more adventurous.

- Use colour as an extension of the client's personality, but do not use too bright or very dark colours on older clients, it can be ageing.

- When a subtle effect is needed always look at the natural base shade carefully, there are usually golden or reddish glints to be seen that can be emphasised and highlighted. When using two or more colours on the hair try to keep within the same colour tones, and use different depths of these tones, e.g. red tones, gold tones, beige tones. This will produce a more natural effect.

- Do not be afraid to experiment with more than one technique on one head. With confidence, you can develop your own personal techniques.

**POINTS TO REMEMBER**

Retouching of highlights should only be needed every three months and then only at the crown, front hairline and any partings. After a further three months, highlighting should be repeated on the roots of the entire head. Avoid the ends of the hair if it is already highlighted by blocking them in a suitable barrier, otherwise the effect will be an overall bleached look.

# Partial highlighting using plastic packets

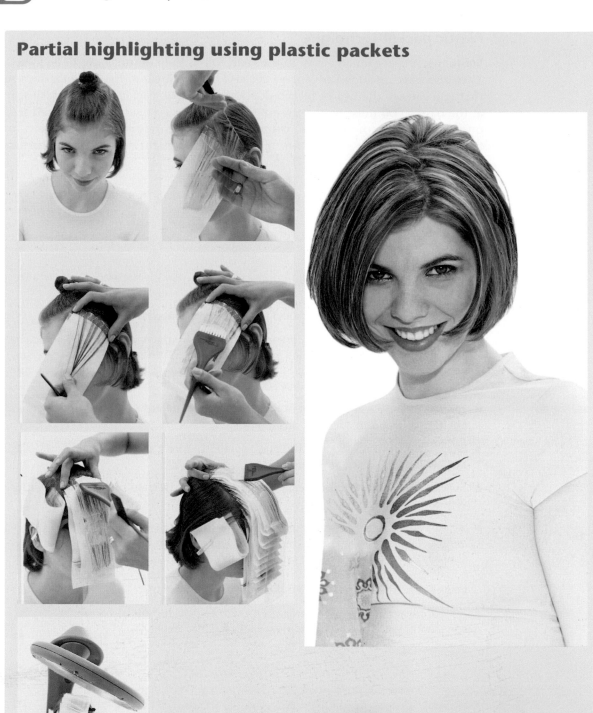

Hair is sectioned where needed then strands of hair are woven out and placed on the white side of the packet. Tint or bleach is applied to woven hair and the packet sealed. Continue until sides, front and crown have been completed then place under a rollerball accelerator to speed development.

## Safety precautions when highlighting and lowlighting

- When using tinfoil to add lights to the hair, make sure there is no seepage at the roots by wrapping a doubled strip of tinfoil around the packet at the root.
- Always discard rubber streaking caps when holes become too large. The bleach or tint can seep through these holes onto the scalp and hair with disastrous results.
- Some of the tinting techniques are so quick that it is a great temptation to tint more of the hair than necessary. Remember that it is better to apply tint to too few areas than too many. It is easier to add new highlights than to remove unwanted highlights.
- The main mistake when highlighting hair is to weave or pull hair through too thickly. This can give too striped an effect and make the hair so light overall that a regrowth can soon be seen.
- Always advise the client on the after-care of their coloration. The condition of the hair is of prime importance, as tinted hair only looks good when it is healthy. The client will also need advice on the upkeep of their colour and on how often salon visits will be necessary.
- Be aware of your responsibilities under the COSHH Regulations.

## Different highlighting effects

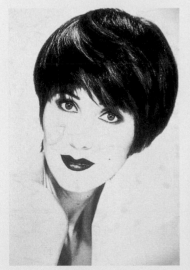 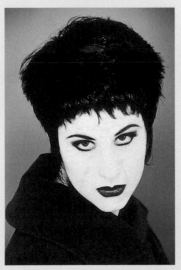 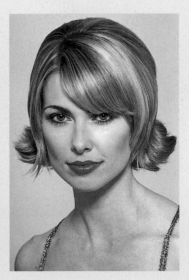

Dramatic hair effects created using lightened slices of hair and semi-permanent colour.

## Solving colour and highlighting problems

| Problem | Cause | Action |
| --- | --- | --- |
| Patchy, uneven result | Sections too large<br>Incorrect mixing<br>Uneven porosity of the hair<br>Uneven application | Spot tint light areas |
| Scalp irritation | Client allergic to tint<br>Peroxide strength too high<br>Sensitive skin<br>Cuts or scratches on the skin | Rinse off immediately with cool water<br>If irritation continues then seek medical aid |
| Poor coverage of white hair or hair resistant to tint | Closely packed cuticle scales<br>Incorrect mixing<br>Tint mixed too soon<br>Incorrect product used<br>Uneven application<br>Insufficient development | Reapply product or spot tint areas not covered<br>Pre-soften hair next time |
| Hair breakage | Hair fragile or overporous<br>Peroxide too strong<br>Wrong choice of product<br>Overprocessing<br>Overlapping<br>Incompatible chemicals on the hair<br>Combing tint through hair too much | Rinse off immediately<br>Use deep penetrating conditioners and restructurant<br>Cut if possible |
| Seepage of product from foil or packets | Holes in cap too large<br>Material applied incorrectly<br>Incorrect tint application<br>Incorrect mixing of product<br>Too much product applied | Spot tint areas too light<br>Condition hair |
| Colour result too yellow after bleaching | Wrong selection of product<br>Underprocessing<br>Base shade too warm for chosen colour<br>Base shade too dark | Take tests of hair<br>If strong enough then rebleach<br>If not, condition and apply mauve toning colour |

## Things to do

1. Weave highlighting with foil or plastic packets is effective but needs lots of practice to become competent. Other equipment for applying colour, such as the streaking gun, can also be used to apply colour. See what is available in your salon and practise with them. You will need:

   - Tuition head and clamp.
   - Tail comb and section clips.
   - Foil, plastic packets and any other equipment used for highlighting/lowlighting available in your salon.
   - Thick conditioner.
   - Rubber gloves and apron.

   Use the tuition head and conditioner to practise the different methods of highlighting the hair. List any problem areas and talk them over with your supervisor or tutor.

2. Look through trade journals and hair magazines for pictures or photographs of hairstyles with different types of colour. Cut out six that you prefer and paste each one onto a separate, plain piece of paper. Under each picture explain how you think the colour was achieved and why. Look in the shade chart and try to match the colours to those on the chart. Under each picture, write what colour you think has been used using just the numbers and letters of the shade chart.

3. Using this textbook, make your own notes (in your own words) on how you would carry out the following:

   (a) strand test
   (b) incompatibility test
   (c) porosity test
   (d) elasticity test

## What do you know?

- List the **four** main types of colouring products.

- What is the **acid** dye used in temporary rinses?

- Give **four** uses of temporary rinses

- Why do you have to take **extra** care when applying colour to porous hair?

- List **four** types of temporary colour that can be applied to dry hair.

- Where on the hair shaft do the **semi-permanent** colour molecules go?

- What is sodium lauryl sulphate and why is it added to semi-permanent dyes?

- List **six** things that you need to consider before applying a semi-permanent.

- Why **must** a client have a skin test before having a quasi tint?

- Give **six** uses of a quasi tint.

- When would you carry out an incompatibility test?

- What is an elasticity test used for?

- What is a skin test used for?

- Briefly describe how you would carry out a skin test.
- Explain what happens to **para dye** colour molecules when they are mixed with hydrogen peroxide.
- What **volume strength** of peroxide is usually used to lighten hair?
- Explain the effect of body heat when tinting a full-head lighter.
- What does ICC stand for?
- What are your responsibilities under the **COSHH Regulations** when colouring hair?
- What are the **four** main features of the Data Protection Act 1984 in relation to client records and information?
- Give **six** health and safety considerations when para tinting.
- What are the main differences between a full-head darkening and a lightening tint application?
- List **five** contra-indications for para tinting.
- Explain the **difference** between highlighting and lowlighting.
- Give a **summary** of the chemical action of bleach.

# 7

In this unit you will learn about:

- Communication: verbal and non-verbal.
- Using the telephone.
- Dealing with client enquiries and client contact in an efficient and effective way.
- Recording appointments.
- Client payment for the services and products supplied by the salon.

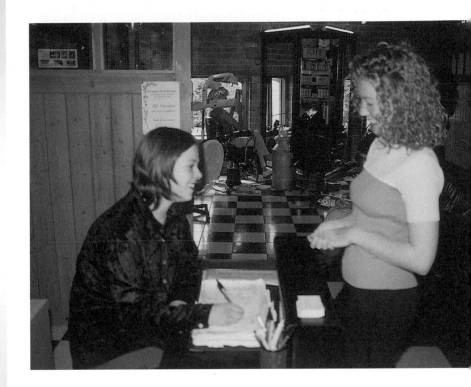

# Salon reception

Clients are fundamental for a salon to succeed and to stay in business. How a client is treated and the quality of the service they receive will determine:

- Whether they return.
- Whether they recommend the salon to others.

## Communication

Good communication is the two-way transfer of information between client and stylist. Communication is not just about what is said (although this is important). The message depends on how it is said and the whole range of body postures and facial expressions which together are called **non-verbal communication**.

Most of us are very good at interpreting non-verbal signals from others and we tend to leak our feelings in this way. First impressions are also very important. Clients expect a reasonable level of welcome to feel they matter to the salon staff.

### Face-to-face communication

The attitude of the staff towards the client and their work is very important. All members of staff should be pleasant, polite and helpful and show enthusiasm for their career. A sulky, sullen stylist makes the client feel unwelcome, uncomfortable and disinclined to return to the salon. Instead, it should be the aim of all staff members to give the client the best possible service and to ensure that a visit to the salon is an enjoyable experience.

Here are a few simple guidelines to keep a good client/assistant relationship.

- Never discuss or gossip about other people with the client.
- Show respect for the client. Be polite at all times and always make them feel welcome. Never be too familiar, nor too distant, as both of these attitudes can make the client feel uncomfortable.
- Do not talk to other members of staff while dealing with the client, unless they are included and involved in the conversation.
- Never sit down, comb your own hair or apply make-up in the salon; it gives an unprofessional impression. Use the staffroom for this purpose instead.
- Never eat, smoke or drink in the salon. Again, use the staffroom.
- Remember that every client is paying for a service. They are entitled to courtesy and respect as well as the best possible service you can give them.

### Confidentiality

Confidentiality is very important. Here are some reasons for this and the possible consequences of breaking the rules governing confidential information.

- Ethical reasons – it is wrong to pass on confidential information without someone's knowledge and consent.
- Legal reasons – the Data Protection Act insists that computerised records are kept confidential.
- To maintain good relationships and the professional image of the salon.

# Activity

A client hears two hairdressers chatting about another client. They realise that the person who is being discussed in a rather negative way is a personal friend of theirs. What is the probable outcome of this? How may this influence the salon as a business?

## Effective face-to-face communication

Effective communication with the client is essential to clarify the service they require and make sure they fully understand the time, cost and processes involved. Misunderstandings, even little ones, are very bad for the salon's reputation. Effective communication involves:

- Active listening.
- Questioning.
- Non-verbal behaviour.

Always discuss fully the client's requirements. Apart from the obvious fact that you need to know this information before beginning any hairdressing service, it also helps to build up a strong client/stylist relationship which strengthens the trust that a client must have in the person who is dealing with their hair.

Never argue with other members of staff while working in the salon and never argue with the client; it is most unprofessional. Beware of argumentative subjects, e.g. politics and religion, as some people have very strong opinions and it is very easy to offend them, even unintentionally.

## Posture and appearance

Correct posture is an important issue for any hairdresser. Incorrect posture can lead to tiredness, inefficiency and physical strain, all of which will mean that the client is not receiving the best service and could lead to long-term problems for the stylist. Incorrect posture can also communicate a poor attitude and approach even when this is not intended. Appearance is a key non-verbal set of signals which speaks volumes about the salon.

# Activity

List the factors which contribute to a professional image, i.e. which make a good impression on clients. It may be helpful to divide the factors into two groups:

(a) salon environment

(b) appearance and attitude of staff

# Communication over the telephone

Although other means of electronic communication are growing and developing rapidly, e.g. e-mail and websites, the telephone remains the most important electronic contact.

The telephone is a vital link with the client and it is crucial that they hear only a voice which is always pleasant and helpful, no matter how busy the salon may be. Time must always be found to answer the phone – if staff are too busy to book an appointment at that particular moment, the name of the salon should be stated and then, if necessary, the client could be asked to hold on. All staff must be trained to answer the telephone and to book appointments, even if the salon employs a receptionist. Bad telephone technique such as an abrupt reply or an unhelpful manner could lose many potential or regular clients.

In some salons, incoming telephone calls for members of staff are not allowed. Therefore, any rules regarding the receiving or ringing out of calls should be clearly indicated to all staff to prevent any unnecessary friction in the salon.

## Telephone services

There are now many operator services available for business use although not all are suitable for the smaller hairdressing salon. New technology has meant that all communication services, including the telephone, are being expanded and updated at a bewildering speed. Consequently, it is often a useful exercise to become reacquainted with the facilities that are available approximately every twelve months or so.

The telephone is a vital link between the salon and the client so any faults should be rectified as quickly as possible to prevent loss of business. If the telephone is completely out of order then the fault should be reported immediately from elsewhere on a 'live' telephone.

## Use of the telephone directory

All the information needed for using the telephone is contained in the **phone book**. This is issued by the telephone provider to all their subscribers free of charge and is written specifically for the area in which the subscriber lives.

The phone book contains far more information than just the names, addresses and telephone numbers of its subscribers. It also gives information on what services are available, how to use those services, the procedure for emergency calls, reporting faults, and how to handle nuisance calls. It provides information on places of interest, call charges and useful numbers within the subscribers' locality. It also gives guidance on how to find the number required and how to make local, national and international calls.

If using British Telecom, some useful numbers to remember are:

- 100 Operator services (including alarm calls, credit card calls, fixed time calls, freephone calls, personal calls, transferred charge and advice of duration and charge (ADC) calls).

- 151 Faults – telephone lines or equipment.
- 192 Directory enquiries.
- 999 Emergency services.

## Using the emergency services

There are three main telephone emergency services: fire, police, ambulance (with coastguard and mountain rescue depending on the location), each of which consists of a highly skilled team used to dealing with all types of disasters.

An emergency usually involves an unusual or frightening situation, so the most important thing to remember is to keep calm even though this may be difficult in the circumstances.

The correct procedure for contacting the emergency services is as follows:

1. Dial **999** or the emergency number shown on the number label.
2. When the **operator** answers, give the telephone number shown on the telephone.
3. Ask for the **service** you need.
4. When the service answers, give the **address** where help is needed.
5. Supply any other **information** which may be of use.

Always try to speak **clearly** to prevent any misunderstandings and to allow the services to react immediately and bring help as quickly as possible.

## Taking messages

Always **write down** a verbal message as it is often difficult to remember the correct information, particularly if the person who is to receive the message is not available at that precise moment. Writing down a message also has the added advantage of acting as a **reminder** to pass on the message at a later time.

The following facts should be included when writing down messages:

- Date and time of message.
- Name of the person giving the message.
- Name of the person to receive the message.
- Exact details of the message.
- Name of the person taking the message.

When these details have been recorded, repeat the message back to the caller to make sure that it has been written down correctly.

# Activity

What are the salon procedures for taking and passing on messages? Is there a message form in use? If not, design one or obtain commercially produced examples from stationery suppliers or shops.

## Booking appointments

A booking should be entered in the appointment book in pencil so that it can be easily removed if the client cancels. The name of the client and the service required must be written **clearly** so that it can be easily read by all the staff; it is very embarrassing to call the client by the wrong name. If your handwriting is poor the information should be printed instead.

When booking an appointment, enough time must be allocated to each service otherwise the stylists become overbooked and clients have to wait; this may give a poor impression of the salon and it causes frustration to all concerned. Different salons operate different systems and some salons employ staff as specialists to carry out certain tasks such as perming or tinting. In this case a client booking an appointment for a perm followed by a semi-permanent colour and cut and blow-dry may have more than three people working on their hair at separate times, and this has to be organised correctly in the appointment book. Thus, it is very important that all the staff know exactly what system is in operation in their own salon and how to dovetail bookings so the salon runs smoothly and efficiently.

### Timing of salon services

Knowing how long a process takes is essential for phasing appointments correctly. Table 2.7.1 lists some common services and the times they may take.

**Table 2.7.1** Duration of common services

| Service | Approximate time needed in minutes |
| --- | --- |
| Shampoo | 5 |
| Cutting | 30–40 |
| Blow-dry | 20–45 |
| Setting | 60–90 (including drying time) |
| Perms | 90 (virgin hair) |
|  | 75 (treated) |
| Colouring | Varies, up to 60 |
| Bleaching | Varies, up to 60 |
| Plaiting | Varies, up to 90 |

### Record keeping

A detailed record should be kept of all hairdressing treatments, particularly those that will be carried out over a period of weeks. This builds up a very clear picture of how the hair is reacting and progressing with the treatments and any modifications made. A typical record card of hair or scalp treatment is shown in Fig. 2.7.1.

Client records may be kept on paper and filed or they may be kept as computer information on disk.

**RECORD CARD**
**HAIR/SCALP TREATMENT**

Name: ............................................................. Tel No: .....................................................

Address:..............................................................................................................................

.......................................................................................................................................

| Hair assessment | | Type | Porosity | Diseases/abnormalities |
|---|---|---|---|---|
| | | | | |

| Scalp assessment | | Skin type | | Diseases/abnormalities |
|---|---|---|---|---|
| | | | | |

| Cause of damage | | | |
|---|---|---|---|

| Date | Conditioner /lotion | Type of massage | Time | Source of heat | Time | Result |
|---|---|---|---|---|---|---|
| | | | | | | |

**Fig. 2.7.1**　Sample record card for hairdressing treatments

## Processing cash and non-cash payments

Most salons will have their own system for keeping records of daily transactions. Computerised cash tills are now commonly used to balance stock control by allowing a constant and immediate check on any items that need reordering. Electronic cash registers (tills) have **clerk keys** which will keep each stylist's takings, and any other sundries such as sales, separate on the till roll; this makes the totalling at the end of the day much easier. However, salons without either of these systems have their own individual procedures which usually involve the checking of daily totals against the cash till receipts, client dockets, sales receipts and appointment book to ensure there are no discrepancies.

Salons also have to have some form of **petty cash** to deal with any small items that may have to be purchased during the working day such as coffee or sugar. This may be in the form of a petty cash box or a book which lists any items purchased with a total at the end of each day. Whatever type of system is operated it is essential to keep a precise record, together with any receipts, of any cash used during the day, otherwise time can be wasted wondering why the day's takings do not add up correctly.

At the beginning of the day a set amount of small change and notes, known as a **float**, is put in the cash till. This is to make sure that there is enough change in the till should the client not give the exact amount for their service. The float must be subtracted from the day's takings when cashing up at the end of the day.

Remember that the handling of cash is always open to abuse by both staff and clients; therefore an efficient and effective system of cash control is essential to maintain a successful business.

## Cash payments

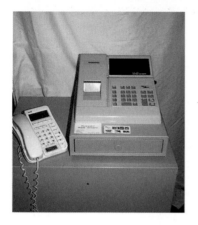

All members of staff must be competent in operating the cash till, receiving cash, giving change and calculating any relevant VAT. It is also essential that staff are familiar with the varying procedures necessary to ensure the validity of client payments made by cheque, credit card, account card or gift voucher as errors in these areas can be extremely costly to the salon.

### Accepting cash payments

Great care must be taken when accepting cash from a client as mistakes can easily happen, particularly during busy periods. The short-changing of a client can cause ill-feeling and loss of future custom.

**Procedure**

1. Inform the client of the charge for the services they have received.

2. Check that the cash received is in the correct currency.

3. Ring up the correct amount on the cash till or computer. If the client needs change, place any paper money on the top before removing the change from the cash till to prevent any misunderstanding as to the amount given.

## Non-cash payments

Non-cash payments include cheques, credit cards and gift vouchers which are all legal tender but must be processed correctly to ensure the salon receives payment for their services.

### Receiving cheques

A cheque is paid directly into a bank account. You should be able to read the writing on any cheque and it must contain the following information, in ink, if it is to be accepted by the bank:

- Correct date.
- Name of the person or salon to whom the cheque is to be paid.
- Amount to be paid in words as well as numbers.
- Signature of the person writing the cheque.

**Procedure**

1. Make sure that the cheque contains the information listed above.
2. Ask to see the client's **cheque guarantee card**. This is a card issued by the bank which, when used with a cheque, ensures that the bank will honour payment up to a certain amount even if the client does not have that amount in their bank account at that particular time.
3. Check that the signature on the cheque matches the signature on the guarantee card and that it is not past the expiry date.
4. Make sure that the bank name, bank code and account number are the same on both the cheque and guarantee card.
5. Write the guarantee card number on the back of the cheque.
6. Return the guarantee card to the client then place the cheque in the cash till.

**Precautions**

Make sure that:

- The writing on the cheque is in ink.
- You can read the writing.
- Any alterations are signed or initialled by the client.
- The correct date has been entered.
- The amount is made out in sterling, i.e. UK currency.
- It is not an open cheque, i.e. it has the name of the person to whom it is payable written on it, otherwise it could be misused by someone else.
- There are no spaces where other words could be added or altered.
- The date on the cheque guarantee card is valid.

## Credit card transactions

Some clients prefer to use credit cards, particularly for large bills, as it allows them to spread payment over a period of time. However, not all salons accept credit cards, particularly smaller establishments, as a charge is made by the bank to the salon for the use of the facility. However, as with a cheque, the bank will honour the payment even if the client does not have the money in their account to cover the debt.

**Procedure**

1. Use the imprinter and relevant voucher to duplicate the credit card details.
2. Using a pen, write in the date, description of goods, amount in words and numbers, your signature and the authorisation code.
3. The client must then sign the form in the space provided.
4. Check that the signature is the same on both the form and the credit card.
5. Check that the date on the credit card is valid.
6. Tear out the carbons then give the top copy to the client for their records and keep the remaining copies in a safe place.

### Electronic funds transfer (EFT) cards

EFT cards fulfil the roles of both bank guarantee card and service card. The client's current account is debited electronically without the client having to write a cheque.

The card is drawn through a special terminal which then stores the details of the transaction. A two-part voucher is supplied which the client has to sign. One part is kept by the client as a record of the transaction and the other is retained by the salon. Always check that the signature on the voucher is the same as that on the EFT card.

Due to the high level of theft and fraud linked to credit cards of all types it is likely that all cards will soon have to include the card holder's photograph. When this becomes common, checks will need to be made on:

- The match between photo and person with the card.
- Any tampering with the photograph.

### Gift vouchers

Gift vouchers are usually in multiples of pounds and are at their most popular during the Christmas season. Each salon will have its own system for processing gift vouchers but usually it is easier to deal with them if they are thought of as paper currency and treated as such. Change is not usually given however.

### Traveller's cheques

Traveller's cheques are another method of non-cash payment. Rather like gift vouchers, if the salon accepts them they can be treated as cash. Check the signature on the cheque with the signature on the traveller's folder.

### Suspected fraud

Fraud is mostly likely to involve non-cash payments as it is very hard to produce counterfeit money. If fraud is suspected:

- Stay calm.
- Stay polite.
- Say something like 'Could you wait a moment please?'
- Get some assistance.

Try not to alert the pearson, although in practice this is very difficult. They are looking out for problems and quickly sense them. Try to get assistance without leaving the area. Some salons have a code for alerting other staff to a potential problem. Always put people before property or money. Don't take risks in what is potentially a nasty situation.

Do bear in mind that not all problems with payments are deliberate. Sometimes there are genuine mistakes or cards are cancelled for all sorts of reasons that the client has not realised.

## Things to do

1. To help you gain a greater understanding of the services which your salon has to offer, make a chart in the format set out below. You can obtain the information contained in the packaging and instruction leaflets of the products, by asking the people who work with you and by watching the various services being carried out in the salon.

   When it is complete, ask if the chart can be put up in your staffroom at work as a reminder while you are learning your reception duties.

| Service | Timing stylists | Timing client | Benefits and effects | Cost to client |
|---------|-----------------|---------------|----------------------|----------------|
| (a) | (b) | (c) | (d) | (e) |

   In column (a) list all the services that your salon has to offer – you may be surprised at how long this list will be! Any large services, such as perming, should be subdivided into the different types as their benefits and costs will be different even if the timing is very similar.

   In column (b) give the timings for the separate stages, particularly large tasks. This will help you to dovetail appointments in the future. In column (c) find out the total time that the client will be in the salon. In column (d) write down the benefits and effects of each service and look at the finished results in the salon. Why and how do you think their hair has been improved? Use your own experience as well as other sources to complete column (d). For example, if you have had your own hair permed or coloured, why do you think that it is better than before and why did you have it done?

   Fill in column (e) by looking at the salon price list.

2. Make a list of the terms used in a salon to cover all the aspects of non-cash payments. Explain how each is used. Explain how non-cash payments are recorded. What is the documentation involved?

## What do you know?

- List the **main** areas involved in dealing with clients.
- Why should bookings be entered in the appointment book in **pencil**?
- Why is a **good** telephone manner important?
- What telephone number would you dial to report a telephone **fault**?
- What action should be taken if a client has to **wait**?
- What are the **main** areas to consider when communicating with a client?
- What is the procedure for contacting the **emergency** services by telephone?
- When writing down a **verbal** message, what facts should be included?
- What is the procedure for accepting **cash** payments?
- Give **eight** precautions or considerations when receiving a cheque from a client.

# 8

In this unit you will learn about:

- Organising your work.
- Adapting to circumstances.
- Being an effective team member.
- Improving yourself within your job role.

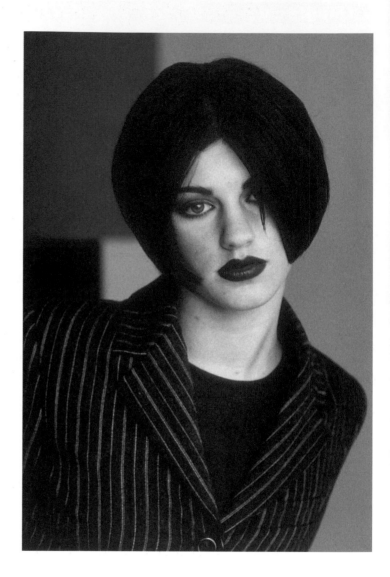

# Teamwork

## Working in the salon team

A good salon has an atmosphere of cooperation between staff, with staff being interested and motivated in their work and keen to offer a top quality service to the salon's clients. People can sense this atmosphere when they enter the premises. What produces this atmosphere? Some of the key factors are covered in this teamwork unit.

### Organising your own work

This is based on the appointments that have been made. Considering the types of appointments booked will produce a plan for activities based on:

- **What** needs to be done or organised for the services requested.
- **When** the client is booked in.
- **How** the services will be carried out.
- **Where** the services will be carried out.
- **How long** the service or services to the client will take.

The plan should make best use of the salon's resources and provide a good efficient service to the client. Unfortunately, the best plans go wrong when the unexpected happens. There are events not anticipated in the planning which can upset the whole thing. What are these events and what action can the stylist take?

### Adapting to circumstances: some examples

#### Client is late

The question is how late? If only a little late there is usually a little slack in the appointments schedule which can allow for this. Use the time productively while waiting. There is always something worth doing, or if not sure, ask. If the client is very late their appointment is probably gone and other clients are being processed. Offer the client another appointment as soon as possible, e.g. later the same day or with another stylist or look to rearranging later appointments (perhaps use more of the salon junior's time for some basic processes).

#### Client is unscheduled

Make sure the client feels welcome and not a liability. Proceed as above by rescheduling, offering a later appointment, etc.

#### Overbooking

Overbooking should not happen. The major cause is someone not writing the appointment down in the appointment book or keying it in. If it does, carry on as you would for an unscheduled client.

#### Client changes their requirements

A client may have booked in for one thing and, perhaps without consulting the stylist, they may then ask for a different salon service. This may need some rescheduling, or more use of junior staff.

### Services take longer than planned

Services often take longer than planned and contingencies like having a little slack time built into appointments can help here. If very prolonged then schedules can be replanned and more use made of junior staff.

### Staff are absent

When staff are absent, clients can be fitted into other stylists' appointments. Junior staff can be used for some basic operations, e.g. blow-drying, to free up stylist time. As a last resort, clients can be telephoned, the position explained and their appointments rebooked.

## Preparation of work areas

Work areas need to be clean and tidy, equipment and products need to be ready for the next client, and everything should be left in good order at the end of the salon service. Routine hygiene practices should be automatic.

## Activity

Make a list of the routine hygiene practices in the salon

## Being an effective member of the salon team

Always remember that all members make a significant contribution to the effectiveness of the team, both in terms of their varying personalities and in their various skills and experience. Good teams work together well. There has been a mass of research into what makes this happen or hinders it. Here is a summary of some key things about effective teams:

- **Interpersonal skills** – treating others with courtesy and respect.

Keeping up good communication is very important. Effective communication is about:

- clear concise messages
- good positive body language and facial expression

Good communication is the oil that keeps effective teams going. Key areas are dispute management and the encouragement of trust.

- **Shared skills and experiences, aims and objectives** – this comes out of good interpersonal skills. Requests for assistance are responded to positively and the help given is encouraging and within the competence of the helper.
- **Being clear about what is expected** in a job role and who is responsible for what, when and to whom to refer problems and requests for help.
- **Supportive supervisor/manager** – good teams need to develop good interpersonal skills and the sharing of skills and experience needs to be fostered,

encouraged and reinforced. Team members need to be encouraged to promote good relations in the team. Development of team members needs to be given a high priority to enable the team members, and therefore the team as a whole, to be more effective in their **job roles**.

## Problems and what to do

There are a whole host of problems that can occur in the salon, these may be technical, personal, or to do with colleagues. As their experience and skills develop, a stylist can manage an increasingly wide range of problems but there will always be some instances where it is sensible to ask for help and advice. In general, if in doubt do ask for help from your supervisor, but remember it is important to learn from the advice and experience of others.

## Providing information when requested

Effective management is about many things but a key process is **communication** between supervisors or managers and their salon teams. There is a variety of information that may be requested in order to monitor and improve salon procedures and processes. These include:

- **Provision of services** – how many, of which type, any problems?
- **Personnel** – is the team working effectively? Can there be improvements? Staff appraisal.
- **Health and safety** – are policies known and understood? Are procedures being followed? Are there any problems? Are they sorted out in a reasonable timescale? Are channels of communication open?

The important thing with requests for information is to be:

- **Prompt** – provide the information quickly.
- **Accurate** – bad information causes bad decisions to be made for the best of motives.

# Activity

Make a list covering your job role in the salon. What are your main duties and responsibilities. What would happen if you did not fulfil your job role properly?

## Self-improvement within the job role

The first step in becoming a more effective member of the team by means of self-evaluation involves being clear as to what the job role actually is. If there is a lack of clarity about this, it needs to be sorted out with the supervisor and/or the salon management. Once the job role is clear, carry out an appraisal review.

The idea of this system is to help salon team members identify their strengths and points for development and to help them plan how this development should take place. This involves setting targets. Targets can be set by the person themselves or by the supervisor. These targets need to be realistic and achievable within a set time period. This period can be short, medium or long. A good, constructive and effective appraisal review needs to follow this procedure:

1. Strengths as well as weaknesses need to be identified and recorded.

2. Improvements need to be agreed, not imposed, and the action plan for your development needs to be:
   - realistic
   - constructive and developmental
   - subject to a review after a fixed time period

3. It is important to be **positive** about the appraisal or review. It is an opportunity to tell your supervisor or manager about what you do. Particularly what you feel you do well and those areas you would like to develop. The appraisal process makes them listen.

Think of a review or appraisal as a **positive** experience. It should support you and the team. It should form part of a general ongoing awareness of opportunities for improvement and it should be supported and encouraged by salon management. The outcomes of the appraisal can be activities based around:

- Advice and guidance.
- Training or other development activities.
- Increased role in salon.

There is always a need for development of staff due to:

- Fashion trends.
- Technology (products, tools and equipment).

The stylist needs to keep abreast of these changes. Information about these areas can be found through sales reps or in:

- Trade journals.
- Exhibitions, presentations and demonstrations.
- Training and update sessions organised in the salon or elsewhere (e.g. local FE college).
- Films and television programmes.

A good team works together by sharing ideas, things they have seen, and the skills or techniques they have picked up from the sources listed above.

## Things to do

1. Get together with other staff members. Have a 'brain-storming' session on 'what makes a good team'. Any and all contributions should be recorded (where people can see them if possible, e.g. on a flip-chart sheet). Next discuss how many points on your list fit a team known to you and how many do not. Then have another session on discussing/planning how a particular team could be made better. Write these down. If appropriate show your points to a manager/supervisor/tutor and ask for their comments.

2. Make a list of problems you feel you could sort out yourself if they occurred in the salon and those you would need help with. Store this and discuss it with your supervisor/manager/tutor and ask for their comments.

3. As a group consider how hairdressers can update themselves on fashion trends, techniques, products, tools and equipment. Which would be the most cost effective? Which would be the most time effective?

## What do you know?

- What are the **main** problems that can occur in the organisation of work in the salon? What should be done if these problems occur?

- What type of information may be **requested** by management?

- What are the **key** aspects of an effective team?

- What are the **main** features of an appraisal or review system?

- List the **main** sources of information that can be used by hairdressers to update and improve their expertise.

In this unit you will learn about:

- The background legislation on health and safety in the salon.
- The practice and procedures for evacuation of the salon.
- First aid and fire-fighting equipment.
- Reporting accidents and seeking help.
- Your personal role in health and safety, e.g. hair, accessories, conduct, lifting techniques, removing and reporting hazards in the salon.
- Salon security and what to do if there are security problems.

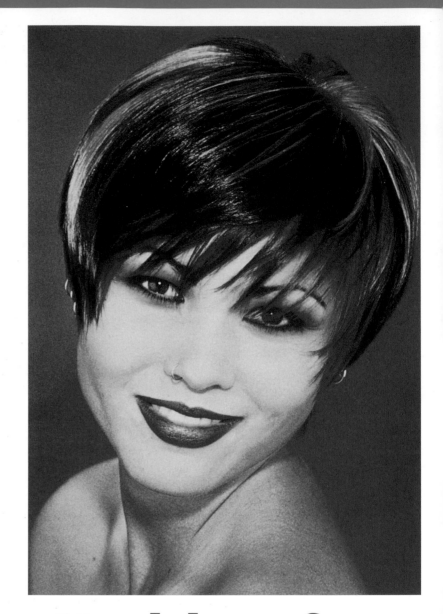

# Health, safety and security

Everyone working in the salon has a responsibility for their own health and safety and that of the salon clients. A well-run salon is efficient and safe. Health and safety is everyone's responsibility both because it is ethically 'right' and because it is legally required.

## Health and safety legislation

Health and safety legislation is also covered in Units 1.5 and 3.6.

## Activity

Draw up a table listing the legislation below. Use Units 1.5 and 3.6 to summarise the key points of your responsibilities to **each** item:

(a)  Health and Safety at Work Act 1974

(b)  The Workplace (Health, Safety and Welfare) Regulations 1992

(c)  The Manual Handling Operation Regulations 1992

(d)  The Control of Substances Hazardous to Health Regulations 1992 (COSHH)

(e)  Electricity at Work Regulations 1992

In addition many salons need to meet local conditions (often called by-laws) and need to be **licensed**. Licensing involves the salon being required to meet particular **standards**. These standards can refer to:

● Evacuation procedures.

● Fire-fighting equipment and fire-retarding construction materials.

● First-aid resources and procedures.

● Toilet and wash facilities.

● Provision of a restroom.

Standards vary from area to area and, like national legislation, they change from time to time. A good source of up-to-date information is the local environment health department (or equivalent). They are listed in the phone book or can be contacted through the local authority. Another useful contact is the regional office of the Health and Safety Executive, also listed in the phone book.

## Emergency procedures

Some hairdressers never encounter emergency situations but they can happen at any time. The main thing is to have **procedures** in place that salon personnel are familiar with. Many emergencies do not provide much time to think and certainly not time to work out what to do from the beginning. These procedures should be:

- Who is responsible for first aid, often called the first aider. This should be clearly identified to all staff and a rota set up to make sure a first aider is available when the salon is open. First-aid certificates for the workplace are provided on successfully completing training courses organised by the St John Ambulance.
- How to evacuate the salon in a safe manner. This includes clients partway through services. Where to assemble outside. This needs to be clearly identified on a notice or notices placed prominently. Turn off electrical equipment. Shut doors and windows (if possible).
- What to do in the event of a fire. Where is the fire-fighting equipment? What type is it?

# Activity

(a) Draw a floor plan of the salon. Mark the evacuation routes and the locations of fire-fighting equipment.

(b) Design a poster for a salon explaining what to do in a fire.

## Fire-fighting

Fire-fighting should only be undertaken if it presents no risk to you. The common means of fighting fires are:

- **Water** – sometimes in water-based fire extinguishers. The main problem here is that water conducts electricity and so water must **never** be used where there is electrical equipment.
- **Carbon dioxide** – common as a fire extinguisher. Carbon dioxide extinguishers are good all-purpose extinguishers but the gas rapidly disperses and the fire can flare up again.
- **Powder** – this coats the burning material with a layer of dry powder, smothering the fire. Powder extinguishers are very effective and worth the mess they make.

## Reporting accidents

Salons need to keep an **accident book** into which details of accidents (and dangerous occurrences) are written. You need to report all accidents and potential accidents (near misses, things you have noticed, etc.) to your supervisor. Do this in writing if necessary. When contacting the emergency services:

- Stay calm.
- Speak clearly.
- Give full details.

## First aid

A detailed account of first aid is beyond the scope of this book. The best course is to complete a programme in first aid training of the type offered by the St John Ambulance. Unit 3.6 covers basic first aid.

# Activity

(a)  Who are the salon first aiders?

(b)  How long is the basic first-aid course offered by St John Ambulance?

(c)  Where is the first-aid equipment located?

## General salon safety

It is good practice to make many health and safety practices automatic. This would include ensuring that

- Work areas are kept clean and tidy and other general hygiene practices are maintained.
- Hairdressing products are used and stored properly.
- Tools and equipment are checked over before use.
- Tools and equipment are kept and used properly.

A good source of help and information on health and safety are local environmental health departments. Good hygiene practices are covered in Unit 1.5.

### Hairdressing products

The storage and use of hairdressing products is covered by a number of pieces of health and safety legislation (Unit 3.6). The main point is that the products are handled, used and stored in a safe manner following:

- Manufacturer's instructions.
- Requirement of legislation

A good example of a legal requirement is the hairdresser's responsibility to the client under the COSHH Regulations 1992.

### Safety tools and equipment

Tools and equipment should be kept clean and in good order. It should be routine to give them a quick check before use. Electrical equipment poses a particular hazard due to the possibility of it becoming damp or wet during hairdressing operations and consequently giving someone an electric shock. Cables to electrical equipment also tend to rub or fray and sometimes they are jerked; this tends to pull the flex out of the equipment and/or the plug, perhaps exposing bare cable. Bare cable could cause someone to receive an electric shock or a burn should it short out with an electric spark.

As with products, the care, maintenance and use of salon tools and equipment are covered by a number of regulations. Particularly important is the Provision and Use of Work Equipment Regulations 1992 (Unit 3.6).

## Personal health, hygiene and appearance

This topic covered in Units 1.4 and 1.5. It concerns standards in:

- Personal appearance.
- Personal hygiene.
- Taking care to maintain good posture.

Here are some other important aspects.

### Personal conduct

Everyone has a responsibility under the Health and Safety at Work Act to act in a way that does not cause a risk to either themselves or others.

- Take care to be safe.
- Think safety.

# Activity

Carry out a **safety audit** on a salon. This involves looking for potential problems, reviewing procedures and finding out the staff's level of awareness of salon safety.

### Infectious condition of salon staff

If someone has a potentially infectious condition such as a cut or graze on their hands or fingers, then it is important that they report this to their supervisor. Small cuts and nicks are not uncommon in hairdressers, especially when training. These are a potential source of infection to others, i.e. they can cause **cross-infection** and should be:

- Cleaned
- Covered with a sterile dressing.

Expert advice on whether the infection (or potential infection) could be a hazard in the salon can be obtained from health clinics or general practitioners.

### Personal protective equipment

The Personal Protective Equipment at Work Regulations 1982 require employers to provide 'suitable and suffient' protective clothing and equipment as and when it is needed. In hairdressing there is the supply of:

- **Protective gloves** – to protect the hands during hairdressing services.
- **Overalls/aprons** – to protect the stylist from spills, clients' hair fragments, which can cause infection.

There is sometimes a tendency not to wear protective gloves, especially if there is a cut or graze on the hands or the early stages of dermatitis. Close-fitting gloves trap sweat and heat and can irritate these conditions. A light dusting with talc can help this and it is worth remembering that exposing sensitive skin to more water, shampoo or chemicals will in the long run lead to a worse situation than the short-term discomfort of wearing gloves.

Many hairdressing products are hazardous – bleaches, perm lotions and permanent tints, for example – and it is very important not to expose the skin to them. Even low-hazard products like shampoos can cause problems due to the long-term repeated exposure to skin contact that shampooing without protective gloves, or at least a barrier cream, produces.

## Safe manual lifting

In the UK more days of work are lost to people being off work with back injury than any other single cause. The human back is vulnerable to the stress and strain put onto it by bending the spine and lifting. The safe method is:

1. Keep back straight.
2. Bend legs.
3. Lift by using legs not the back.

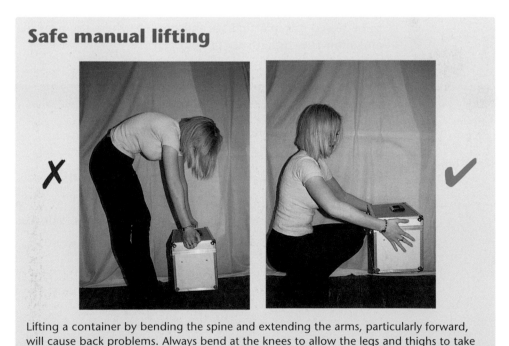

### Safe manual lifting

Lifting a container by bending the spine and extending the arms, particularly forward, will cause back problems. Always bend at the knees to allow the legs and thighs to take the strain.

## Hazards in the salon

In additional to products, processes, tools and equipment covered earlier in this unit, other potential hazards include:

- Faults or damage to equipment, tools, hairdressing products, fixtures and fittings.
- Spillages.
- Slippery floors.
- Obstructions preventing easy access or escape to parts of the salon and/or exits.

In most cases these can be dealt with by the stylist by cleaning up spills, washing floors made slippery and moving obstructions, etc. Sometimes there are recurrent hazards where something keeps happening. Report these to your supervisor, in writing if necessary.

## Waste disposal

A number of potentially hazardous waste materials are produced by a hairdressing salon, these include:

- Tissues/swabs, etc., used in chemical treatments.
- Neck strips.
- Hair clippings.
- Sharps.

These need to be disposed of safety. All sharps, such as razor blades, must be disposed of safely in accordance with the salon's procedures. All other waste needs to be sealed into plastic bags and not left where the bags may become damaged and allow the contents to spill out.

## Salon security

Salon security includes:

- Clients, staff and their possessions.
- Salon equipment, products, tools, fixtures and fittings.

Security is about preventing harm, damage or theft by **prevention**. It also involves what to do if there are security problems. Salon security is treated in detail in Unit 3.6.

# Activity

Carry out a **security audit**. Put yourself in the place of someone who wishes to steal or damage salon or client property. How would you do it? Where is the salon vulnerable to break-ins? Is there an alarm system? Do staff know the procedures to follow if there are security problems?

## Things to do

1. List routine hygiene practices in the salon. Explain how each protects staff and clients.

2. Design a poster encouraging safety in the salon.

3. Find out and list a salon's emergency procedures for:

   (a) accidents – to staff and/or clients
   (b) emergencies – such as a fire or bomb alert

## What do you know?

- Why is personal appearance and hygiene important in the salon?

- Where can a hairdresser get advice about infectious conditions?

- Where can a hairdresser get advice about health and safety legislation?

- List some possible **hazards** in the salon. What can be done to reduce them?

- List some possible salon **emergencies**. Explain what procedures should be followed in each case.

# 10

In this unit you will learn about:

- The tools and equipment needed to cut men's hair.
- The techniques used to cut men's hair.
- Types of hairstyles and neckline shapes.
- How to prepare the client for cutting.
- How to cut men's hair into a variety of styles.
- The health and safety aspects of cutting men's hair.
- Male pattern baldness and how to deal with it.

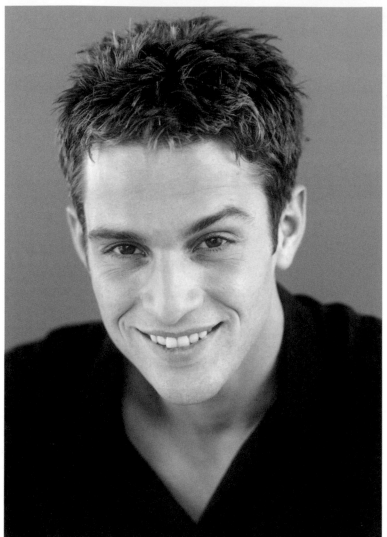

L'Oréal

# Men's haircutting (barbering)

## Cutting men's hair

Similar skills are needed for cutting men's and women's hair. However, although there are similarities there are also many differences. Overall, men's hair tends to be shorter and, because of their larger face shape, it is thought to be more masculine if the shape of the finished style is more 'square'. Several tools are used to cut men's hair.

### Cutting tools

#### Scissors

The preferred scissors for cutting men's hair have longer blades and are usually heavier than those used for cutting women's hair. This lets the barber cut the hair more quickly as more of the hair can be cut across when it is lifted out from the head. Aesculap (thinning scissors) are used to blend in weight lines on graduated hair by cutting into the ends of the hair where the weight is.

#### Razors

Razors are used a great deal in men's hairdressing. They are quick to use and can thin out the hair at the same time as taking off the length. Razors are used to remove stray neck hairs and clean up the nape area after a haircut.

#### Clippers

Clippers are also used extensively in men's hairdressing. They are electric, either with or without a cord. The cordless type are especially useful when cutting beards and moustaches. They have attachments which allow the hair to be cut to various lengths. Keep clipper blades free from hair and well oiled with antiseptic clipper oil.

#### Combs

Cutting combs are used for most of the cutting techniques. Combs that are used to cut very short cuts around the ears and neckline are called **barber's combs**. They are thinner and more pliable (bend more easily) than other combs. This allows them to bend to the shape of the head so that the hair can be cut nearer to the scalp.

#### Neck brush

Hair attracts bacteria and germs – they stick to the grease. So it is important to use the neck brush throughout the haircut, and then immediately after, to make sure the client and his clothing are free from all cut hair. (See Unit 2.4 for how to look after your scissors, razors, clippers, combs and neck brush safely and hygienically.)

## Haircutting techniques

The same basic techniques are used to cut both men's and women's hair (Table 2.10.1). They are sometimes applied differently in men's cutting to create a slightly different, more masculine look.

### Club cutting

Cutting the hair straight across using either the scissors or clippers. Club cutting can be carried out on either wet or dry hair. This technique keeps thickness and weight on the ends of the hair, therefore it helps to discourage curl and keeps the hair as thick as possible.

### Taper cutting

This is a slicing movement which thins the ends of the hair while removing the length. It is usually carried out with a razor on wet hair and scissors on dry. It will encourage any curl as it has removed some of the weight from the ends of the hair.

#### Taper cutting dry hair

Hold a section of hair firmly between the first and second fingers. Then, using a slithering action with the open blades of the scissors near to the crutch, direct the scissors from the points of the hair to the middle lengths. The blades should be closed very slightly during the stroke towards the scalp, then opened again drawing the scissors away from the scalp. Never completely close the scissors during the stroke towards the scalp as this could remove too much hair and create 'steps'.

#### Taper cutting wet hair

Take the section of hair to be cut and, with the razor blade held at a slight angle, make light slicing movements from the mid-lengths to the points of the hair, either on top or underneath. The pressure on the blade will determine how much of the hair is cut away and the length of the stroke will determine the amount of taper (Fig. 2.10.1).

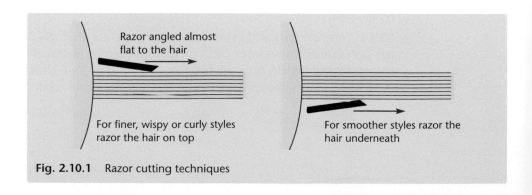

Razor angled almost flat to the hair

For finer, wispy or curly styles razor the hair on top

For smoother styles razor the hair underneath

**Fig. 2.10.1**  Razor cutting techniques

## Thinning

As its name suggests, this type of cutting thins the hair. It does not remove lengths from the hair but because it removes weight the hair will curl more easily.

## Scissors and clipper over comb

This technique can cut the hair very short. Using a barber's comb, the hair is combed upwards from the nape neckline and the hair that protrudes between the teeth of the comb is cut off. The scissors or clippers should rest along the length of the comb and should open and close quickly while the comb is moving up the head. If the scissor movement is too slow then this could produce steps in the haircut. The angle at which the comb is held will determine the length of the hair – the further away from the scalp the longer the hair will be. If the client wants his hair cut very short then you will need to hold the comb next to the scalp.

**Table 2.10.1**  Techniques for cutting men's hair

| Cutting techniques | Tools used | Wet or dry hair |
|---|---|---|
| Club cutting | Scissors | Wet or dry |
| Taper cutting | Scissors or razor | Dry with scissors Wet with razor |
| Thinning | Scissors, razor or aesculap scissors | Wet or dry |
| Scissors and clipper over comb | Scissors or clippers | Wet or dry |

## Haircutting effects

There are two main effects created by the various cutting techniques used in men's hairdressing:

- uniform layer
- graduated layer

**TECHNICAL TIPS**

Read Unit 2.4 for more detailed information on:

- Cutting tools.
- Cleaning and sterilising tools.
- Cutting techniques.

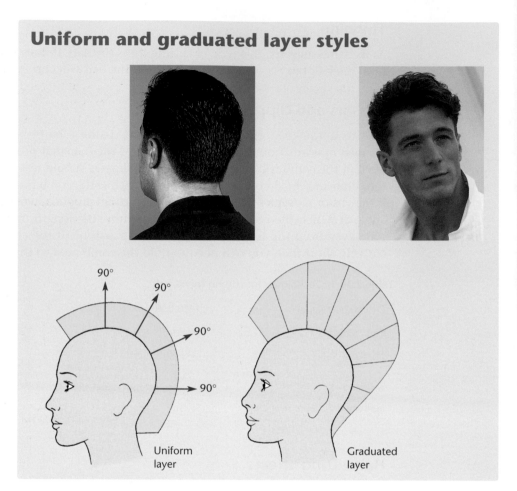

# Uniform and graduated layer styles

Uniform layer

Graduated layer

## Critical factors

Talk to the client. Always carry out a thorough consultation and look at the factors listed below. You need to disguise any blemishes and this can sometimes be very difficult if the finished hairstyle is quite short.

### Face shape

You need to look at the thickness of the neck, the cheekbones and prominence of chin and forehead. You also need to take note of the size of ears and whether they are even on both sides of the head.

- A **rounded** face with softer contours looks better with straight, hard lines.
- An **angular**, squarer face needs the edges of the haircut softened with fine graduation.

## Head shape and body size

Make sure that you allow for the shape of the **occipital bone** at the back of the head. It is not as prominent as a woman's but if you cut the hair with the weight line **above** the occipital bone it will create the wrong shape and the hair will stick out. The haircut must be in proportion to the client's body size, so take note of this when they walk into the salon. A tall, angular man would look better with weight left in the hair if possible.

## Hair growth patterns and hairline

Try to make the most of what you've got and camouflage the areas that create difficulties. Here are some of the common things you will come across (Fig. 2.10.2):

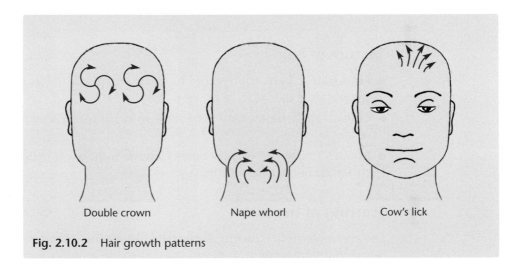

Double crown          Nape whorl          Cow's lick

**Fig. 2.10.2**   Hair growth patterns

- **Cow's lick** – leave the hair longer here and style it in the direction that the hair grows.
- **Receding hairline** – if it has just started receding and the top hair is still full, then the areas behind where it recedes, you may have to leave them a bit longer to compensate. If the hair is starting to thin on top or there is baldness, the hair looks better if it is cut short.
- **Baldness** – extreme baldness looks better if the hair is cut short all over the head. Try to dissuade the client from growing the back and sides long in a effort to cover up a bald patch as it emphasises rather than camouflages it.
- **Double crown** – if you cut the hair too short on the crown then it will stick up.
- **Napeline hair growth patterns** – a nape whorl or uneven hairline needs to be tapered into the neckline or left long enough for the hair to be cut round it (Fig. 2.10.3). Consider the growth patterns before deciding on a neckline shape.

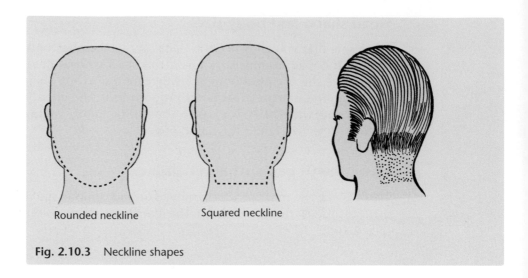

Rounded neckline          Squared neckline

**Fig. 2.10.3**   Neckline shapes

## Texture of hair

- **Fine hair** – keep the weight by club cutting it. Be careful when cutting straight, fine hair as it 'steps' very easily,
- **Thick, coarse hair** – may need to be thinned with either the aesculap scissors or razor.
- **African Caribbean or very curly Caucasian hair** – is better cut freehand with either the clippers or scissors.

## Scarring of the skin

The correct term for scarring is **cicatrical alopecia**. Check the scalp for any scars before you start cutting. Scars will show through hair if it is cut very short.

## Preparation of the client

### Client consultation

You must find out from the client exactly what they want before you begin cutting. You may have to show style books or magazines to the client. You also need to give him advice on what is suitable for his hair. While you are talking to the client you also need to be thinking about the critical factors in the previous section.

### Client protection

Make sure that the cutting gown and towels fully protect the client. A cutting collar is also useful to prevent small hairs going down the neck.

## Hair preparation

Comb through the hair to disentangle it. If you are cutting the hair wet, you will need to shampoo it with a suitable shampoo then towel it dry.

## Types of hairstyle

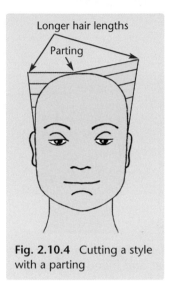

**Fig. 2.10.4** Cutting a style with a parting

### With or without a parting

With a parting the hair is usually left longer on either side of the parting (Fig. 2.10.4). This means that the hair has to be held at 45° to create this length. Styles without a parting are often more layered. They can be worn off or forward onto the face or to either side.

### With or without a fringe

Be careful when you cut the guideline for a fringe – you need to allow extra length and cut the hair freehand with no tension. Remember that the hair will kick back slightly and look shorter when dry. As a rough guide, try cutting the guideline by combing the hair forward, rest your fingers on the bridge of the nose and cut the hair to just below this level. Hairstyles without a fringe can be left either longer or shorter on top depending on how the client wants the finished style.

### With or without ears showing

You need to allow for **ear protrusion** when cutting styles without the ears showing. This means leaving the hair longer over the ears by cutting it freehand without tension in this area. Styles with the ears showing have the hair cut off around the ear against the natural hairline. Check that the ears are even both sides. You will also have to ask the client how he wants the sides to be shaped. There are three main shapes (Fig. 2.10.5).

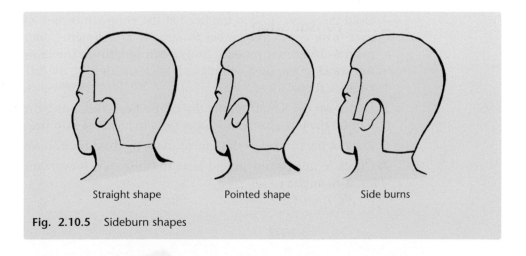

Straight shape          Pointed shape          Side burns

**Fig. 2.10.5** Sideburn shapes

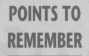

**TECHNICAL TIPS**

You can remove hair outside of the desired shape by:

- Outlining the side of the neck with the scissors, razor or clippers.
- Turning the clippers over onto their cutting edge to cut a straight line at the sides or to produce a square neckline.

**POINTS TO REMEMBER**

Check whether the client is wearing any added hair before starting the haircut. If he is you will need to take care that you don't catch your comb in the base of the added hair and it will have to be blended into the rest of the haircut very well.

## How to cut a traditional short back and sides

Any barber must be able to cut this classic haircut as many of the new styles evolve from it. Take into consideration any balding areas and blend the hair in.

### Procedure

1. Protect the client with gown and towels, comb through the hair.
2. Place a no. 1 cutter head attachment to the clippers. Use a higher number attachment if the hair length needs to be longer.
3. Run the clippers up the neck to below the crown to approximately level with the top of the ear, round the ear and up the sideburns. Just below the required line, ease the clippers away from the head in an outward curving movement to bevel the hair and prevent a hard line.
4. Hold the comb close to the head at the clipper line and, using scissors or clippers over comb (remember to remove attachment), increase distance from head to blend but produce longer hair length on the crown. Cutting the hair too short in this area will make it stick up and the overall finished shape will be wrongly balanced.
5. Decide on the length for the top of the head and, using this as a guide, cut the hair on the top, crown and upper sides to blend in with the short clippered hair.
6. Remove the hair below the haircut shape by shaving clean with razor or clippers.
7. Check in mirror and around head that the style is even and correctly balanced from all angles.

## Cutting a short back and sides

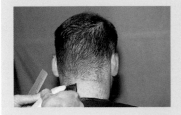
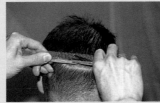
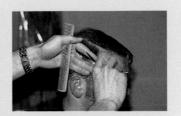

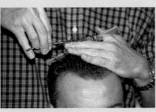
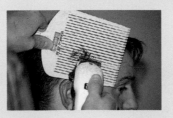

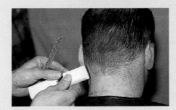
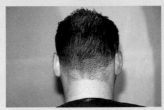
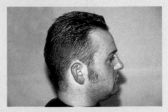

The hair at the nape is cut with clippers using a no. 1 attachment then back hair is scissor-over-combed to the crown area. The sides are graduated to leave more length and weight, then the top hair is club cut with the front hair pulled back slightly to leave extra length at the front. The sides are blended with the top using a 'flat topper' and finally the haircut is outlined with cordless, outlining clippers. The finished haircut has a squared neckline and longer sideburns.

8. Clean client free from hair and advise on after-care of the cut. Dispose of any sharps safely and complete a record of work carried out.

## How to cut a crew cut or flat top

These haircuts come from the old German 'Boche' cut. Before starting to cut the hair talk to the client to find out whether the hair is to be 'squared' or 'rounded' at the sides. The flat top is very squared whereas the crew cut can be either.

### Procedure

1. Assess the hair and scalp, determine whether the finished shape is to be rounded or squared.
2. Cut the back and sides quite short, as with a short back and sides cut. Alternatively, the hair may be left the same length as the top with graduation at the nape only.

3. Make the hair on top of the head stand upright using either brushes or wax. Insert a comb at the front of the head towards the back. Make sure that the comb is level then remove the protruding hair with either scissors or clippers.

4. Repeat this process all over the top of the head to make sure all the top hair is cut to a uniform length. Use the mirror to check the shape continually.

5. Blend the top hair with the nape and sides using scissors or clippers over comb. Clean stray hairs from the nape and side areas with either clippers or razor.

6. Check in the mirror and around the head to make sure that the style is even from all angles. Clean client free from hair. Dispose of sharps safely and complete a record of work carried out.

## Health and safety

- **Disposal of waste** – sharps (razor blades, cutting tools) must be disposed of in a special sharps bin in accordance with your salon's procedures and any local by-laws. It is dangerous to leave sharp objects about, if the client or a member of staff cut themself they could seek legal action against you. Hair must be swept up straight away and put in the correct bin.

- **Correct use and storage of electrical equipment** – always check wires and plugs before you start. Don't let the wires trail or someone may trip. Switch off the power at the plug when you have finished then clean the equipment and put away in the salon's designated place.

- **Correct use and storage of other cutting tools** – use them only for what they are supposed to be used for. Carry scissors carefully and close the blades when not in use. Clean all tools after use and keep in the salon's designated place.

- **Sterilisation of tools and equipment** – to help prevent cross-infection or infestation, all tools and equipment should be cleaned and sterilised after use. Workstations should be kept clean and tidy at all times.

- **Safety laws** – you must know what responsibilities you have under these laws. The main law for cutting is the Electricity at Work Regulations.

- **Protection of the client and yourself** – make sure that the client's clothing is well protected and that there is a minimum risk of sharp, cut hairs piercing the skin. If you should cut the client, wear rubber gloves and stop the bleeding with a styptic pen. Seek assistance and medical aid if the wound is deep.

**POINTS TO REMEMBER**

The **Electricity at Work** Regulations state that you must:

- Know how to use your electrical equipment.
- Only use the equipment for what it is intended for.
- Always check that it is safe to use before you start (loose or frayed wires, etc).
- Switch off at the plug when you have finished.
- Keep clean and store safely in the correct place.

## Dealing with baldness

Men can be very sensitive about their loss of hair and it is therefore important to be very tactful during the consultation process. Always try to style and cut the hair to underemphasise thinning or hair loss by blending the haircut well with any bald areas and advising the client on a suitable style.

Some men prefer to disguise their loss of hair by the addition of false hair such as a wig or toupee. These must be well cut and of a colour to blend with any existing hair. Unfortunately, because the hair does not 'grow out' it becomes discoloured by sunlight and the atmosphere and may need recolouring from time to time. It is also easy to tear the base of the wig or toupee if it is not treated correctly. Always give your client plenty of advice and guidance on the care and maintenance of their added hair.

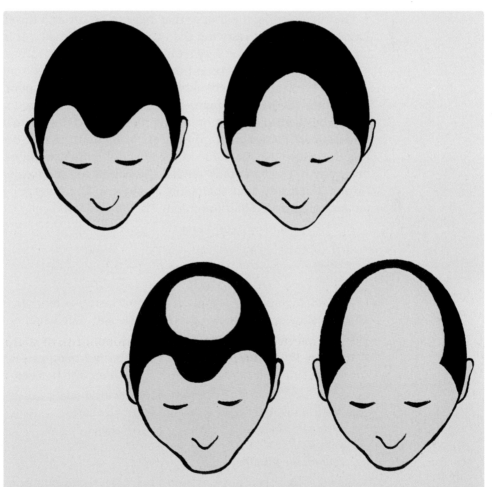

**Fig. 2.10.6** The hair begins to recede both sides at the front, then at the front itself until the hairline becomes much further back. Often the crown area also begins to thin. The hair loss area increases in size until the hair completely disappears from the crown and front areas to leave a horseshoe shape.

## Securing added hair (toupee) to the head

Before placing the toupee on the client's head, the scalp should be clean and free of grease to allow it to stick to the scalp. Draw the toupee over the scalp from the front hairline towards the back, making sure it is in the correct position by checking in the mirror. Attach to the client's scalp with double-sided adhesive tape. Clients with some hair on the top may have the toupee clipped into position and there are now various types of added hair which have been designed with snap-on clips for rigid fastening.

Gently comb the hair into position, blending in the edges of the toupee with the existing hair, taking care not to snag or pull its base. Check that there are no hard edges and that the front hairline is styled to make it appear as natural as possible. This part of the toupee is the most noticeable to others, so it is always worthwhile paying special attention to make sure it is not combed either too far forward or too far back.

On initial fitting, the toupee may have to be cut into the shape of the existing hairstyle. If it needs restyling then this must be carried out by an expert as mistakes at this stage can be very costly.

When the toupee has been fitted, make sure that it feels comfortable and that the client is happy with the result. Demonstrate to the client how to attach and remove the hairpiece and give advice on its maintenance. Explain how the hair should be combed to prevent tearing the base and that the base must be kept dry (unless specially designed otherwise). Stress that the hair does not grow, therefore the colour may fade due to the effect of natural sunlight and that it may be necessary to professionally refresh the colour (or add extra white hairs) in the future. Make sure that the client is aware of the need for professional maintenance of all added hair to prolong its 'life'.

## Things to do

1. Collect photographs or pictures of different hairstyles for men. Stick them neatly onto a plain piece of paper. Label each one and state whether the style is a uniform layer or a graduated layer.

2. Practise the scissor movement over comb for five minutes each day for a week. You will be surprised how much easier it becomes with practice.

3. Collect as many leaflets as you can about electrical safety at work and put them in your file. Useful places to look for this information are:
   (a) electricity board
   (b) libraries
   (c) your local authority

4. Make your own style book of men's hairstyles using photographs and pictures from trade journals or magazines.

## What do you know?

- List the **five** main tools used when cutting men's hair and give their uses.
- Name the **four** techniques used when cutting hair.
- Which type of cutting can **only** be done on wet hair?
- What are the **two** main effects that can be created on men's hair?
- List **five** critical influencing factors when cutting men's hair.
- What are the **five** difficult hair growth patterns? Briefly state how you would camouflage each one.
- What is the **correct** term for scarring the skin?
- What **precautions** would you take when cutting a fringe?
- How can you remove hair **outside** the desired shape?
- List your **responsibilities** under the Electricity at Work Regulations.

In this unit you will learn about:

- Preparing the client for a shave and massage.
- The tools and equipment needed to carry out a shave and massage.
- Honing and stropping an open razor.
- How to shave the face and neck.
- Massaging the face and the massage techniques used.
- Vibro massage.
- Adverse skin conditions.
- How to work safely and efficiently.

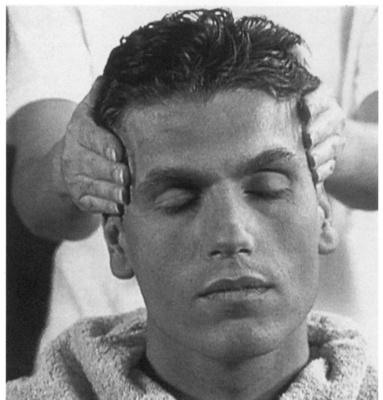

L'Oréal

# Shaving and face massage

## Shaving

Shaving is a specialised art and you will need lots of practice to make sure you are able to work safely. Here are some of the tools and equipment.

### Gowns and towels

The client must be well protected during the shave. The gowns used in shaving often fasten at the back and the towels are white and smaller than those used for shampooing.

### Barber's chair

The barber's chair is hydraulic so it can be adjusted to the right height for the client and barber. It has a neck rest which is locked in position to allow the head to be placed horizontal for ease of shaving.

### Shaving mugs and brushes

The shaving mug is filled with hot water and is used with a shaving brush. The brush is dipped in the hot water then rotated quickly round the shaving soap to produce a creamy lather.

### Steamers

Steamers are special steaming cabinets that hold the towels and steam them. If the salon does not have a steamer then the towels have to be steamed manually with hot water. If you do have to steam the towels in this way, take care not to burn your hands.

### Razors

There are various types of razor that can be used to shave the beard. Traditionally, **open razors** have been used by barbers to shave beards. However, for safety and hygienic reasons, **safety razors** with disposable blades are more commonly used as each client can have their own new, sterile blade for each shave. Some local by-laws also prohibit the use of open razors in salons. The most recently developed safety razor has special blades which can be inserted and removed without the operator having to handle any part of the blade at all.

For those salons that prefer to use open razors, extreme care must be taken to make sure that the razors are kept clean, sharp and sterile and that all possible precautions are taken to prevent cuts to the skin and cross-infection.

### Open razors

Open razors (Fig. 2.11.1) have a 'fixed' blade and are made of steel with a bone, vulcanite or celluloid handle. There are two types (Table 2.11.1):

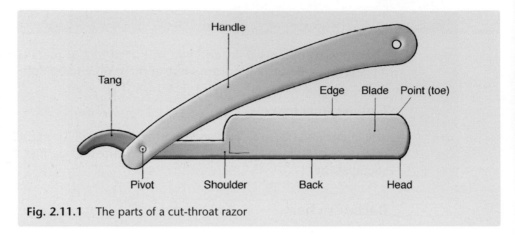

**Fig. 2.11.1**    The parts of a cut-throat razor

- **Hollow ground** (English or German) – these are fine, pliable and quick to 'set'. If an open razor is used in the salon then these are the ones most commonly used.
- **Solid** (French) – these are rigid but kinder to sensitive skin. They can also be used for cutting hair on the head.

When magnified, the edge of the razor is like the teeth of a carpenter's saw which becomes worn down with use. To make the edge sharp again, they are sharpened by honing and stropping:

- **Honing** restores the worn edge by creating a new row of teeth. The honing process is often called setting and is done on a stone known as a **hone**. If it is carried out correctly it will give a perfect cutting edge to the razor's blade.
- **Stropping** is used between honing to help preserve the edge for as long as possible.

**Table 2.11.1**  The two types of open razor

| Type | Advantages | Disadvantages |
|------|-----------|---------------|
| English/German hollow-ground | Durable, pliable, quicker to set and lighter to handle | Too hard for sensitive skin types. Will damage cuticle of the hair if used for haircutting |
| French solid | Smooth and soft to the skin therefore good for thin, fine skin. Suitable for haircutting | Has to be ground and stropped more frequently than hollow-ground as the metal is softer |

## Honing

**Honing a hollow-ground razor (Fig. 2.11.2)**

1. Place the hone on a tissue. Wipe the surface of the hone so that it is clean.
2. Sprinkle lubricant (oil) over the surface of the hone and spread evenly with the back of the razor.

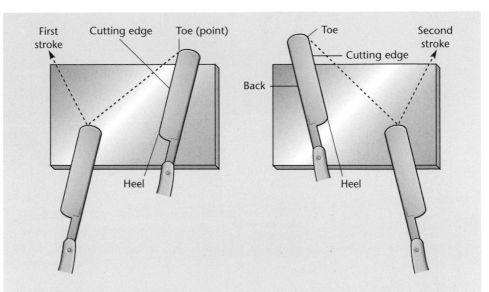

**Fig. 2.11.2** Setting a razor hone: the razor is stroked down and up the hone in a V-shape; the razor is then turned to sharpen the other side of the blade by stroking it in a V-shape in the opposite direction

3. Stroke the razor blade diagonally across the hone, leading with the cutting edge of the razor. Start with the heel and finish with the toe. The blade should be kept flat on the surface and equal pressure used on the razor at all times.

4. Turn the razor on its back to start the second stroke. Use your fingers to roll the razor over and not your wrist. As the razor turns over, slide it from the bottom to the top of the hone so the heel is on the hone again.

5. Next draw the razor diagonally across the hone with the cutting edge leading.

6. Repeat this figure-of-eight movement until the razor is set, i.e. the cutting edge has been restored. The lubricant will darken during the honing process as the steel is removed from the blade.

7. After setting, wipe the blade on a tissue (along the back to avoid cutting the fingers). Clean the hone and store away carefully with the surface protected so that it does not become chipped.

### Honing a French solid razor (Fig. 2.11.3)

The steel of a French solid razor is softer than the steel of a hollow-ground razor and must therefore always be set on a fine grain hone with thin oil as a lubricant.

**TECHNICAL TIPS**

When honing any type of razor the edge can be blunted and damaged if the razor is turned on its edge instead of its back.

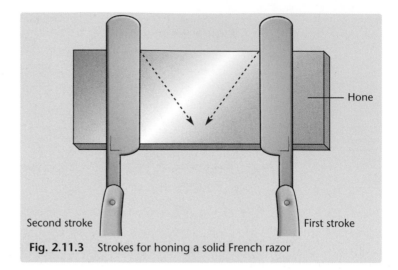

**Fig. 2.11.3**    Strokes for honing a solid French razor

The strokes should be shorter than those used for the hollow-ground razor with only the razor edge resting, almost flat, on the hone. The strokes resemble a V-shape with the razor turned on its back at the end of each stroke. As the strokes progress they become steeper and steeper until they are almost at a 90° angle.

### Testing the razor

Testing is done by pulling the razor across a moistened thumbnail:

- A perfect or **keen** edge will dig into the nail with a smooth, steady grip.
- A blunt or **dull** edge will pull smoothly across the nail without dragging or cutting.
- An **overhoned** edge will stick to the nail with a harsh, grating sound.
- A **nick** in the razor will feel uneven when it is drawn across the nail.

## Stropping

Stropping is done to keep the cutting edge of the razor between settings. It cleans the razor's edge and realigns the teeth. It is carried out on a leather strop which can be either:

- **Hanging strop** – has a canvas back: used for hollow-ground razors.
- **Solid or hand strop** – used for solid French razors.

### Stropping a hollow-ground razor

1. Place hanging strop on a hook and hold out in a horizontal position. Hold the razor between the first finger and thumb of the other hand to allow the razor to be revolved easily during stropping.
2. Lie the razor flat and stroke it, with the back leading, away and down the strop.

3. About two-thirds of the way down the strop, turn the razor on its back and bring it back up in the opposite direction.
4. At first, the strokes should be slow and careful – speed only comes with practice. Twelve strokes are usually enough (six forward and six back) to sharpen the edge.

**Stropping a French solid razor**

1. Place solid strop in horizontal position on a workstation.
2. Hold razor between thumb and first finger.
3. Place **back** of the razor slightly off the strop with the edge resting flat.
4. Stroke the razor down the strop as before.

**POINTS TO REMEMBER**

Before being used for the first time, a new strop must be treated by smearing it with plenty of oil and leaving it to soak overnight. The canvas side of a hanging strop should also be treated by rubbing soap into the canvas. After treating, both surfaces are then rubbed with a round, glass bottle until a glazed surface is obtained. Always store strops away from dust, damp and hair cuttings as any damage to the surface will spoil the cutting edge of the razor.

**Sterilising razors**

- Wash open razors in hot, soapy water then put in disinfectant or use the autoclave.
- Safety razors need a new blade for each client. Clean other parts of the razor in hot, soapy water then put in disinfectant or an autoclave.

## Shaving

A good shave should not be felt by the client and should result in smooth skin. It can be:

- On the whole face.
- Partial, leaving out moustache or sideburns.
- Used to clean outline shapes at the nape and sideburns.

Shaving has **three** separate phases: preparation of the client, lathering and shaving.

### Preparation of the client

1. Wash your hands and nails.
2. Make sure the client's beard is free from dirt and grease.
3. Carry out client consultation.
4. Prepare reclining chair with clean paper towel over headrest.
5. Seat client and protect with gown and a towel placed across his chest, tucked into the neck.

6. Position client's head well back so that you can work easily on his chin and lower face. Place paper towel, tissue or shaving square near neck.

7. Examine face looking for any critical factors.

**Critical factors before shaving**

- **What the client wants** – talk to the client and listen carefully to what he has to say. This is also an opportunity for you to offer help and advice.

- **Hair growth patterns** – beard hair can have strong growth patterns in the same way as hair at the nape. If you are unsure, ask the client as they usually know where these areas are. You will have to take extra care to shave against the growth pattern for a close shave.

- **Unusual features** – this can be anything from skin scars to cysts or other abnormal growths or skin pitting. Make sure that the skin is not too sensitive in these areas and watch the angle of your razor when you are shaving.

- **Adverse skin conditions** – you cannot carry out a shave if there is any risk of cross-infection or harm to the client or yourself. The table on p. 295 lists infectious and non-infectious skin conditions. If in doubt, ask your supervisor or tutor for guidance.

## Lathering

Lathering is carried out to soften the beard and prevent the shave being painful. Lather is produced by soap and water. Shaving soap can be obtained as foam, powder, cream or liquid.

**TECHNICAL TIPS**

Block or tablet soap is not recommended for lathering because it would be unhygienic to use the same block for a large number of clients

**How to lather**

1. Place a sterile, steamed towel over the beard area. Do not cover nose to allow client to breathe. If an open razor is to be used, strop while face is steaming.

2. Replace the cooled towel with a second steamed towel. Fill a shaving mug or bowl with hot water.

3. Remove the towel.

4. Mix the lather by dipping the shaving brush into the mug of hot water then put a small amount of soap into the centre of the brush bristles. Rotate the brush vigorously (almost like whisking an egg) in the bowl of the shaving mug until a lather is produced.

5. Place brush under tip of client's chin and rotate over chin, cheeks and neck until all beard is well covered.

6. Lather upper lip by placing finger in the centre of the brush bristles to spread them. This prevents lather from going up the nose or on the lips.

7. Keep brush warm by dipping it into the hot water.

**POINTS TO REMEMBER**

Any shaving will remove a fine layer of the epidermal (top) skin so the angle of the razor and the direction of the razor strokes must be correct.

When shaving, the blade of the razor must be wiped clean of hair and lather between each razor stroke. It is *very important* to wipe the razor on its back, avoiding the edge otherwise the operator may cut their fingers quite badly and blunt the razor edge.

The temperature of the water should be kept warm. Cold water will cause the razor to drag while hot water swells the face and prevents a close shave.

A good lather will make the beard easier to shave.

**TECHNICAL TIPS**

Always stretch the skin taut when stroking with the razor as this will hold the hair up to the razor and allow it to be cut more closely and will also help to prevent cuts to the skin.

## First time over shave

The first time over shave is always done in the same direction as the hair growth, **with** the grain of the hair. When stretching the skin for this shave, place your fingers behind the razor instead of in front, as it is very difficult to get a firm grip on the skin when the face is slippery with the lather.

### How to first time over shave

1. Hold razor loosely with your thumb on the blade. The position will vary with the different strokes.

2. Dip razor into hot water.

3. Begin the shave on the side nearest to you. Start by holding the dry, unlathered skin at the sideburn area to prevent your fingers slipping. Pull it taut.

4. Move razor in a slicing motion following the movements shown in Fig. 2.11.4.

**TECHNICAL TIPS**

A right-handed barber should stand and start on the right-hand side while a left-handed one should stand and start on the left.

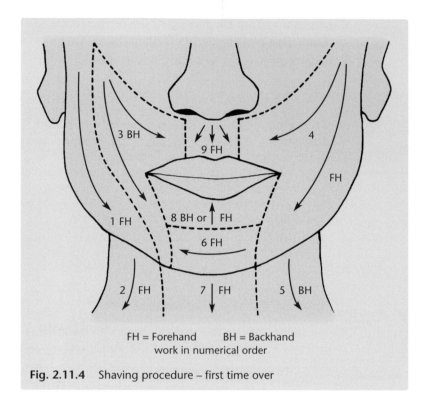

FH = Forehand        BH = Backhand
work in numerical order

**Fig. 2.11.4**    Shaving procedure – first time over

**TECHNICAL TIPS**

It is important to start any razor stroke before a bony prominence to prevent cutting the client.

5. Completely shave one side of the face together with the side of the upper lip area. Leave just the centre section, which is then shaved upwards while pressing the tip of the nose upwards to tighten the skin.
6. Turn client's head towards you and shave the other side, leaving centre chin until last.
7. To shave the point of the chin, pull skin tight between the finger and thumb then use the middle of the razor blade to shave across the chin.
8. Finish by shaving the neck downwards.

## Second time over shave

This cuts the hair **against** the growth in an upward movement to make sure that the beard is cut as closely as possible. The result should be smooth and clean. A dark-haired, strong-growth beard may need another **sponge shave** after the second time over. To do this you will need to soak a sponge in hot water then drag it across the face with the razor following.

How to second time over shave

1. Relather face as before.

2. Begin the shave at the collar area. Move upwards in backhand strokes, completing one side of the face before starting the other as for the first time over shave. See Fig 2.11.5 for the order and manner of strokes.

3. Clean the face with damp, warm towel or sponge. Gently pat dry with another clean towel.

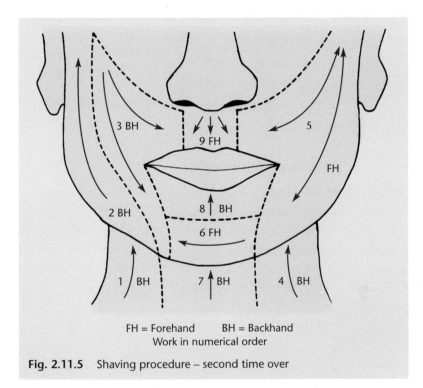

FH = Forehand        BH = Backhand
Work in numerical order

**Fig. 2.11.5**    Shaving procedure – second time over

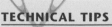

## TECHNICAL TIPS

Juvenile beards are quite soft and may not need shaving against the growth with upward strokes.

## POINTS TO REMEMBER

Any cuts or punctures to the skin should have a new styptic pencil for each client applied to stop the flow of blood. However, for hygienic and health reasons extreme care must by taken to avoid contact with blood, so wear rubber gloves.

4. Apply a small amount of talcum powder to dry the skin; this is to prevent chapping.

5. Finish with an after-shave lotion to close the pores, reduce the risk of infection and leave the skin feeling fresh and clean.

6. Dispose of any sharps (razor blades, etc.) safely in accordance with the salon's health and safety policy and local by-laws.

## Men's face massage

The massage is usually carried out after shaving to:

- Help skin elasticity.
- Tone the facial muscles.
- Encourage natural excretion of waste products.
- Relax the client.

### Massage movements

- **Effleurage** – a slow, stroking movement with the flat of the fingers.
- **Petrissage** – a slow, kneading, rotating movement that moves the skin over the bones of the face with fingers in a claw-like position.
- **Tapotement** – a gentle tapping movement with the tips of the fingers. Used mainly on fleshy areas and double chins. (See Units 1.1 and 1.2 for more detailed information.)

### Preparation for massage

- Protect client's clothing and hair.
- Assemble all equipment and products. Arrange without causing hazards or obstruction to others.
- Wash hands and nails.
- Position client comfortably with head flat and resting on a paper towel on the headrest.
- Steam the face with two hot towels to open pores, relax client and stimulate blood flow.

# How to massage

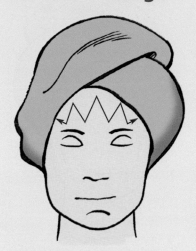

**1** Stand behind client. Apply massage cream with **effleurage** massage movements. Place flat of fingers on forehead at eyebrows. Stroke fingers back towards front hairline.

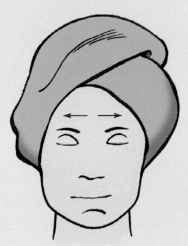

**2** Stroke across forehead in gentle **effleurage** movements to relax client.

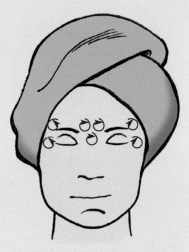

**3** Rotate skin at corner of the eyes with **petrissage** movements then move to above the nose. Gentle **tapotement** used under eyes to prevent skin pulling.

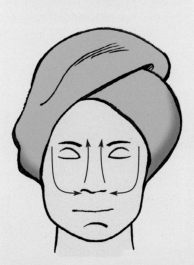

**4** Stroke from temple down to cheekbone and side of nostril base. Turn hands with backs together to carry movement up the sides of nose to between eyebrows.

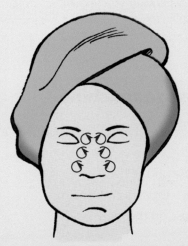

**5** Place third finger of each hand on the side of nostrils, use small, circular petrissage movements up the sides to help to unblock the pores.

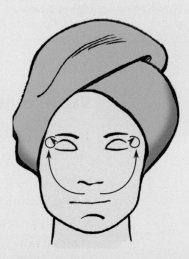

**6** Tips of fingers together, stroke from the upper lip sliding the fingers sideways and diagonally upwards towards the outer corner of the eye, finishing with a circular petrissage movement around the bony part of the eye socket.

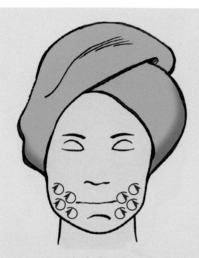 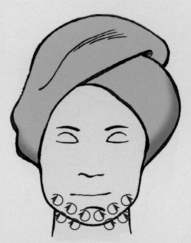 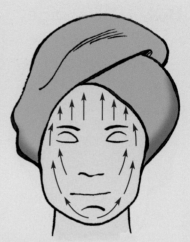

**7** Massage lower part of face in a circular petrissage movement from the mouth out towards the ear then from below the mouth to under the ears.

**8** The top of the chin and jawline are massaged by petrissage movements but tapotement is more suitable for fleshy or double chins.

**9** Finish the massage by rolling the skin upwards between the thumb and the forefinger from the chin to the forehead.

**10** Finish treatment with another hot towel followed by a cool towel and/or an astringent to close the pores, tighten the skin and reduce the risk of infection.

**11** Apply a light dusting of powder, cream or lotion depending on the client's preference.

**12** Clear away all tools and equipment. Leave workstation clean and tidy.

## Vibro massage machine

The vibro massage machine is used to provide a mechanical massage. It has three main applicators:

- **Spiked** – for use on the scalp.
- **Flat vulcanite** – for use on the skin.
- **Sponge** – for use on the face.

### Using vibro massage

The vibro massage gives strong tapotement movements. It can be used in place of a manual hand massage but it is only suitable for the fleshy areas. Take care when you are using the vibro on bony areas such as the jawline and forehead. It can be very uncomfortable for the client and must never be used on the nose and around the eyes. If you are using the vibro to replace some of the hand massage movements, use it in the same order and direction as the massage movements it is replacing.

Always be aware of the comfort of the client and use the vibro carefully and gently. If it feels too strong for the client then use the attachments over the hand.

## Adverse skin conditions

These are also covered in detail in Unit 3.1.

| Condition | Infectious | Carry out shave? |
| --- | --- | --- |
| Impetigo | Very | No, not under any circumstances |
| Acne vulgaris (common acne) | Yes | No, there is a danger of spreading infection |
| Boils | Yes | No, there could be a danger of spreading infection |
| Facial alopecia (facial hair loss) | No | Yes, but with medical permission |
| Psoriasis | No | No, unless condition is mild otherwise the raised skin causes problems. Medical permission might be needed |
| Moles | No | No, it is not recommended to remove hair on or near moles |
| Scars | No | Yes, but must be at least six months old. Risk of cutting client if skin is raised |
| Warts (verrucae) | No | No, if a wart is cut there may be severe bleeding |
| Sunburn | No | No, if the skin is still red it would be too sensitive |

## Adverse skin conditions

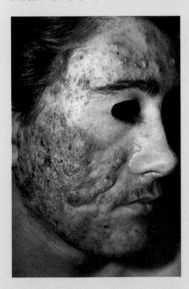
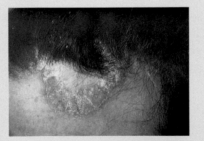
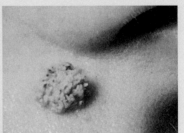
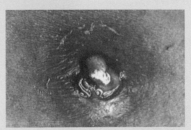

Shaving should not be carried out if any of these conditions were present on the lower face: very severe acne vulgaris (common acne), psoriasis, wart and a boil with pus-filled centre

# Health and safety for shaving and massage

- Protect client with clean gown and towels.
- Handle razors and scissors carefully.
- Always wipe razors on their back not their cutting edge.
- Dispose of waste products safely in the correct place.
- Dispose of sharps in accordance with your salon procedures and local by-laws.
- Keep workstation clean and tidy at all times to prevent cross-infection.
- Use disposable paper towels on chair headrest.
- Wash your hands and nails before shaving and massaging.
- Check for adverse skin conditions before you start.
- Take care when handling steamed towels – they could burn your hands.
- Clean and sterilise all tools and equipment after use and store safely.
- Know and understand your responsibilities under the COSHH Regulations and any local by-laws about the use and disposal of razors and sharp objects.

## Dealing with cuts

1. Tell client what has happened – be tactful.
2. Tell your supervisor, tutor or other relevant person what has happened.
3. Wear rubber gloves to wipe the blood.
4. Apply styptic pencil to the wound. Use new one for each client to prevent cross-infection.
5. Apply antiseptic and dressing from the first-aid box.
6. Write up what has happened in the accident book.
7. Clear away soiled items and put them in a sealed plastic bag. Some items may need to be cleaned in bleach, others will have to be disposed of safely in accordance with your salon's procedures.
8. Put any soiled towels or gowns for laundering separately.

## Things to do

Shaving the face is a skilled operation which improves with practice. It is, however, the hairdressing operation most likely to cause bleeding and it is important to know what to do if this happens. This assignment is designed to help you develop your practical skills and hygiene operations.

1. Using an inflated balloon of about head size, lather and shave as you would a face. You know instantly if you have cut into it! You can use a peach instead of a balloon but this lacks the realistic size.

2. If you cut a client while shaving (or at any other time):
   (a) Use a styptic to stop the bleeding; put the styptic onto a tissue and give this to the client for them to hold on the cut.
   (b) If any blood has fallen onto surfaces, wipe with neat bleach and wash off with plenty of water and detergent.

   Explain each of these steps.

3. Collect pictures and photographs of shaving tools and equipment (trade journals and your local wholesalers may have some). Cut them out and stick neatly onto a piece of paper. Write a brief account of:
   (a) what each is used for
   (b) how you would clean and sterilise each one
   (c) the salon procedure for safe handling and storage

   Put in your file for future reference.

## What do you know?

- How is the razor edge tested for sharpness?
- What is the **difference** between stropping and honing?
- What are the **three** phrases of shaving?
- List **seven** points when preparing the client for shaving.
- List **five** adverse skin conditions.
- Why is the face lathered before shaving?
- Give **five** critical factors.
- Why is the skin stretched **taut** when stroking with the razor?
- How often is the razor wiped clean when shaving?
- How is the razor wiped and what could happen if it was wiped along its edge?
- What type of shave may a dark-haired, strong-growth beard need and how is it done?

- Name **four** reasons for carrying out a face massage.
- Name the **three** massage movements for the face.
- Which type of massage movement is used first to **relax** the client?
- What type of movements are more suitable for fleshy or double chins?
- Why is an astringent used after a massage?
- What is the vibro massager suitable for?
- Where must the vibro massager **never** be used?
- What can be done to aid client comfort if the vibro feels too strong for the client?
- Give **ten** health and safety precautions for shaving and massage.

In this unit you will learn about:

- The tools you need to cut beards and moustaches.
- The methods of sterilisation for these tools.
- How to prepare a client before cutting a beard or moustache.
- How to trim and shape a beard.
- How to trim and shape a moustache.
- The health and safety precautions you need to take.

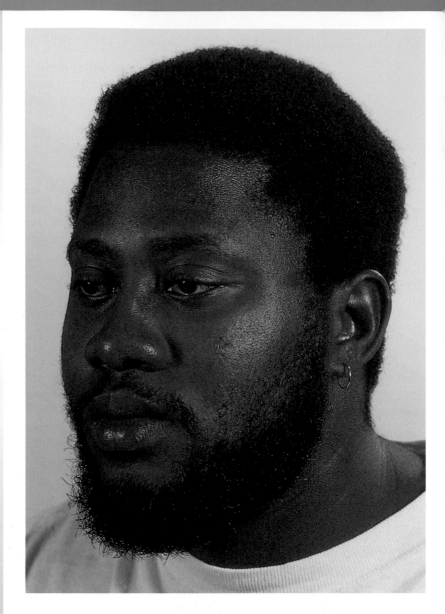

# Beards and moustaches

## Trimming tools and techniques

A beard should suit the client's face shape and size of head. It should also balance the hairstyle giving a 'total' look. Client consultation is very important before starting the beard trim to find out the shape and length of beard that the client wants.

Clippers and attachments are often used for very close beards, for example, 'designer stubble' or when a very short uniform look is wanted.

### Tools

- **Scissors** – store and handle safely, sterilise by wiping with spirit after each client. Clean in hot, soapy water then place in disinfectant or the autoclave.

- **Clippers** – store and handle safely taking care not to damage the teeth. Store with the guard on. Brush out hair from blades, wipe over and use antiseptic oil after each client (Fig. 2.12.1). Clean by wiping with spirit. Check plug and flex before using. Switch off at the socket when you have finished.

- **Clipper attachments** – come in various sizes which are numbered. The higher the number the longer it will leave the hair. A no. 1 attachment will cut the hair very short whereas a no. 8 will leave it much longer. After each client, wash in hot, soapy water then put in disinfectant or the autoclave.

- **Razors** – handle and store carefully. Keep all razors closed when not in use and preferably in a safety pouch. Clean in hot, soapy water then place in disinfectant or the autoclave.

- **Combs** – should be the correct size for use. Fine flexible barber's combs are used to cut the hair close to the skin. Clean after use then place in disinfectant, autoclave or sterilising cabinet. It is good hygienic practice to keep combs in a bactericidal jar when they are not being used.

- **Neck brush** – remove cut hairs after use. Clean in hot, soapy water then place in the sterilising cabinet.

### Techniques

The techniques are the same as used for cutting men's hair. Usually you will need to use a few techniques together on one client to get the result you want (Figs. 2.12.2 and 2.12.3):

- Scissors over comb.
- Clipper over comb.
- Clipper with attachment.
- Freehand.
- Razoring.

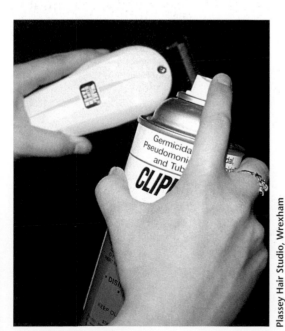

Plassey Hair Studio, Wrexham

**Fig. 2.12.1**  Antiseptic oil is sprayed onto the clippers after they have been used

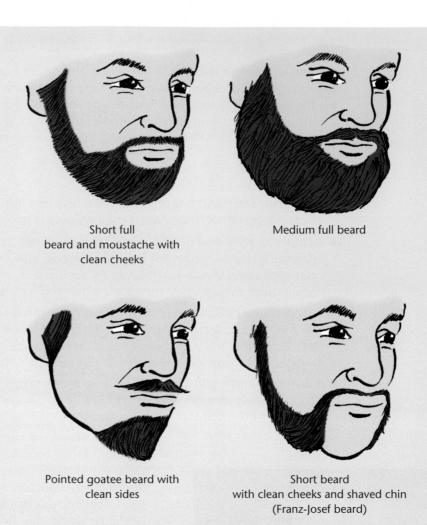

Short full
beard and moustache with
clean cheeks

Medium full beard

Pointed goatee beard with
clean sides

Short beard
with clean cheeks and shaved chin
(Franz-Josef beard)

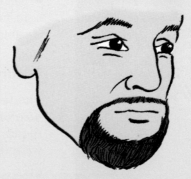

Short rounded
beard and moustache with clean
cheeks and jaw

**Fig. 2.12.2**    A variety of beard shapes

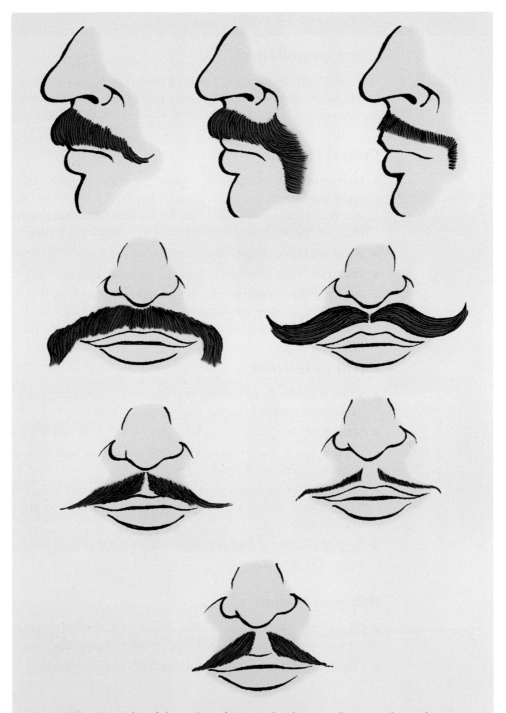

**Fig. 2.12.3**    Examples of the variety of moustache shapes a client can choose from

## Preparation of the client

### Client consultation

Use your communication skills to find out what the client wants before you begin. Offer suggestions and advice if it is needed – remember that consultation is a two-way process which helps to build up trust between you and the client.

### Critical factors

- **Hair growth patterns** – hair grows in different directions on the face in the same way as on the head. Usually the hair will grow down and slightly outwards but sometimes there may be a whorl or strong growth pattern under the chin on the neck. You need to cut into the growth pattern if the hair is short.
- **Head and face shape** – the beard should suit both the head and face shape.
- **Hairstyle** – the beard must balance with the hairstyle to give a total look.
- **Adverse skin conditions** – you must only cut hair if it is safe to do so. The same adverse skin conditions apply to trimming beards and moustaches as they do to shaving. Look at the table of adverse conditions on p. 295.

### Client protection

- Short, cut hair is very sharp and can easily penetrate the skin. It is also full of bacteria so may turn septic if it enters the skin.
- Make sure you protect the client well with gown and towels.
- Offer a small cloth for the client's eyes or ask him to keep them shut while you are cutting the hair.
- Adjust the chair height so that both you and the client are comfortable. His head should rest on a paper towel on the headrest to prevent any neck strain or cross-infection.
- Keep the client as free as possible from cut hair and sweep up immediately at end of the service.

### Hair preparation

- Check that the hair is free from grease and dirt. Dirty, greasy hair will stop the scissors cutting properly and clog up clipper blades.
- Comb through in a downward direction to disentangle.

**POINTS TO REMEMBER**

A beard must be trimmed to suit the face and match in with the hairstyle. Different face shapes suit different beard shapes. Here are the most common:

- **Round face** – to make the face appear thinner: cut the beard close, or shave the sides and shape the hair to be longer at the chin; shave under the neck.
- **Narrow face with hollow cheeks** – to widen the face and fill out hollows: leave the sides full and create a round shape at the chin; leave the hair a medium length under the chin and just above the collar line.
- **Long chin** – to create the illusion of a shorter chin: cut the beard in a square shape across both the sides and chin area.

## Trimming a beard and moustache

### How to do it

1. Place the client in a reclined position.
2. Cut the beard using the scissors or clipper over comb method, combing the beard upwards.
3. Take small sections and keep the comb moving as you cut. Remember that the further away from the face the comb is held, the longer it will leave the hair.
4. Take extra care when trimming under the chin and around the lips as it is easy to tickle the client and could cut the skin (Fig. 2.12.4).
5. Outline the moustache, supporting the scissors with the first finger to prevent cutting the lips, then cut the hair freehand.
6. Outline the final shape using a razor/shaper or clippers (Fig. 2.12.5).

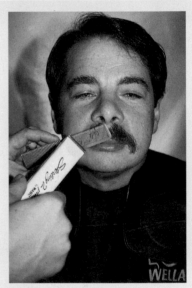

**Fig. 2.12.4** Cutting a moustache using clippers and comb

**TECHNICAL TIPS**

Small, bristly beard cuttings are sharp, dangerous and can cause infection; therefore it is extremely important to protect the client as much as possible.

7. Remove the beard clippings from the client with a brush and show him the result in the mirror.
8. Tidy and clear away tools and equipment. Clean the workstation.

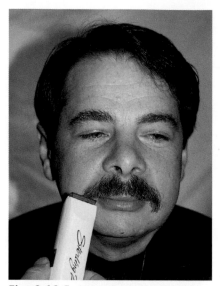

**Fig. 2.12.5** Using a cordless outline to create the outline shape at the sides of the moustache

## Precautions to take

- Always carry out a consultation before you start, to make sure that the client's wishes are taken into consideration.
- Check whether the client wants the finished beard 'blended' into the neck or prefers a definite outline shape.
- Longer beards are sometimes cut freehand, remember to comb the hair into shape before cutting.
- Beards can be thinned out with the razor, but take care not to make the finished result too wispy.
- Take strong hair growth patterns into consideration when cutting the hair.
- Always dispose of sharps safely in the correct place and according to local by-laws.

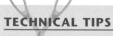

**TECHNICAL TIPS**

Facial hair can have strong hair growth patterns. If a close-cropped beard is required it is necessary to cut hair against its growth pattern.

## Health and safety

- Make sure that both you and the client are well protected.
- Make sure the client is comfortable without any strain on his neck.
- Protect the client's eyes with a small cloth or ask him to keep them closed.
- Check all electrical equipment you may use before you begin. Better still, use cordless clippers.
- Do not have any trailing wires and keep tools and products well organised.
- Take care not to cut the client's skin, especially around the lips and under the chin.
- Keep the workstation clean and tidy to prevent cross-infection.
- Clean and sterilise all tools and equipment after use; store them safely in the correct place.
- Sweep up any hair immediately you have finished.
- Switch off any electrical equipment at the socket.

● Dispose of any sharps or waste products in the correct place according to salon procedures and local by-laws.

● Know and understand your responsibilities under the Electricity at Work Regulations 1989.

## Things to do

1. Look up and read about the Electricity at Work Regulations 1989. Discuss with your supervisor or tutor your responsibilities under these regulations. Write a brief summary on:
   (a) what the regulations are
   (b) what you need to do to work safely with electricity at work

   Keep your summary in your file for future reference.

2. Collect pictures and illustrations of different beard and moustache shapes. Stick them neatly onto an A4 size piece of plain paper and draw a border round them. Place in your file for future reference or use in the salon as examples for your clients to see.

3. Read up about adverse skin conditions in Unit 2.11. Discuss with your supervisor or tutor what you would say to the client if he had one of these conditions. Write a brief account of how you would tell the client.

## What do you know?

● How would you clean and sterilise razors?

● Which type of comb allows the hair to be cut close to the skin?

● Name **five** cutting techniques you could use for trimming a beard.

● Give **four** critical influencing factors for beard and moustache trimming.

● How would you shape the beard for a client with a long chin?

● How is the hair prepared for beard trimming?

● Why should you take extra care when you are cutting around the lips?

● Why is it important to dispose of sharps safely?

● What are your responsibilities under the Electricity at Work Regulations?

# *13*

In this unit you will learn about:

- The effects of humidity on hair.
- What happens within the hair when it is dried.
- The tools, equipment and types of products you will need for drying and finishing hair.
- Preparation of the client.
- Critical influencing factors and other considerations when drying hair.
- The techniques used when drying and finishing.
- How to work safely and efficiently when drying and finishing.

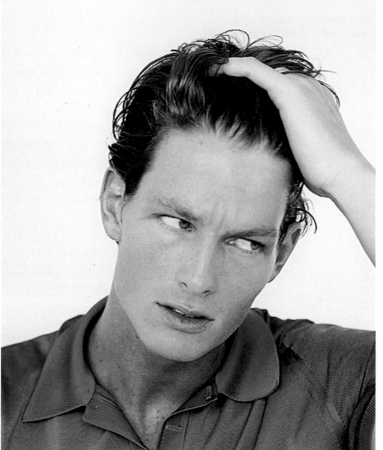

L'Oréal

# Drying and finishing men's hair

## Drying and finishing men's hair

A good haircut needs to be dried and finished well to make it look at its best. Similar techniques are used to dry men's hair and women's hair and they are covered in detail in Unit 2.3. The effects of humidity and what happens inside the hair when it is dried are also covered in Unit 2.3 but here is a summary.

### What happens in the hair when it's dried

Hair is elastic and therefore it will stretch. It stretches more when it is wet than when it is dry. When hair is in its natural, unstretched state it is called **alpha keratin**; when we wet it and stretch it during drying it becomes **beta keratin**. Hair will then stay as beta keratin until it reverts back to its natural unstretched, alpha keratin, when style 'drops'. Alpha is the Greek letter A and beta is the Greek letter B, so what we are really saying is that when hair is wet, stretched and dried it goes from A to B.

### How humidity affects the hair

Hair contains a lot of water which it absorbs from the atmosphere (atmospheric moisture). Because of this, the hair starts to revert back to its natural state, alpha keratin, which makes the hairstyle drop. To try to avoid this, and to make the style last longer, we use various products such as mousses, gels and waxes that will put a coating barrier on the hair to stop the atsmopheric moisture being absorbed.

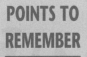

**POINTS TO REMEMBER**

Another way to say that hair absorbs moisture is to say it is **hygroscopic**.

### Types of product

There are many different products you can use when drying and finishing the hair, and different manufacturers have their own ranges. You need to find out which ones are used in your salon and how to use them correctly. Products can be used before drying or after drying.

**Before drying**

- **Mousse** – foam in an aerosol can. Place the size of a golf ball in the palm of your hand and apply evenly to the hair. Comb through. Suitable for most hair types, usually has firm and normal hold. Can be mixed with gel to give more hold.
- **Blow-dry lotions** – sprinkle evenly onto hair, comb through. Suitable for most hair types.

- **Gel** – place amount need on palm of hand then rub through hair, comb through. Stronger than lotion and mousse and good for spiky styles or where hair needs to be given texture or moulded. Gel is also used when hair is dry to 'strand' it.
- **Moisturisers** – these add moisture to the hair. Apply as blow-dry lotion. Use on very dry hair or chemically damaged hair.
- **Activators** – keep the hair more supple and help maintain the curl in permed or naturally curly hair. Do not use on greasy hair.

### After drying

- **Wax** – solid in a jar. Put a small amount of wax on hands then rub them together vigorously. This heats the wax and melts it slightly. Apply sparingly to break up the outline of a style or strand it. It is very greasy so use carefully.
- **Dressing creams** – lighter than wax, they help to reduce static electricity, put a shine on the hair and replace natural oils. Apply sparingly, they can make the hair greasy.
- **Sprays** – these hold the hair in place. Can be spray or aerosol. They put a plastic coating on the hair so the atmospheric moisture cannot penetrate as easily and the style keeps longer.

## Tools and equipment

- Brushes of various sizes.
- Combs.
- Hairdryer and attachments, including diffuser.

## Preparation of the client

### Client consultation

Even though you may have done this before with the previous process, you still need to make sure that you understand what the client wants. Tell the client what products you are going to use on the hair. This gives them the opportunity to disagree with your choice and for you to give them advice on how to maintain their style at home.

**POINTS TO REMEMBER**
Use all your interpersonal skills when carrying out any consultation. This includes non-verbal as well as verbal communication – no pulling faces. Smile and be pleasant instead and use your listening skills to really listen to what the client is telling you he wants.

## Critical factors

- **Haircut and hair length** – work with the shape that has been cut into the hair, you can only work with what you've got.
- **Hair texture** – finer hair may need smaller brushes and lotions that give volume to the hair. Thicker hair will need larger brushes or just finger drying.
- **Head and face shape** – the finished style should flatter these. See Unit 2.10 for more information on suitable styles for face shapes.
- **Hair growth patterns** – if you dry the hair against its natural fall, it will stick up and the style will not hold. You may want this for some spiky styles.

## Client protection

Protect the client's clothing with towel and gown. Remember that the equipment used to dry hair produces heat, so make sure sensitive areas like the neck or ears are well protected. Be careful when applying products, don't let them go on the skin or in the client's eyes.

## Hair preparation

Hair has usually been shampooed before you dry it. If not, it should still be clean before you start. Choose suitable products to use by thinking about:

- How you want the style to be.
- Texture, porosity and elasticity of the hair.
- What the client wants.

## Techniques for use on men's hair

Barbers use similar techniques as for women's hair, they are just applied differently. You can use a combination of techniques on one head. Read Unit 2.3 for more information on some of the techniques listed below.

### Finger drying

Finger drying is using fingers instead of a brush (Fig 2.13.1). Mould the hair in the direction of the final style and lift the hair to dry underneath at the roots if you need lift. Good for unstructured looks or on the very short hair of some styles.

### Blow-drying

Blow-drying is drying the hair with a hand dryer with or without a nozzle. Using the nozzle concentrates the airflow in one area, using the dryer without the nozzle diffuses the airflow. Remember that, unlike women, men usually prefer a squarer outline shape with not too much lift, especially at the sides.

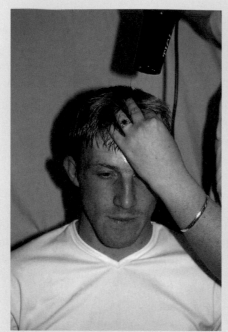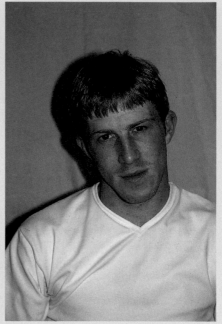

L'Oréal

**Fig. 2.13.1**  Finger drying

## Blow-waving

Blow-waving is drying the hair to create waves and movement in the style – usually only used in men's hairdressing. Hair is dried using a flattened nozzle attachment to direct the flow of air against it to form movement:

1. Start at front hairline and follow the natural growth direction.
2. Insert coarse end of comb in hair and push back to form wave crest.
3. Use half-strength airflow to direct air onto centre of wave in opposite direction to held comb.
4. Move dryer along hair to avoid burning the scalp.
5. Continue until areas needing waving are completed.

## Health and safety

### Electrical tools

Most equipment for drying hair is electrical. You must know how to use it safely and hygienically. The Electricity at Work Regulations state that to do this you need to:

● Know how to use equipment.
● Make sure it is not used for anything other than what it is intended for.
● Always check wires and plug before you start.

- Switch off at the socket when you have finished.
- Store safely in the correct place.

## Other safety

- Keep your workstation clean and tidy to help prevent cross-infection.
- Organise the products and tools you use so that you can work efficiently and without being in the way of others.
- Make sure the client is well protected.
- Use products in accordance with the manufacturer's instructions.
- Direct the airflow so it doesn't burn the client's scalp.
- Clean and sterilse all tools when you have finished.
- Store all tools and equipment safely and in the correct place. Wires should not be left trailing where someone could trip over them.
- Tell the relevant person if the stock levels of the products you have used are low, then you won't run out in future.
- Dispose of any waste products in the right place.

## Things to do

1. Read Unit 2.3 and take notes on:
   (a) The tools and equipment used for drying and finishing.
   (b) What humidity is, its effect on the hair and what changes take place inside the hair when you are drying it.
   (c) What you need to do before, during and after a blow-dry.
   (d) Any differences between drying and finishing men's hair and women's hair.
   Keep the notes in your file for future reference.

2. Find out what drying and finishing products are used in your salon then:
   (a) Read the instructions for each.
   (b) Make your own notes on how they should be used and what they should be used for.
   (c) Keep in your file for future reference.

3. Read about the different methods of sterilisation in Unit ?. Write a brief account on how you would clean and sterilise:
   (a) brushes
   (b) combs
   (c) work surfaces

## What do you know?

- What do **alpha** and **beta** keratin mean?
- What is the **correct** term for hair absorbing moisture?
- List **eight** products that can be used when drying and finishing hair.
- Give **five** influencing factors that you need to consider before drying hair.
- Explain **briefly** how you would protect the client before drying the hair.
- What do you need to think about to help you **choose** the correct product for the hair and the final result?
- Give **three** techniques for drying hair.
- What are your **responsibilities** under the Electricity at Work Regulations?
- List **seven** non-electrical safety considerations.

# Level 3

# 1

In this unit you will learn about:

- Client consultation.
- Maintaining an effective working relationship with clients.
- Dealing with client complaints.
- Hair and scalp conditions that influence or prohibit salon services.
- Health and safety aspects of certain hair and scalp condition.
- Selling and promoting after care procedures.

The key role of effective communication is stressed throughout. The unit also looks at after-care services and products and how to promote them with clients. Finally, it considers how to improve salon services, particularly by encouraging feedback from the clients.

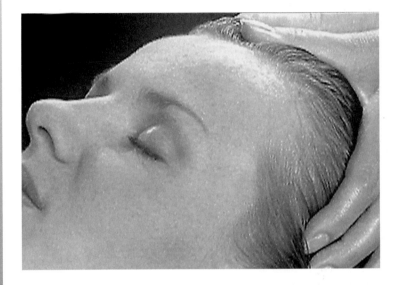

# Maintaining and improving client services

## Client consultation

Always remember that clients are indispensable to your business and your behaviour towards them should show that you value them and their custom. Talking to the client before their treatment will not only help you know their specific needs but will also help to develop a positive relationship between you and the client.

Listen carefully to find out exactly what the client requires and check your understanding by repeating their request. Talk to them in a language they understand – using specialist terminology is fine as long as everyone understands what is being said. Mistakes can easily be made through the differing perceptions of both client and stylist.

In addition to finding out the client's wishes, any consultation should include an examination of the head and face shape, and also the texture, length and condition of the hair to make sure that what the client actually wants is compatible with their hair type and facial features. When diagnosing the hair before carrying out a chemical treatment, it is very important to determine which, if any, chemicals have been used previously on the hair. This can be done through feeling and looking at the hair and also by questioning the client. Sometimes a client may be less than truthful due to embarrassment or not realising how long a product will remain on or in the hair. If in doubt, always carry out a suitable test – not only does it prevent harmful mistakes, it also shows professionalism and saves any argument as to the suitability of the required service.

Clients are not always aware of the range of products and services that the salon has to offer, so a discussion of their relevance and the benefits, along with their cost, can highlight your expertise and make the client feel that they are receiving individual attention.

Client consultation is an ongoing process and, although the major part of the diagnosis will be carried out before the service, there should be continuing dialogue with the client both during and at the end of the service. All staff should be familiar with the range of products used and sold in the salon to enable them to offer advice and guidance on which after-care products would be suitable for home use. Up-to-date records should be kept of all client services and products used or recommended, to help with future consultations.

## Effective working relationships with clients

A salon cannot exist for long without clients. Hairdressing is a highly competitive service industry and success depends on developing and keeping a good client base. What makes a client return to a salon? What makes a client recommend the salon to someone else?

The key to success is communicating a **positive attitude.** Is the salon a welcoming, friendly place? Will a client feel valued? Will they feel they have experienced a thoroughly professional service? Here are two situations that may create difficulties.

### Referring clients to other services

The need to refer clients to other services, hairdressing or non-hairdressing (such as medical) will arise from time to time. This may well be as a result of client consultation and assessment of the condition of a client's hair and scalp. The outcome of the hair and scalp assessment may be relatively unimportant (such as using a different type of mousse) or it may be more sensitive (such as the presence of head lice). Sometimes a client will have a hair or scalp condition which is beyond the salon's ability to help. In this case the person may be referred to professional medical treatment. Scalp ringworm is an example of such a condition. On other occasions referral to other professionals such as trichologists may be appropriate (psoriasis is an example).

On any occasion requiring referral of a client, the key word is **tact**. The information is confidential; treat it so. Talk quietly, be positive, listen to the client, reassure them. Explain that they will:

- Need expert opinion to confirm the diagnosis.
- Be welcome to return to the salon if the condition turns out to be non-infectious.
- Understand the need to suspend hairdressing operations (should this be necessary) in order to prevent infecting others.

## Dealing with a client complaint

Most people, if dealt with pleasantly and correctly, are easy to please, but there will always be one client who has some grievance, whether real or imagined. Tactful dealing with the client is essential to keep their goodwill and create a good impression of the salon. It is very tempting to feel that the salon would be better off without this type of client but remember that when a client is lost, the salon also loses many more potential clients because the unsatisfied client will almost certainly give a bad impression of the salon's service to others. The best practice is to **anticipate** problems. Most people will 'leak' their dissatisfaction in a non-verbal way. Look out for:

- Body movements
- Body posture
- Facial expressions

which indicate that the client is not very happy.

If a complaint does occur it must be dealt with immediately, whatever the cause. If it is a complaint against the service, it should be dealt with to their complete satisfaction. For example, in the case of an unsatisfactory perm – it is no use trying to persuade the client that it is satisfactory. Instead, you should deal with the incident without fuss and reperm where necessary, giving a quiet explanation as to the failure. This is a far more professional attitude and more acceptable than an argument, which does not solve anything.

If a client is loud in their protests and embarrassing to yourself and other clients, you should take them quietly to a private part of the salon to rectify the complaint. If it concerns another member of staff, it must be rectified with that member of staff present.

Even in the best-run salons, mistakes sometimes happen. A colour does not come up to expectations or a perm may be limp. If this occurs it is often the best policy to tell the client, before they complain, that you are not satisfied with the result and will rectify it immediately. This promotes goodwill and the client will have more trust, feeling that the stylist cares about their hair and will not be satisfied with second-best results. Their recommendations to others could win many new clients and is an extremely effective way of advertising.

Looking after clients is good business. The wages of the staff depend upon clients returning regularly to the salon. If a client has enjoyed their visit and feels that they have had a first-class service, they will almost certainly return.

## Hair and scalp: conditions that can influence salon services

Hair and scalp conditions include:

- Diseases of the hair and skin.
- Infections caused by micro-organisms.
- Infestations by animal parasites.
- Non-infectious hair and skin problems.

Both infections and infestations are caused by parasites. These terms are explained below:

- A **parasite** is a living organism which lives off another living thing, called the parasite's **host**, but with only the parasite benefiting.
- A body **infection** is caused by a disease-causing, or **pathogenic micro-organism**, living on the body, feeding from it and producing the signs or symptoms of the disease. These parasites, commonly called **germs**, involve many different sorts of living things, but they all share the characteristic of being too small to be seen with the unaided eye.
- A body **infestation** describes an invasion by larger animal parasites which are visible to the unaided eye and mostly live at or near the surface of the body.

A summary of the main infections and infestations is given in Table 3.1.1.

### Transmission

Both pathogenic micro-organisms and the larger animal parasites need to be passed or transmitted from one person to another. This transmission may take place in two main ways, which are either by contact or through the air.

#### Transmission by contact

Contact means that physical touching causes the transmission of the parasite. If a parasite can be passed in this way it is described as being **contagious**. This contact can be direct or indirect. Touching lips during kissing can transmit the micro-organism which causes **cold sores** (**herpes**) from one person to another. Touching heads allows the **head louse** to walk from one head to another. Both of these examples involve direct contact.

Indirect contact often involves inanimate objects which have been in contact with one person and are then touched by another; cold sores, for example, can be spread on damp towels, face cloths, etc., which have been in contact with one person and then used by another. Head lice may be transmitted from brushes and combs from one person to another.

### Transmission through the air

This only involves the parasitic micro-organisms. If a parasite is passed from one person to another in this way it is described as **infectious**. The micro-organisms which cause the common cold and influenza (flu) are spread by tiny droplets released by coughing and sneezing being breathed in by someone else. The micro-organism which causes **ringworm** (**tinea**) is often spread in minute **skin flakes** released by an infected person (or animal) which settle onto someone else.

## Infections caused by micro-organisms

### Skin and scalp conditions caused by bacteria

Many skin and scalp conditions are caused by bacteria normally found living on the skin. Two groups in particular, **staphylococci** and **streptococci**, will turn up several times as the cause of bacterial skin and scalp conditions. Both of these can also cause wound infection, or **sepsis**, which involves reddening, inflammation, swelling and pus formation.

#### Impetigo

*Cause*
The skin bacteria staphylococci and streptococci.

*Major symptoms*
Blisters which contain a clear fluid and eventually form yellow crusts on the skin. Common on face and scalp, where the infection spreads rapidly.

- Impetigo is commonly caused by bacteria invading skin broken by scratching, e.g. as a result of head lice or itchmite infestation. This is called **secondary infection**.

- It is very contagious and spread by both direct and indirect contact. Hairdressing operations should not be started, or if they have, the stylist should stop and take care to sterilise with disinfectant any tools and equipment used.

- A different form of impetigo occurs in children (called Bockhardt's impetigo) which is caused by staphylococci bacteria invading scalp hair follicles and causing them to become inflamed, i.e. producing folliculitis. The condition appears as small red spots in the skin at the base of the hair with a head of pus. The client should seek medical aid.

### Boils (furunculosis)

*Cause*

A staphylococci bacteria invading a hair follicle or sebaceous gland and producing severe inflammation.

*Major symptoms*

A red raised area of the skin, very tender, with a central 'core' containing pus.

- Boils are common where clothing rubs, e.g. back or side of neck in males, where a shirt collar may rub. Staphylococcus aureus, which causes boils, is found living in the noses of between 10 and 30 per cent of the population. So it is possible to infect someone by coughing and sneezing. Sometimes a group of neighbouring follicles become involved, and this is called a **carbuncle**.

- Do not start hairdressing operations (or stop if already started) if a boil is in the area involved, e.g. scalp or beard. If the boil is not in such an area, take great care not to touch it with the tools, equipment, towels, etc. This will be painful for the client and there is the possibility of picking up, and thus spreading, the bacteria.

### Barber's itch (sycosis barbae)

*Cause*

Staphylococci bacteria invading the hair follicles in the beard area in males.

*Major symptoms*

Inflammation and pus formation in some of the beard hair follicles. Pain and itching in these areas.

- Barber's itch can be spread by indirect contact on shaving brushes, razors and towels.

- If scalp operations are intended, take great care not to touch beard area involved with tools, equipment or towels and gowns. Sterilise all these items after use. Do not start shaving or beard-trimming.

### Folliculitis

*Cause*

Staphylococci bacteria.

*Major symptoms*

Infected hair follicles producing yellow spot with hair in centre. Itching and scratching.

## Fungi

The fungi group ranges in size from mushrooms and toadstools down to microscopic varieties. Most live off dead organic material where they cause **decay**. Some microscopic types are parasites and cause skin and scalp conditions called ringworm.

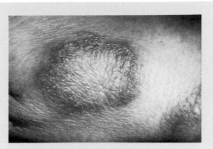

**Fig. 3.1.1** The appearance of ringworm on the hand

## Ringworm (tinea)

Ringworm (Fig. 3.1.1) can be found as:

- Ringworm of the **scalp** (tinea capitis) – covered in detail below.
- Ringworm of the **body** (tinea corporis) – similar symptoms to scalp ringworm but most often caught from domestic animals.
- Ringworm of the **foot** or athlete's foot (tinea pedis) – a common condition, where the fungus grows through the skin between the toes causing reddening and itching (and possibly skin cracking). Commonly contracted by indirect contact through wet floors, e.g. changing rooms and swimming pools.

### Ringworm of the scalp (tinea capitis)

*Cause*
The microscopic threads of the parasitic fungus growing through the cornified (horny) layer of the skin epidermis and through any hair shafts it encounters.

*Major symptoms*
Bald patches on the scalp with a stubble of broken-off hairs (due to weakening of the hair shaft as the fungus grows through it). The bald patches are often circular and the skin inflamed.

- It is highly contagious by both indirect and direct contact and is infectious in that skin flakes breaking off from an infected person can land on another, and if they lodge for long enough they can grow from the flake into the other person's skin. It can be contracted from domestic animals.
- It is most common in children.
- Do not start (or stop, if already started) hairdressing operations. If operations have been started then disinfect tools, equipment, gowns, towels and seating.
- Sweep up (or better, vacuum) any hair clippings; place in sealed plastic bags and preferably dispose of by burning outside the salon.

## Viruses

Viruses are the smallest of all the micro-organisms and unlike bacteria, moulds, yeasts and fungi, they cannot survive for long outside living cells. A common form of transmission of viral diseases is by **droplet infection**. When someone coughs or sneezes, hundreds of tiny droplets of liquid are blown into the air. These may contain living viruses which can survive as long as the droplet persists. In damp air (air with a high relative humidity) the droplets evaporate slowly and this increases the chances of someone else inhaling the droplets and becoming infected. In dry air (air with a low relative humidity) the droplets evaporate quickly and the viruses die. The common cold and flu (influenza) are spread in this way. Because of the large amounts of moisture entering the air in hairdressing salons (due to hot water being used, the large amount of drying, etc.) the air tends to have a relatively high humidity, unless the ventilation system can cope with its removal. This is one reason why an efficient ventilation system is important in the salon.

The various skin conditions caused by viruses are cold sores (herpes simplex) and some types of wart.

### Cold sores (herpes simplex)

*Cause*

A virus which lives in the germinative layer of the skin epidermis (present in about 90 per cent of the population) and develops when a person's general resistance is lowered, e.g. by another disease.

*Major symptoms*

Often begins as a small crack in dry skin in the corner (or corners) of the mouth. It spreads rapidly with some blistering and develops into an oozing crust (like a soft scab).

- It is very common, especially in children.
- It can be passed by direct or indirect contact; therefore, care should be taken to sterilise cups, etc., used by clients or towels likely to have touched the face. If persistent, suggest the client sees a doctor. Often clears up spontaneously, but is carried in the body until the next time conditions favour its growth.

### Warts (verrucae)

*Cause*

A virus (called papova virus) which lives in the germinative layer of the skin epidermis, where it triggers a large amount of cell division in a small area. This produces the lumps characteristic of common warts. On the feet the pressure causes the wart to grow inwards, which produces a plantar wart (commonly called verrucae).

*Major symptoms*

1. **Raised warts** – may be rough and rise some distance above the skin (common warts) or be smaller and smooth-topped (plane warts – common in children).
2. **Plantar warts** (verrucae) – grow into the skin on the feet, where the pressure caused by the weight of the body is greatest, e.g. on the ball of the foot.

- Unless a client feels strongly that the size and position of the wart necessitates removal, they are best left alone. If removal is desirable, then recommend they see their doctor and do not use the proprietary 'wart removers' on the market.
- Warts often clear spontaneously as the body eventually becomes immune to the virus which causes them.
- They can be transmitted by direct or indirect contact, so take reasonable precautions.
- Plantar warts (verrucae) are spread by indirect contact in places with damp or wet floors, e.g. changing rooms and swimming pools.

### Aids and hepatitis B

Aids is short for acquired immune deficiency syndrome, which is a very dangerous disease that could possibly be transmitted in the salon. The chances of this happening are very small but it is worth taking reasonable precautions. The virus that causes Aids can be transmitted in body fluids and therefore could pass from one person to another in blood, such as someone being nicked with a razor, the razor not being cleaned and then someone else being nicked with the same razor. The current advice for any blood spillage is to use neat bleach on the blood and then wash away with lots of water and a detergent.

Hepatitis B is another very serious illness which can be transmitted like Aids and so the precautions are the same.

Information about Aids and Hepatitis B can be obtained from local environmental health centres, health education authorities and the Department of Health.

## Eye infections

Eye infections can spread rapidly by indirect contact with damp towels in the salon. The two main kinds are:

- **Blepharitis** (or sties) – where staphylococci bacteria infect the eyelash follicles, causing soreness, reddening and swelling.
- **Conjunctivitis** – which can have a variety of causes, e.g. bacteria like staphylococci and some viruses. Conjunctivitis is the inflammation of the outer, protective layer on the front of the eyeball and can be spread by indirect contact with damp towels; some forms are very infectious. Because of the high risk of transferring the micro-organisms onto towels, hairdressing operations should be stopped and the client advised to see their doctor.

## Infestations caused by animal parasites

Larger parasites are visible to the unaided eye and feed off the human body. Important examples in hairdressing are:

- Lice (especially the head louse).
- Fleas.
- Itchmites (which cause scabies).

Anyone can become infested and it is not a reflection on personal hygiene to have picked up these parasites. In fact, head lice prefer clean scalps to dirty ones.

Lice and fleas are insects and have six legs. Both have special jaws which can pierce the person's skin and then suck blood (the mouths work rather like the hollow needle of a hypodermic syringe used to take a blood sample at the hospital). When the person's skin is pierced, the animal injects a small amount of **anticoagulant** into the tiny wound to prevent the blood from clotting. It is this action that:

- Produces the skin reddening and itching associated with lice and flea 'bites'. The scratching of these areas often breaks the skin surface and allows invasion by bacteria, producing a secondary infection, e.g. **impetigo**.
- Can lead to other infections passed on by the parasite. This is unlikely in the UK, but fleas can pass on plague and lice can pass on typhus.

Itchmites belong to a branch of the spider family and have eight legs. They are the smallest of the animal parasites with the female mite less that 0.5 mm long (the male is almost half that size). The female digs tunnels into the skin and lays her eggs there. Chemicals released by the mites can cause intense irritation and itching and a common name for scabies is 'the itch'.

## Lice

Infestation of the body by lice is called **pediculosis**. The head louse is the most important type in hairdressing:

### Head lice (pediculus capitis)

About 4 per cent of the population have head lice at any one time and they are often first noticed by the hairdresser. The adults are about 3 mm long and have flattened bodies. Each leg has strong claws at the end, used to grip hair shafts. The flattened bodies and the claws make it difficult to dislodge adult lice and any lice which fall out of untreated hair are dying (due to injury or old age).

Lice pierce the skin and suck blood, causing a certain amount of irritation. Lice only have a lifespan of about 30 days and events during this time are outlined in Fig. 3.1.2.

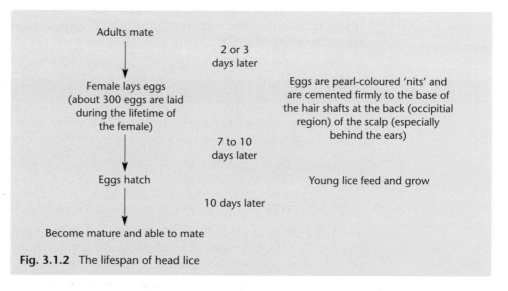

**Fig. 3.1.2** The lifespan of head lice

Only a few of the eggs laid survive to maturity and a typical head infestation involves about 20 adult lice.

Head lice are contagious and can be transmitted from one person to another by direct head-to-head contact or indirect contact from pillows, upholstery, etc. Lice cannot jump or fly and any seen off the scalp are usually dying or dead.

### Symptoms

The client will probably have noticed some itching but may be unaware of its cause. The infestation is often first noticed by the presence of the eggs or nits glued to the bases of the hair shafts (Fig. 3.1.3) and sometimes the adults are visible.

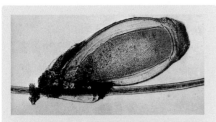

**Fig. 3.1.3** A head louse egg (nit) attached to a hair follicle

- Reassure the client that contracting head lice is nothing to do with personal hygiene (many people are horrified when they are told) and that it is easy to eradicate (the community health councils hold a range of very useful pamphlets on skin disorders and body parasites, including the head louse, and these are available free from your nearest office which will be in the phone book).
- Do point out that others in the family are likely to be infected and that expert advice, e.g. doctor, health visitor or local health clinic, should be sought.
- Because head lice are contagious, do not begin (or stop, if started) hairdressing operations. Take care to disinfect tools and equipment thoroughly, wipe down with disinfectant and vacuum the upholstery of chairs the client has used.
- The eggs or nits can sometimes be mistaken for flakes of dandruff. If in doubt, try to rub the flake off the hair. Dandruff flakes are easily removed, nits are not.

## Non-infectious or non-contagious hair problems

In addition to the infectious and contagious conditions there are a number of non-infectious or non-contagious hair conditions.

- **Fragilitis crinium** – commonly known as split ends where the hair points are split lengthways. The only cure is to cut the ends off.
- **Trichorrhexis nodosa** – where hair is fragile due to splits along the hair shaft.
- **Monilethrix** – a very rare condition where the hair shaft has a beaded appearance due to distorted growth. Treatment for both trichorrhexis and monilethrix involves using **restructurants** and **protein treatments** (see below).
- **Damaged cuticle** – the most common cause of damaged cuticle is chemical treatment, but it can be caused by vigorous brushing or combing. The cuticle is important for hair condition (the cuticle in good condition makes hair shine) and porosity (in extreme cases hair is so porous that even permanent tints wash out).

A very common feature of damage to the cuticle (even relatively little damage) is hair becoming tangled. There is no treatment as such, but protein-based and other types of 'restructurants' in shampoo and/or conditioning treatments can help. These add to the hair in the porous areas; in other words, they are **substantive**. They automatically enter the hair where needed.

Some conditions are caused by hair in areas that are normally **vellus** becoming secondary hair. Examples are **hypertrichosis**, where this happens in certain areas, and **hirsutism**, which is more general across the whole body.

A summary of non-infectious hair conditions is presented in Table 3.1.1.

**Table 3.1.1** Summary of the main infections and infestations

| Name of condition | Caused by | Major symptoms | Infectious or contagious? | Stop hairdressing operations? | Medical advice needed? |
|---|---|---|---|---|---|
| Impetigo | Bacteria | Blisters and yellow crusts | Yes (very) | Yes | Yes |
| Boils (furuncles) | Bacteria | Red, raised area in skin. Very tender. Central pus | Yes (if pus released) | Only if boil in scalp area | Yes, if persistent |
| Barber's itch (sycosis barbae) | Bacteria | Swelling and pus formation in beard hair follicles | Yes | Yes, on beard area (avoid contact in this area) | Yes, if persistent |
| Folliculitis | Bacteria | Yellow spot with hair in centre | Yes | Yes | Yes, if persistent |
| Ringworm (tinea) | Fungus | Round bald patches. Stubble of hair, skin may be inflamed | Yes (very) | Yes | Yes |
| Cold sores (herpes simplex) | Virus | Weeping scabs around mouth | Yes | No, but take care to prevent transmission | Not usually, but yes if persistent and extreme |
| Warts (verrucae) | Virus | Lump in skin (rough or smooth) | Yes | No (but avoid nicking with scissors) | Not usually, unless removal wanted |
| Conjunctivitis | Bacteria or virus | Inflamed eyes, possible weeping of fluid | Yes | Yes | Yes |
| Head lice (pediculus capitis) | Head louse | Itching, eggs (nits) glued to base of hair. Sometimes adults seen | Yes | Yes | Yes (but advice can be given by hairdresser) |
| Flea (pulex irritans) | Human flea | Red spots surrounded by pink patches. Itching | Yes | Yes | Yes |
| Scabies | Itchmite (sarcopies scabiei) | Intense itching, especially in joints and at night (burrows sometimes visible) | Yes | Yes | Yes |

## Non-infectious or non-contagious skin conditions

### Psoriasis

Psoriasis is an inherited condition and therefore is commonly found among members of the same family. The cause of psoriasis is not known for certain, but it may be caused by a defect in the chemical reactions taking place in the **germinative** (or basal) layer of the skin epidermis.

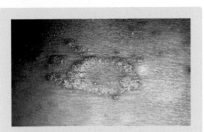

**Fig. 3.1.4** The appearance of psoriasis

### Symptoms

Patches of thickened silver-coloured scales with the underlying skin appearing red. There is no hair loss associated with the condition (Fig. 3.1.4).

- The appearance and extent of psoriasis varies and scalp psoriasis, if extensive and severe, can be distressing to the client. They should be tactfully encouraged to seek expert advice and help.

- There is a coal tar based shampoo for this condition.

A summary of non-infectious skin conditions is presented in Table 3.1.2 (see p. 333).

## Dermatitis and eczema

Both the terms 'dermatitis' and 'eczema' are used interchangeably to describe an inflammation of the skin surface. Distinctions can be made on the basis of:

- Whether the condition is dry or releases a fluid, i.e. weeps, where dermatitis is used for the dry condition and eczema for the weeping variety.
- What causes (or triggers) the development of the condition.
- Dermatitis is thought to be caused by internal and external factors and eczema by only internal factors.

### Contact dermatitis

As its name suggests, contact dermatitis may be produced in the skin due to contact with a chemical or chemicals. Some chemicals will produce a dermal rash on first exposure and this overreaction can be called an **allergy**. People may be allergic to many different substances, a common one being pollen grains in the air, causing hay fever. All allergies involve the body defence system overreacting to a substance.

Thus, the external factor involved is the contact with the chemical and the internal factors determine the person's reaction to that chemical. Other substances can produce dermatitis after a number of exposures. This is a major problem in hairdressing as the actual number of times a person needs to be exposed to a substance until they get dermatitis varies with different individuals. Substances which may eventually produce a reaction are called **sensitisers**. The chemical in para hair tints is a fairly common sensitiser and the reason for the skin test which should be carried out 24–48 hours before using such a tint is to check whether previous exposures have sensitised the client.

### Symptoms

These are very variable, but include:

- Inflammation of the skin surface.
- Cracking of the skin and possibly weeping of fluid.
- A certain amount of itching.

The risk to the hairdresser involves the hands in 90 per cent of cases.

The risk to the client tends to be on the face. Dermatitis triggered by the para dyes tends to involve the skin of the eyelids, ears and neck.

### Prevention

There is no cure once someone has developed a sensitisation to a substance, and the only action is to avoid contact with it. If a hairdresser develops a high level of sensitisation to a commonly used hairdressing chemical, often the only course of action is to leave hairdressing altogether. The best prevention is protection, particularly by using rubber gloves for all hairdressing operations involving chemicals. Barrier creams offer some protection but are not as effective as a pair of rubber gloves.

Protection of the client involves taking care to prevent hairdressing products, especially those known to be sensitisers, from touching their skin.

## Seborrhoea

Seborrhoea is the general name for the overproduction of sebum by the skin's **sebaceous glands**. The surplus of natural oil makes the hair greasy and the skin oily. This condition is common in people at **puberty**, where the sudden rise in the level of **sex hormones** in the blood triggers the overproduction of sebum.

Seborrhoea is involved in the development of acne and in some kinds of **dandruff**. If the dandruff is linked to an inflammation of the scalp, this is called **seborrhoeic dermatitis**.

### Dandruff (pityriasis)

Dandruff, or scurf, is a common scalp condition caused by the **flaking** of the cornified (or horny) layer of the skin epidermis. This flaking of the outermost skin layer occurs all over the body, all of the time and each person loses millions of these tiny flakes per day. The main reason for this general flaking is to remove skin bacteria, and thus keep the numbers of bacteria on the skin under control.

On the scalp, the hair tends to trap these flakes and they build up, or accumulate, into the large flakes which are characteristic of the condition. The damp, warm conditions under these flakes favour the multiplication of **bacteria** and **yeasts**.

At one time it was thought that dandruff was caused by bacteria. It is now known that it is not and that some people have a tendency to produce a large number of skin flakes on the scalp, whereas others do not. Whether bacteria are involved in the itching which often accompanies severe dandruff is not clear at the moment, but antiseptics are included in many medicated or anti-dandruff shampoos to keep the number of bacteria under control. These shampoos also contain substances like **selenium sulphide** and **zinc pyrithione**, which reduce the flaking by reducing the activities of the germinative layer of the skin epidermis.

The most common form of dandruff is where the flakes fall freely from the hair when brushed or combed (this is called dry dandruff or **pityriasis capitis**). If dandruff occurs in connection with seborrhoea (an overproduction of sebum) then the oil tends to make the flakes stick to the scalp (this is sometimes called oily dandruff or **pityriasis stearoides**). This can lead to seborrhoeic dermatitis. In this case the client should be referred to their doctor.

### Sebaceous cysts

Sebaceous cysts appear as raised areas on the skin and are caused by a blockage in a sebaceous gland. The sebum normally released onto the hair and skin in that area accumulates and causes the swelling. This type of cyst is sometimes called a **wen** and they are harmless.

## Baldness (alopecia)

The most common type of baldness is **male pattern** baldness, which affects about 40 per cent of males by the age of 40. This condition is inherited and is not as common in females as in males. The necessary trigger for the hair loss is the presence of the male sex hormone and this is the reason that this type of hair loss is relatively rare in women. Older women may suffer a version of this balding as their levels of female hormones fall after the **menopause**.

How the male hormone triggers the condition is not known. For no apparent reason the hair follicles start to die when they reach the end of **telogen** in the hair growth cycle. Because of this, no new hair grows to replace the old when it falls out of the follicle. For this reason, this type of balding is a gradual process, with the hair thinning and disappearing from around the crown and above the forehead. Whether high frequency treatment has a positive effect is not clear. At the moment it is not possible to prevent the hair follicles from dying, and the only effective treatment is a hair transplant.

Male pattern baldness accounts for about 90 per cent of hair loss encountered by the salon. The other 10 per cent is made up of conditions where the balding tends to be patchy or scattered; here are some of them.

### Alopecia areata

Alopecia areata is the appearance of roughly circular bald patches on the scalp. (Fig. 3.1.5). The skin of the area is soft, smooth and has no hair. These features are important in distinguishing alopecia areata from ringworm. With ringworm, the bald patches have a stubble of broken-off hairs running across them and the skin is often red and inflamed. There is no itching with alopecia areata and the condition also has 'exclamation mark' hairs around the borders of the bald patches.

Exclamation mark hairs are caused by the hair breaking and the hair root breaking down. Hairs are wider and darker near the broken end and about 0.5 cm ($\frac{1}{4}$ in) long. They are easily pulled out and appear like an exclamation mark.

Alopecia areata usually disappears in two to three months, but may recur at intervals. Figure 3.1.6 shows an example of hair regrowth following a bout of alopecia areata – the new hair has grown back white. The precise reasons for the development of the condition are not known.

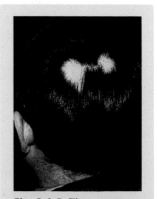

**Fig. 3.1.5** The appearance of alopecia areata

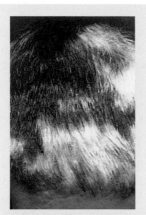

**Fig. 3.1.6** New hair growth following alopecia areata

### Diffuse alopecia (alopecia diffusa)

Diffuse alopecia describes a general thinning of the scalp hair, often most noticeable at the crown and along the parting. It can occur in young women, who find it very distressing, due to hormonal changes after childbirth and sometimes as a result of oral contraception. It can also occur after serious illness and drug treatments. The hair usually regrows. Another type of thinning is **alopecia senilis**, associated with old age.

### Traction alopecia

Traction alopecia is a general term used to describe hair being pulled out of the scalp (Fig. 3.1.7). This can result from the tension caused by tight rollers or the hairstyle adopted, e.g. tight plaits or hair rolled into a tight bun. It can also be caused by a nervous twisting of the hair around the fingers. If the cause of the tension on the hair is removed, then the hair usually grows back.

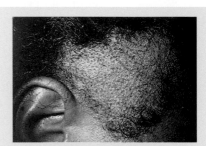

**Fig. 3.1.7** The appearance of traction alopecia

### Cicatrical (scarring) alopecia

Cicatrical alopecia results from skin damage and scarred areas in which hair will not grow. There is no treatment available.

## Health in the salon

### Preventing the transmission of disease in the salon

Preventing the transmission of infections and infestations depends on two main factors:

● General salon hygiene.
● The ability of the salon staff to recognise which skin and scalp conditions are infectious or contagious and which are not.

### Hygiene

The transmission of the parasites which cause infections and infestations can be limited by good hygiene in the salon. Good hygiene involves a number of things but they can be summarised in three points:

● The routine practice carried out by the hairdresser, e.g. sterilising brushes and combs, using a new neck strip, etc., for each client.
● Salon management practice, e.g. regular laundering of uniforms and gowns, regular cleaning of surfaces, training staff to carry these out.
● Salon design features which help hygiene, e.g. choice of wall and floor coverings, type of upholstery on seating, type of ventilation system.

**Table 3.1.2** Summary of non-infections hair and scalp conditions

| Condition | Symptoms | Notes |
|---|---|---|
| Split ends (fragilitas crinium) | Splitting of the hair at the points | Often occurs at the points of long hair with a tendency to be dry. Breaks can occur along the length of the hair and there is no real cure. Restructurant conditioners can be used but the only real answer is to cut off the split ends |
| Trichorrhexis nodosa | Swellings occur along the hair | These are weak points and the hair tends to break. It can be caused by rollers or by strong alkaline chemicals. Can use 'restructurant' to help prevent breakage |
| Damaged cuticle | Hair rough and dull and tangles easily. Difficult to untangle | Caused by chemical treatment. Use 'restructurant' to help make hair more manageable |
| Monilethrix | Bead-like swellings along the hair shaft | A very rare condition that is inherited and appears mostly in children. Tendency for hair loss as the hair tends to break off near the scalp |
| Hypertrichosis | The growth of thick secondary (terminal) hair in an area which usually shows only the fine downy (vellus) hair | Can occur on a facial mole for example |
| Hirsutism | Where male type secondary (terminal) hair growth patterns occur in females | Includes bearded ladies, of which a there are several medically certified cases |
| Psoriasis | Silver-coloured scales and reddened skin | Inherited condition. Tends to clear up and recur |
| Dermatitis and eczema | Swelling of skin. Sometimes cracking and weeping of fluid | Terms are used interchangeably. Contact dermatitis is the major occupational risk to hairdressers |
| Seborrhoea | Greasy hair and skin | Caused by overproduction of sebum. Implicated in acne |
| Dandruff (pityriasis) | Flaking of scalp | Can be dry or oily. Not caused by bacteria. Some people more prone than others |
| Sebaceous cyst (wen) | Appearance of roughly circular lumps on the skin | Caused by a blockage which prevents release of sebum onto the skin. Sebum accumulates under skin |
| Baldness (alopecia) | Hair loss | Most common in male pattern baldness. Inherited and triggered by male hormone. |

## Sterilisation and disinfection

Sterilisation means the destruction of all living things including the harmful micro-organisms that cause disease (germs). These micro-organisms can be passed from one person to another and transmitted in the salon on tools and equipment, particularly razors, scissors and clippers. There is some risk with all tools and equipment such as brushes, combs, clips, towels, etc .

Sterilisation is only really possible by using an autoclave. Autoclaves work by using steam under pressure (like a pressure cooker) at high temperatures, 125 °C for example, which is sufficient to kill all micro-organisms in about five minutes. Autoclaves have not been widely used in salons but their use is spreading as cheap automatic autoclaves enter the market.

Disinfection means reducing the chances of infection and techniques for this are widespread in hairdressing.

## Methods of disinfection

### Chemicals

Chemicals can either destroy or retard the growth of micro-organisms. A chemical which destroys micro-organisms is called a **disinfectant** (bactericide or germicide). The problems with disinfectants include:

- They rapidly go off and cease to work efficiently.
- They become overloaded and cease to work efficiently.
- Some are poisonous to humans.
- Some attack tools, particularly metal tools.

If they are used for washing down walls, upholstery and surfaces, the best type to use are **alcohol** based but this can cause problems as alcohol is a fire risk as it is flammable. Sterilising cabinets are still used in some salons but they suffer from all the problems listed for disinfectant.

Current thinking is that disinfectants are not recommended for reducing the risk of infection by tools.

### Ultraviolet rays

Ultraviolet rays are used in ultraviolet 'sterilisers'. The cabinet contains a mercury vapour tube situated at the top of the cabinet. The ultraviolet rays that it gives off sterilise equipment placed in the cabinet. As the rays cannot penetrate the equipment, items must be turned to ensure complete destruction of the bacteria.

Ultraviolet radiation can cause burns to the skin with continual exposure; therefore most of these cabinets have some form of lid that shields the hands of the operator when tools have to be removed from the cabinet.

### Heat

Very high temperatures are used in the **autoclave** which is the *only* current method of efficiently sterilising tools and equipment. Other methods which use lower temperatures to 'disinfect' rather than sterilise are:

- **Dry heat** – used in glass bead sterilisers which are useful in the salon. The higher the temperature, the shorter the time tools need to be left in and the time to reach their operating temperature. Only the part of the tools covered by the beads will be treated and although good for tools such as scissors, they are less effective with clipper blades.
- **Moist heat** – used in autoclaves and boilers/steamers. Autoclaves work at very high temperatures and are very effective at killing micro-organisms. Boiling or steaming works at a lower temperature and may not kill all pathogens. Tools should be boiled or steamed for at least ten minutes.

## Salon staff

The transmission of infections and infestations can also be reduced by the salon staff knowing:

- How to recognise the various scalp and skin conditions and to know which of them are contagious (spread by contact), which are infectious (spread by the air) and which are neither infectious nor contagious.
- How to deal with the client if a scalp or skin condition is thought to be of an infectious or contagious type.
- What steps to take in the salon to prevent transmission from happening.

### Recognising skin and scalp conditions

This is very much a job for an expert. Few hairdressers have the training or experience needed to be able to determine exactly what the many skin or scalp conditions are. Some are relatively easy and hairdressers have an important role to play in often being the first to notice the condition and be in a position to advise the client. An infestation by head lice is a good example of this, where the client may have noticed the itching, but may be unaware of the cause. Other skin conditions involve rashes, skin scaling, crusting or weeping and these can be due to a variety of causes, some infectious or contagious and others not.

This unit covers them in outline, but the rule should be:

**If in doubt do not start hairdressing operations (if they have started, then stop) and advise the client to see their doctor.**

### How to deal with the client

The key word here is tact. The hairdresser is in a difficult position and there are no rules for dealing with the client. Here are some general guidelines.

- Talk quietly to the client and, if possible, speak to them alone. Find out whether they have seen a doctor about the condition. If they have not, strongly advise them to do so.
- Even if the condition has been identified, do not be too certain when discussing it with the client. It is far better that an expert confirms the nature of the condition.
- Stress that the condition is nothing to do with personal hygiene (this is particularly important with infestations) and that anyone can contract it.

- If hairdressing operations are not possible, explain to the client the risk of infecting other clients (even if you are not sure which condition they have).
- Explain that if the condition is diagnosed by experts as non-infectious/contagious they will be welcome to return to the salon. If it is infectious or contagious, they will be welcome when it has been successfully treated.
- Stress that there are few hair or skin conditions which cannot be successfully treated.

### What to do in the salon

If an infectious or contagious condition has been provisionally identified then:

- Carefully sterilise any tools or equipment used on the client.
- Take gowns, towels, etc., used on the client and soak in a strong disinfectant solution.
- Wipe down chairs they have used with a disinfectant solution (and vacuum clean if possible).
- Carefully sweep or vacuum up any hair clippings and dispose of them immediately outside the salon, by burning if possible.

## Other factors influencing salon services

Here are some other factors that influence client services. Try to match them to the client's wishes.

- Incompatibility between intended service and previous treatments.
- Head and face shape.
- Problem features.
- Hair growth patterns.
- The lifestyle of the client and the intended final image.

## Supplementary information: supervising client consultation

### Training

Carrying out a consultation with a client requires good interpersonal skills on behalf of the trainee and these skills usually have to be taught if they are to form the basis of a good relationship between the client and the salon staff. All salons have their own image and will expect a certain standard of conduct from their personnel. However, it is unrealistic to expect staff to know exactly what is required of them without their being fully briefed so it is essential that they are all given training on how the organisation expects them to behave in a client/staff relationship. The actual training plan will usually be devised by the manager or employer but it is often the role of the supervisor to oversee the actual training and ensure that employees reach the required standard. A clear induction of new staff is very helpful, outlining the salon 'ground rules' with regard to customer care, together with regular practice sessions (for junior staff) which encourage the use of role-play to rehearse their interpersonal skills.

Consultation also includes giving advice and guidance to the client. This is impossible without a thorough knowledge of the products and services used in the salon. The more a product is used, the greater the understanding that staff acquire of its possible uses and effects. Encouraging staff to use the products as frequently as possible, insisting that the manufacturers' instructions are read and carried out correctly, and asking the manufacturers to demonstrate their products in the salon are all means of increasing product knowledge and understanding.

### Keeping up to date

Hairdressing is a rapidly developing industry and in a state of constant change. Good methods of being aware of developments are:

- Trade journals.
- Magazines.
- General television and other moving media.
- Special events such as shows seminars and the wide range of trade-based events.
- Representatives of companies selling hairdressing products and equipment.

### Points to include in training for client care

Good client care begins with personal attitude. All trainees need to be made aware of the importance of the client, and their attitude towards the client should reflect this. Without clients the salon cannot function and it is therefore vital to provide an environment in which the client can relax and enjoy their visit. A client may book an appointment for a technical service but in reality they are also booking a salon 'experience' in which the relationship between the stylist and the client is of paramount importance. Indeed, most clients continue to return to the salon not only because of the skill and expertise of the stylist but also because of the way they are treated and valued as a person.

Building up a relationship of trust is not easy and requires a combination of good interpersonal skills, sound product knowledge and a genuine empathy with the client's requirements. Offering the client help and advice is all part of the hairdressing service and, as has been mentioned in previous units, the advice given must be based on a sound understanding of the client needs combined with expertise gained through experience and thorough product knowledge. Remember that what you recommend for the client should do what it is supposed to do – if it does not then the client has every right to mistrust your judgement and will probably seek future advice elsewhere.

Client care should be an integral part of any training programme and should be constantly reinforced by the example set by senior stylists in the way they themselves treat their clients. However, it is well worth regularly reminding trainees, and possibly all staff, of the following ten points which will help to focus client care at the forefront of their work.

- Remember that the client is essential to the business.
- Develop a trusting relationship with the client.
- Find out **exactly** what the client requires and make sure that you are able to give it.
- Always **listen** to clients and try to understand their points of view.
- Make sure that your behaviour tells clients that you value them and their business.
- Try not to keep clients waiting and **never** ignore them.
- Check that clients are happy with the outcome of their visit.
- Treat all complaints seriously – deal with them courteously and **immediately**.
- Always record and analyse any complaints to enable you to improve future services.
- All staff members should apply 'client care' to each other within the salon as well as to those outside.

## Monitoring progress

While they are acquiring the skills necessary for client consultation, it is important to encourage the trainees to practise these skills as frequently as possible. The more the trainee is exposed to different hair types, face shapes and abnormalities, etc., the more adept they will become in identifying them. Allowing trainees to practise under supervision and monitoring their progress will ensure they learn as quickly as possible to the standards expected by the organisation.

Supportive help and guidance should be given – it is a good idea to apply customer care to 'customers' *within* the organisation as well as outside. Judgements are inevitable when supervising the trainee's performance but any criticism should be constructive and carried out in private in a debriefing session. Emphasis should be placed on the confidentiality of any consultation, the importance of good interpersonal skills, accurate record keeping, and the health and safety requirements of manufacturers, the salon and current legislation.

**POINTS TO REMEMBER**

- Listen to what the client is saying, not just the words but the implications and body language.
- Carry out a thorough diagnosis of the hair, face, scalp and total image of the client.
- When in doubt always test the hair.
- Keep clear, precise and up-to-date records.
- Treat any client consultation with confidentiality.

## Promotion of after-care procedures and selling

Giving the client advice on how to look after their hair at home, and the other services available to them, helps to increase salon business and maximises the potential of their hair. To do this effectively you need to know your salon's products. Always read the manufacturer's instructions and practise using the products until you know exactly what they will do. The main principles of selling are:

- Correctly identify client needs and a sale opportunity.
- Match the client needs against the product or service.
- Explain the main features and benefits of the product service.
- Follow up any positive client response to close sale.

To be effective, you need to keep-up-to-date with all new products and services. Keeping ahead with new technology and the latest trends can be done through:

- Trade magazines
- Hair and fashion magazines and journals
- Films and television
- Attending seminars, shows, trade fairs and short courses

The key points to summarise are that after-care is important:

- To the **client** – in terms of knowing what to do and what not to do with their hair following a salon service.
- For the **salon** – due to the importance of after-care advice in the professional image and operation of a salon.

This is an important factor in client satisfaction and helps develop return custom and positive personal recommendation – both of which are **very** important to the salon business.

After-care products and services can involve:

- Use of particular shampoos and conditioners.
- Styling and finishing products.
- Use of equipment –  at home or in the salon

# Activity

Go back and remind yourself about:

(a) promoting the salon image and salon services

(b) selling goods

(c) providing clients with information about the salon

Now summarise the main points involved in product promotion and selling.

## Maintaining and improving services

### Obtaining feedback from clients

Obtaining feedback from clients is very important in evaluating the quality of a person's experience of the salon and its services. At the end of their treatment the client is asked something along the lines of 'Are you happy with that?'. If a client is very dissatisfied they will let the salon staff know. Many people, however, if only slightly unhappy say 'fine' or something neutral and then leave. Very few salons obtain structured feedback by using a questionnaire. This is well worth considering. Questionnaires can be short (even 'tick the box' types) and are anonymous and confidential. The idea is to pick up lower levels of dissatisfaction and people's general impressions of the way they have been treated. By being quick to complete and anonymous it is hoped that clients will be more honest than if they are asked by the stylist outright. Other forms of feedback which are more often used are the client:

- Returning to the salon.
- Recommending the salon to other people.

Both of these are good indicators of the client's perception of the salon's service.

## Activity

Design a shore 'tick the box' questionnaire for use in a salon. Explain how you would encourage clients to fill this form in and colleagues to use it (both clients and staff). How would confidentiality be protected?

### Managing feedback from clients

Having gathered and recorded feedback, the next step is to implement improvements. This may be:

- **Directly** – within the limits of a supervisor's responsibility.
- **Indirectly** – by recommendations made to management.

To ensure that feedback is used constructively, it is a good idea to discuss this at team meetings in an open and supportive way. The key point is **improvements** which are realistic and achievable. This allows even negative feedback to be used in an effective way to improve salon services.

Client complaints are discussed earlier in this unit (page 319). Being able to successfully manage negative feedback and problem areas is a feature of good teams and effective team leadership.

## Things to do

1. Every professional product used in the salon is accompanied by a detailed set of instructions. The information contained in the instructions covers the company in case there are any problems with the product, e.g. reaction to the client's skin. Read and collect as many different manufacturers' instruction leaflets as you can, covering the following services:
   (a) perming
   (b) colouring
   (c) relaxing
   (d) retail products
   (e) cutting tools
   (f) hairpieces and extensions

   Make notes on any important points which need to be brought to the attention of the other trainees and staff members. Hold a briefing session or meeting to share the information.

2. Take an example of a client complaint. This could be simulated but a real example is better. Make out a report, including a **portfolio** of information about the incident.

## What do you know?

- List what should be included in a client consultation.
- Give a brief account of how and when you would explain the benefits and uses of the range of products and services the salon has to offer.
- Give **three** ideas for ensuring that junior staff reach the required standard for customer care.
- Which areas need to be emphasised to the trainee regarding consultation procedures?
- Explain how you would supervise a trainee carrying out a client consultation.
- Why does a salon need clients?
- Give **two** reasons why it is important for clients to have a positive impression of the salon and its services.
- How can feedback be obtained from clients?
- Explain why non-verbal communication is so important in the salon.
- List **two** strategies that will make a client feel valued.
- How should a client referral to other services be handled?
- List the key points in dealing with a client complaint.
- How may client satisfaction with the salon and its services be measured?
- Explain the importance of client consultation.
- List **three** non-verbal signs of client satisfaction.

In this unit you will learn about:

- The preparation needed before restyling hair.
- Techniques for fashion cutting hair.
- How other salon services can enhance the restyle.
- How to work safely and efficiently.

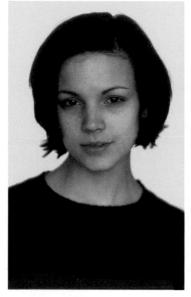 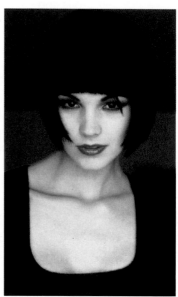

Sabre Europe Ltd

# Fashion cutting and restyling

## Fashion cutting

Fashion cutting techniques are just ways of solving problems – the problem being how to achieve a certain effect with the hair. Several techniques may give the same effect showing that the problem can be approached from different angles. Before attempting any new techniques, you must have a good understanding of the basic methods of cutting hair and the principles of shape, texture and balance. Once you have learnt these basic principles, it is possible to increase your knowledge through practice and experimentation. Being able to create different shapes and textures in the hair comes from knowing and understanding the basic cutting methods then having the courage to mix these methods together to create new shapes and styles.

### Basic cutting shapes

- **Solid form** – when the hair is cut to a perimeter line, all the same length. Gives a chunky squared effect.
- **Uniform layering** – when all the hair is cut at a 90° out from the head so that the hair layers throughout the haircut are all the same length. This produces a rounded silhouette shape which mirrors the shape of the head.
- **Low graduation** – when the top layer of hair is much longer that the underneath layers but still lies above them. The silhouette shape created by low graduation is triangular.
- **Increased graduation** – when the top layer of hair is much shorter than the underneath hair and therefore lies well above it. Creates very steep graduation and can be used when cutting longer hair to give height on top of the head.
- **Reverse graduation** – when the top layers of hair lie *below* the underneath layers. Used for pageboy styles.

### Basic cutting techniques

- **Club cutting** – cutting hair straight across. Keeps the weight on the ends of the hair and reduces length only.
- **Thinning** – removes weight and bulk from the hair but not length. Will increase the hair's natural tendency to curl.
- **Scissors/clipper over comb** – removes length only and allows hair to be cut very short.
- **Freehand cutting** – cutting the hair without holding it in place. Used on fringes, neckline, etc.

**POINTS TO REMEMBER**

All basic cutting shapes and techniques are covered in detail in Unit 2.4. Read through this unit to make sure that you fully understand the basic haircutting principles before starting more advanced, specialised techniques.

## Specialised cutting techniques

### Bevel cutting

Bevel cutting means cutting the hair on a curve. The section of hair is held between the fingers and then bent up and towards the scalp, thus curving the hair round. The hair is then cut straight across, creating graduation on the ends of the hair. This is a useful technique to use with low layering to soften and prevent a definite line or step of the edges of bobbed or wedged hair (Fig. 3.2.1).

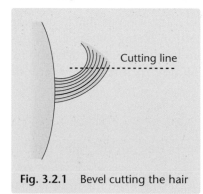

Cutting line

**Fig. 3.2.1    Bevel cutting the hair**

### Slide or slither cutting

This technique is used to blend extremes of hair lengths, e.g. very long outer perimeter line and short layered hair. A fine section of both the short and long hair lengths are taken and the scissors or razor blades then slide down the section without cutting the length of the longer hair, blending the two lengths together (Fig. 2.10.1, page 268).

**SAFETY TIPS**

Remember to be very careful when using the points of the scissors near the eyes and ears.

### Taper cutting

Tapering thins the hair at the same time as removing the length. This removes weight from the hair and helps it to curl more easily. Hair can be tapered either wet or dry. The scissors are used in a slithering movement to taper dry hair. Take care when taper cutting wet hair with the scissors as they can tear the hair and may also cause 'steps' because of the hair's tendency to stick together when wet. Wet hair is usually tapered with a razor.

#### Taper cutting dry hair

Hold the section of hair to be cut firmly between the first and second fingers. Then, using a backcombing or slithering action with the open blades of the scissors near to the crutch, direct the scissors from the points of the hair to the middle lengths. The blades should be closed very slightly during the stroke towards the scalp, then opened again drawing the scissors away from the scalp. Never completely close the scissors during the stroke towards the scalp as this could remove too much hair and create 'steps' in the haircut.

#### Taper cutting wet hair with a razor

Take the section of hair to be cut and, with the razor blade held at a slight angle, make a light slicing movement from the mid-lengths to the points of the hair, either on top or underneath the hair. The pressure on the blade will determine how much of the hair is cut away and the length of the stroke will determine the amount of taper.

## Texturising

Texturising, as the name suggests, gives visual texture to the hair. It removes bulk without length and by cutting selected areas shorter, the cut hair acts as a support for the longer hair, giving lift and volume to the style. Removing weight encourages any natural movement as well as giving a non-uniform effect. There are many ways of texturising the hair. Here are some of them.

### Chipping in

Chipping in removes weight from the ends of the hair. The points of the scissors are held at a 45° angle to the hair, which is then chipped in to give a softer outline to the hairstyle. This technique can also be used on fringes to soften or spike the front outline (Fig. 3.2.2).

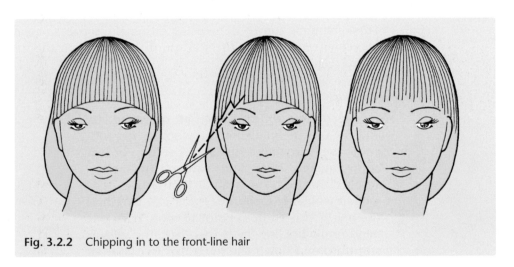

**Fig. 3.2.2**   Chipping in to the front-line hair

### Channel cutting (scaffolding)

This is the drastic removal of hair to produce a spiky effect. A grid of shorter hair is cut to support the longer hair lengths. The hair is cut first one way and then across the other to create the grid effect.

### Weave cutting

The hair to be left long is woven out using either a tail comb or the closed scissors. The hair is then held out of the way while the remaining hair in the section is cut. It can be drastic or subtle depending on how much of the hair is woven out and the effect you are trying to achieve (Fig. 3.2.3).

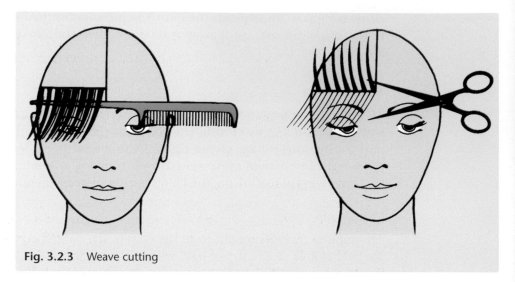

**Fig. 3.2.3**  Weave cutting

### Undercutting

The underneath sections of hair are cut shorter to support the longer lengths. This technique can be done using either the scissors or a razor in a scooping movement underneath the section of the hair from the roots up towards the points (Fig. 3.2.4).

### Twisting

This technique will thin the hair out generally and is a very useful method of 'wisping' and softening the hair around the face. A section of hair approximately 2 cm (1 in) square is taken and combed out from the head at right angles. The section is then twisted until the whole length of the hair is twisted from point to root. With one hand firmly holding the twisted hair, the scissors snip into and down the length of twists at an angle. Care must be taken not to cut the hair straight across by mistake.

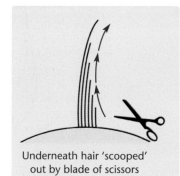

Underneath hair 'scooped' out by blade of scissors

**Fig. 3.2.4**  Undercutting the hair to texturise

## Perimeter lines and shapes

The perimeter line is the outside line or shape of the haircut. When designing the finished style, it is important to make sure that the shape is complementary to the facial features, body size and head shape of the client. Here are some common terms to describe perimeter lines and shapes.

### Baseline

This is the perimeter edge or the line to which the hair is cut. A haircut can have more that one baseline and interesting effects can be achieved by incorporating several baselines and a variety of techniques on one head.

### Symmetrical

This is when a haircut is evenly balanced and each part is in the same proportion. A basic bob is an example of a symmetrical hairstyle with each side being similar.

### Asymmetrical

The haircut is balanced but is not evenly balanced, so instead of each side being similar they are usually of different lengths or style.

### Concave

Sometimes known as an inversion or inverted shape, the term 'concave' means rounded inwards, thus the haircut curves in the opposite direction to the curve of the head. A concave shape at the nape of the neck is the reverse of a natural napeline and is shorter in the centre nape, curving round to longer at the side.

An inversion or concave shape need not be limited to the hairline alone, it can be cut into any part of the hairstyle to produce unlimited effects on both short and long hair. If a concave shape is cut into the top hair, the centre will be the shortest point. Hair will always fall away from its shortest point, therefore width will be created just above the temple area, giving a 'squared-off' shape.

### Convex

A convex shape is the opposite of a concave shape. Therefore, when cut into the nape, it will follow the hair's natural hairline and will be longer in the centre, curving round to shorter at the sides. A convex perimeter line gives a 'rounded' shape which can sometimes be more flattering for mature clients than the more angular shapes.

## Restyle cutting

A restyle is intended to give a completely new image. This means that the client needs to know that the finished style could drastically alter the way they look and they will also need advice and guidance on choosing and managing their new style.

### Advice and guidance

- **Be honest and sincere** – don't mislead the client with false claims and promises. If you are unsure about something then admit it. If the client wants something that is unsuitable or impossible to achieve, explain why and offer alternatives.
- **Be tactful** – you may have to disappoint the client if their needs are unrealistic. Try to explain without upsetting the client.
- **Be direct and factual** – don't waffle; state the facts and show visual images from books and magazines to illustrate what you mean.
- **Be clear** – keep checking that the client fully understands and that there are no misunderstandings between what the client wants and what you think they want.

## Consultation and influencing factors

Before starting a restyle, always assess the client and their hair carefully and discuss what they want in detail. To be successful, the finished style should complement the client's personality, appearance and lifestyle. Factors that influence decisions about cutting tools, cutting techniques, products and finishing techniques will include:

- Client requirements.
- Hair texture and density.
- Amount of curl in the hair.
- Hair growth patterns.
- Head and face shape.
- Finished image or look to be achieved.

## Final image: three main looks

Hairstyles can be broadly divided into three main 'looks':

- Classic.
- Current fashion.
- Avant garde.

### Classic

Classic looks withstand the test of time. A good example of this type of timeless style is the bob. The bob of the 1960s looks just as good in the 21st century. Mature or business clients often prefer smart, classical styles which flatter their image.

### Current fashion

Current fashions are the look of the moment and can change quite quickly. Interestingly, classic haircuts can usually be adapted to meet new fashion trends.

### Avant garde

Avant garde looks are new and unusual ideas; they are the forerunners of current fashion styles. Not usually suitable for the quiet, shy type of client.

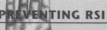

**PREVENTING RSI**

Make sure you keep up to date with the most recent innovations in design. There may be a better design for scissors that will allow for improved hand position and less strain. When such a design surfaces, you want to know about it. The same applies to your other tools, appliances, supplies and equipment.

## Sectioning for restyle cutting

There are no hard and fast rules for sectioning the hair and it should be sectioned as and where needed. Often the hair is sectioned down the centre of the head, from the front through to the nape, but any partings, fringes, etc., should be taken into consideration and sectioned off separately.

## Steps when restyling hair

1. Assess the client and their hair.
2. Carry out a thorough consultation to make sure that you both understand what the final outcome will be.
3. Make decisions on cutting techniques and tools to use.
4. Protect your clothing and the client's clothing. Assemble tools and equipment.
5. Shampoo hair if necessary. Hair usually needs to be kept wet to see the shape more easily and to use its natural hair growth pattern to best advantage.
6. Section hair if necessary then carry out haircut. Check hair length and shape throughout the cut and evaluate progress with the client. Make sure the client's head is in the correct position throughout the haircut.
7. When the cut is finished, check through to make sure the shape and texture of the cut is correct for the finished look.

**POINTS TO REMEMBER** Encourage all staff to keep salon workstations clean and tidy at all times. Encouraging effective and efficient working practices not only makes the salon look professional, it actually saves time in the long run. If everything is kept in its place then everyone knows where to find it.

## How to cut a restyle

All the following restyles use a combination of cutting techniques. The shape of the cut is then emphasised with colour to give the client a totally new image. Long hair does not always have to be cut shorter to give the client a new image.

## Additional salon services

Do not be afraid to use and advise the client on other salon services such as colouring, bleaching and perming. Used creatively, they will enhance the finished style by:

● Giving greater definition to the shape of the haircut.
● Improving the texture and volume of hair.
● Helping the hair to be more manageable.
● Achieving a certain look that the client wants.

# Restyle 1

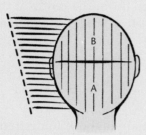
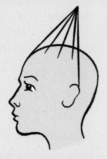

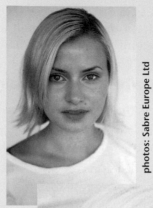

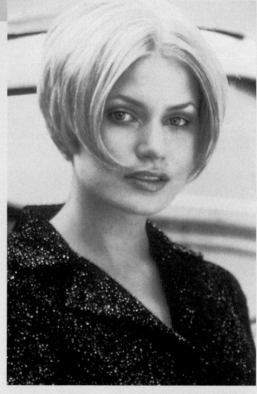

photos: Sabre Europe Ltd

**1** Cut the hair at 90° vertically from occipital to nape. Blend crown vertically with nape in same pattern as A

**2** Overdirect the top to previously cut top crown and blend

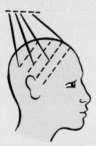
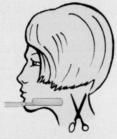

**3** Overdirect sides to the top of the crown and blend. Sides may not blend with the back

**4** Point cut the outline shape. Lightly razor cut around the hairline and continue to the fringe area, leaving the front or the fringe long. Dry with a spray gel and a round paddle brush. Finish style with light hairspray

# Restyle 2

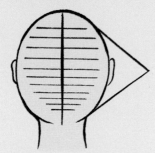

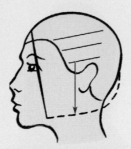

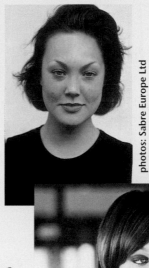

**1** Graduate each section 1 to 2 fingers in the nape. Slowly decrease elevation and start to build the weight

**2** Cut sides keeping first section on the skin, then elevating each section slightly until the part is reached

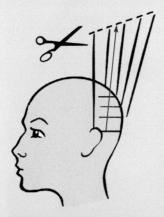

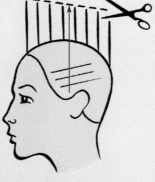

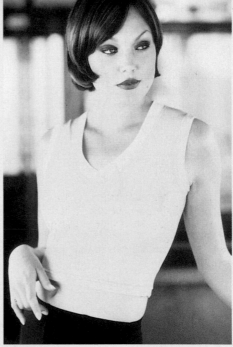

photos: Sabre Europe Ltd

**3** From a guide in the crown, cut from short to long, overdirecting all sections in the back to guide

**4** Repeat the same procedure in the front

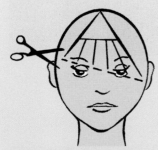

**5** Cut small fringe at an angle. Dry hair with mousse then finish with a light hairspray

## Restyle 3

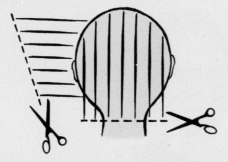

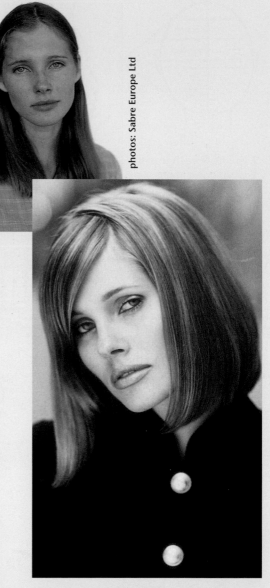

**1** Cut crown vertically so length sits in the nape. Cut length so it blends with hairline

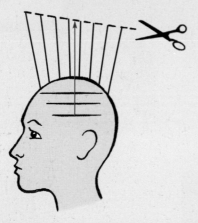

**2** From crown, cut a guideline to front. Overdirect all sections to that guide

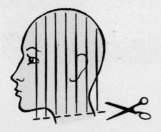

**3** Cut length just above chin

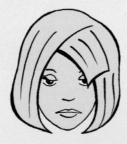

**4** Slice through hair to create light fringe and angle to side. Dry hair with a round brush

# Restyle 4

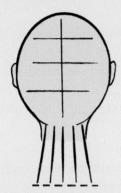

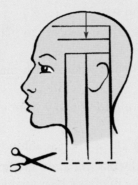

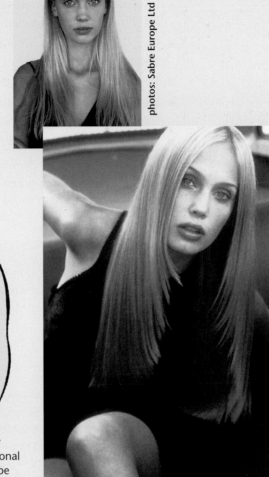

**1** Cut the back section horizontally. Be sure not to round the corners

**2** With the head in the upright position, bring side section down to the same length as back

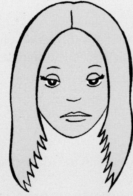

**3** Without overdirecting the sides forward, bring down diagonal sections. Cut a step angle to just forward of the ear (can be slide cut)

**4** Exciting use of colour gives a three-dimensional look to a simple bob shape

photos: Sabre Europe Ltd

## Health and safety when cutting hair

- Adequately protect client and self.
- Check wires and plug on electrical clippers to make sure they are safe to use. Switch off at the sockets after use.
- Prepare tools and products in accordance with manufacturer's instruction and only use them as intended.
- Keep blades and tips of cutting tools away from eyes. Take care when cutting hair onto the skin.
- Remove all cut hair from the client and the salon floor and place in a bin.
- Dispose of any sharps safely by placing them in a special rigid container. Putting sharp objects with other waste in plastic bags could cause serious injury.
- Dispose of any waste materials safely in the correct place.
- Clean and sterilise tools after use. Make sure they are stored in the correct place.
- Clean the work area when finished to keep the salon looking smart and professional and to help avoid cross-infection.

## Things to do

1. Read the relevant section in Unit 2.4 for details on how to sterilise haircutting tools, then write a brief description of how to sterilise:
   (a) scissors
   (b) clippers
   (c) razors
   (d) neck brushes
   (e) combs

2. To make sure that you fully understand the requirements of current legislation and the policy of your organisation:
   (a) Collect information regarding health and safety at work.
   (b) Find out local by-laws regarding the disposal of sharps and industrial waste.
   (c) Write a brief summary of **your** responsibilities.
   (d) Write a brief description of the **employer's** responsibilities.
   (e) Place in your file for future reference.

3. Design a poster for the staffroom on the safe disposal of waste and sharps.

## What do you know?

- Name the **five** basic cutting shapes.
- Give a brief description and use of:
  - (a) bevel cutting
  - (b) slide cutting
  - (c) taper cutting
  - (d) texturising
- List **four** basic cutting techniques.
- Explain, in detail, **three** specialised texturising techniques.
- Name the perimeter lines and shapes.
- Explain the difference between a symmetrical shape and an asymmetrical shape.
- Explain the difference between a concave napeline and a convex napeline.
- What are the main points to keep in mind when giving the client advice and guidance?

- Give a definition of a baseline.
- What would you include in a client consultation before carrying out a restyle?
- List the **seven** steps needed when restyling any type of hair.
- Explain how other salon services can enhance the finished hair style.
- Give a brief summary of what is meant by the following looks:
  - (a) classic
  - (b) current fashion
  - (c) avant garde
- Name the salon services that could be used to enhance the total look.
- What health, hygiene and safety procedures would be necessary when cutting hair?

In this unit you will learn about:

- The effects of perming and neutralising on the hair.
- Preparing the hair and client for perming.
- Factors that influence decisions on choice of products and techniques.
- Creative perming techniques.
- When perming should be avoided.
- How to identify and correct perming problems.
- The importance of working safely, hygienically and efficiently.

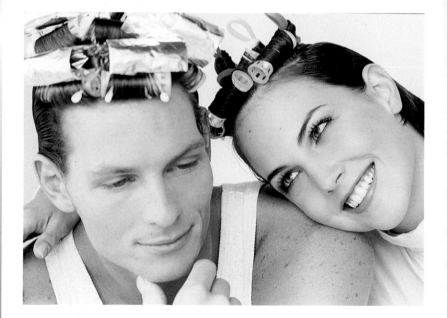

# Creative perming

## Creative perming

To be creative you first need to have a good understanding of the basic perming principles. Read through Unit 2.5a to make sure that you fully understand the basic techinques and what happens to the structure of the hair when it is permed and neutralised.

**POINTS TO REMEMBER**

Traditional, alkaline perms contain ammonium thioglycollate, an alkali with pH of 9 to 9.5. Acid perms contain glycerol thioglycollate, an acid with a pH of about 4, but they are mixed before applying to make the solution alkaline. In both cases the following chemical reactions take place in the hair:

- **Softening** – the cortex has polypeptide chains which are held in place by cross-linkages. The alkalinity of the perm swells the hair and opens the cuticle scales. Water in the perm lotion, and when shampooing, breaks the weaker, water-breakable cross-linkages. The perm lotion then begins to break (60–70 per cent) the stronger, sulphur cross-linkages, known as sulpur bonds, by forcing the sulpur atoms to link to the perm lotion's hydrogen atoms instead of each other.

- **Moulding** – tension is applied to the hair when it is wound around the rods; this causes the polypeptide chains to slip past one another slightly, altering the shape. When enough bonds are broken, the perm lotion is rinsed from the hair.

- **Fixing** – the neutraliser, containing either hydrogen peroxide or sodium perborate, releases oxygen which combines with the hydrogen from the sulphur bonds to form water ($H_2O$). The sulphur bonds can then reform in their new position and the hair is fixed in its new, curled shape.

The adding of hydrogen atoms in the softening stage is called reduction and the perm lotion is known as a reducing agent. The removal of hydrogen atoms in the fixing stage is known as oxidation and the neutraliser is known as an oxidising agent.

Creative perming should enhance the final image of a haircut or style. The curl should be created only where it is needed and this can be anywhere along the hair length as well as throughout the head. By treating each head as unique and really thinking about what you want to achieve, it is possible to combine several techniques on one head and even evolve techniques of your own. Consider the following points:

- Decide on how you want the final image to look before you start.
- Only put curl where it is needed.
- Wind with water then post-damp so that you can begin the wind anywhere on the head (unless the manufacturer states otherwise).
- Decide whether it will be easier to cut the hair before or after perming.
- Section the hair where needed; this keeps it under control and helps you to work more efficiently.
- Use the wealth of available products to make sure the hair is kept in optimum condition.

## Preparation for perming

1. Carry out a thorough consultation and hair/scalp analysis.
2. Give advice and guidance to the client on the products available and their possible effects. Use visual aids such as style books, magazines and photographs.
3. Carry out any necessary tests on the hair. These may include:
   - elasticity
   - porosity
   - incompatibility
   - pre-perm test curl

4. Protect yourself and the client with suitable protective equipment.
5. Shampoo hair with suitable shampoo, usually soapless.
6. Apply any necessary pre-perm treatments.
7. Towel-dry the hair and cut into style if necessary.
6. Assemble tools and equipment.

## Pre-perm treatments

Pre-perm treatments are used before perming to even out the porosity and maintain the moisture content of the hair. They are applied after shampooing and are left in the hair. If in doubt, always use a pre-perm treatment as it will make sure the perming process causes minimum damage to the hair. Pre-perm treatments are available as:

- Gels.
- Sprays.
- Liquids.

## Pre-perm test curl

If in doubt about the hair's overall porosity or elasticity, always take a preliminary test curl:

1. Isolate and section two small sections from damaged areas.
2. Wind sections then protect around them with cotton wool.
3. Apply perm lotion and develop, testing frequently.
4. Rinse and neutralise as per manufacturer's instructions.
5. Check elasticity while neutraliser is still on hair.
6. If hair feels strong enough, rinse and perm remaining hair.
7. If hair feels slimy or breaks under pressure, relax the movement in the hair with gentle combing then rinse neutraliser from hair.
8. Restructure and give a course of deep-penetrating conditioning treatments.

## Factors to consider

- **Amount of curl needed** – this may only be on partial areas instead of the whole head or hair length and will influence the perming technique you select.
- **Hair condition** – apply pre-perm treatment or postpone the service if the hair is too damaged or fragile.
- **Hair texture** – coarse hair will need a stronger product than finer hair.
- **Hair growth patterns** – try to work with the hair growth patterns by directionally winding the hair.
- **Shape of cut and hair length** – put the curl only where needed to give volume to the style. Longer hair usually needs a slightly tighter curl than required to allow for loosening of the curl because of the hair's weight.
- **Temperature** – heat speeds up the perming process. A cold salon will decrease the development time.

**POINTS TO REMEMBER**

Follow the manufacturer's instructions on how frequently to take a development test curl. Look for a firm S-bend with **alkaline** perms and stranding and separation with **acid** perms. Rinse the hair thoroughly in warm water and time the neutraliser accurately to allow enough sulphur bonds to reform and prevent hair damage. Apply a pH balance conditioner to the hair after final rinsing to return hair to its natural, acidic pH state, replace lost moisture and prevent further oxidation.

**SAFETY TIPS**

Permanent wave reagents are potentially hazardous chemicals and due care and attention must be paid at all times to health, hygiene and safety procedures to satisfy current legislation, manufacturers' guidelines, and salon guidelines.

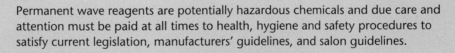

## Health and safety

- Protect yourself and the client throughout the process.
- Assemble tools and equipment in a safe, accessible position.
- Be aware of potential hazards and follow manufacturers' instructions.
- Take care when applying products to the hair. Protect the eyes and skin.
- Make sure that perm rods and bands are positioned correctly to prevent hair breakage.
- Use clean, sterile tools and equipment.
- Clean up any spillage immediately and keep work area clean and tidy.
- Dispose of waste products and materials safety in accordance with salon policy and local by-laws.
- To keep hair in good condition, advise client on after-care and suitable products for use on permed hair.

## Root perming and partial winding

### Root perming

This technique is used to give support and lift to shorter hairstyles. It is not usually suitable for longer hair as the weight of the hair pulls out any lift.

Lift at the roots can be achieved by various methods, for example, winding the hair with water and coating the mid-lengths and ends of the hair with hair gel or oil, then wrapping this part of the hair in tinfoil to prevent penetration of the perm into these areas. The hair should then be post-damped with the perm lotion, allowing the root area only to be affected.

Manufacturers have produced a gel perming lotion which is applied after winding is complete. Because of its viscous nature, this type of perm lotion does not penetrate through the hair mesh and is therefore active on the root area only.

However, it must be remembered that the intended effect of a root perm is to give support and *not* curl to the hair. It is therefore not advisable for clients who need a substantial amount of curl or body in their hair.

### Partial winding

As the name suggests, only some areas of the head are permed to create volume and texture where required. There are unlimited variations to this type of wind and it is a method that can be used on long or short hair.

Figure 3.3.1 shows two partial winds: the first creates volume at the front of the head; in the second example the top and fringe areas are left straight while the back and side areas are permed. In both cases the rods may be placed in any direction and wound by whatever method necessary to produce the desired style.

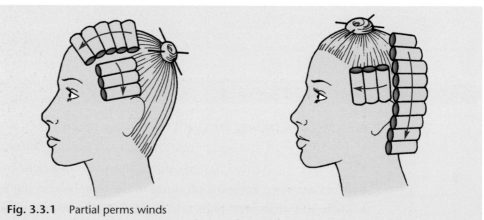

**Fig. 3.3.1**   Partial perms winds

### TECHNICAL TIPS

It is often better to apply the reagent after winding to prevent overprocessing and to give a more even curl.

## A selection of techniques

There are many techniques to choose from and these have evolved to meet the changing needs of fashion and the client. The following selection can be used on their own or in combination, depending on the required result.

### Candlestick wind

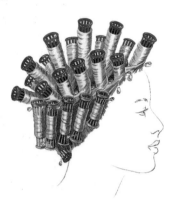

**Use**
Produces a soft, natural spiral curl with good root movement.

**Method**

- Take a triangular section the same diameter as the rod.
- Wind hair spirally down the rod.
- At the roots, turn the rod vertically so that it stands on it own base.
- Secure with plastic pins through the base.
- May be pre- or post-damped.

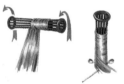

L'Oréal

**TECHNICAL TIPS**

The candlestick technique is most commonly used on the crown area only.

### Weave wind

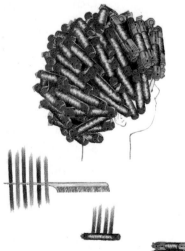

**Use**
Creates a natural, undisciplined textured look on shorter or mid-length hair. Can be used to blend in unpermed, straight nape hair when partial winding.

**Method**

- Section hair as usual.
- Take section of hair same size as the rod and weave out fine strands of hair (Fig. 3.3.2).
- Clip strands out of the way and wind remaining hair.
- Continue winding in this way throughout the head.
- Wind woven hair onto a larger rod, so rods sit on top of one another.
- For less curl, leave the woven strands out altogether.

L'Oréal

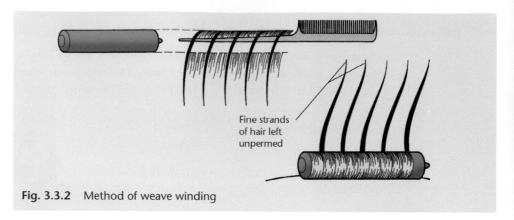

**Fig. 3.3.2**    Method of weave winding

Fine strands
of hair left
unpermed

## Wind and leave

### Use
Gives soft volume and curl. Good for coarse hair with a natural wave.

### Method

- Wind hair without lotion in the direction required.
- Protect alternative rods with either foil, cling film or plastic packets.
- Apply perm lotion to unprotected rods.
- Develop and neutralise as normal.

## Double-decker wind

### Use
Produces lift at the roots with more curl on the ends of the hair. Usually used on the crown area only and in combination with other techniques.

### Method

- Wind with lotion in style direction.
- Wind hair down to where a softer curl is needed.
- Put second rod under the first rod and wind hair with both rods together, down to the roots.

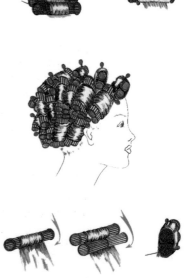

L'Oréal

L'Oréal

## Piggyback wind (Fig. 3.3.3)

### Use
On long hair to give an even curl along the hair length.

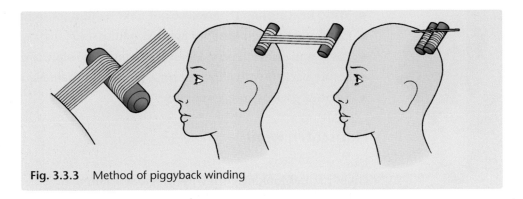

**Fig. 3.3.3**    Method of piggyback winding

### Method

- Taking normal sections, wind hair from mid-lengths down to the root, leaving the ends of the hair out.
- Wind the ends on another rod, down until it sits on the first rod.
- Secure the rods together with a plastic pin.
- Varying the rod sizes creates endless possibilities.

## Root and extension wind

### Use

On long, fine hair to give an even, soft curl throughout the hair length. Similar to the piggyback wind but hair is spirally wound instead of like a croquignole.

### Method

- Section hair at nape.
- Taking small sections, place rod against scalp and wind hair around it leaving out the ends. Fasten the band.
- Wind remainder of hair on a second rod of the same size, down to the first rod and secure.

## Perm and colour wind

### Use

On shorter hair to enhance the colour or for clients who do not have the time to have both services done separately.

L'Oréal

### Method

- Wind hair in brick pattern, without water, starting at the front of the head.
- Wind one or two rods then take a section and weave out hair for highlights. Use foil or plastic packets and apply tint to woven hair.

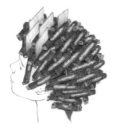

- Wind next section then weave out next section for lights.
- Continue through head for approximately six to eight packets.
- Post-damp hair with perm lotion 10–15 minutes before colour is developed.
- Secure packets with clips and rinse perm from hair. Neutralise.
- Remove packets and gentle rinse.

## Hopscotch wind

**Use**
Gives natural-looking curls with irregular volume.

L'Oréal

# Hopscotch wind

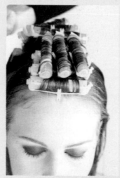

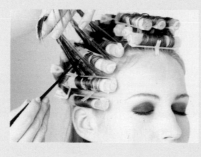

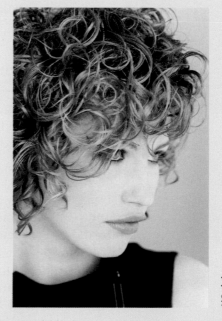

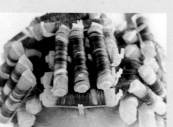

L'Oréal

Four of five sections on the crown are weave wound, then the protruding hair is wound vertically to sit on top of the previously wound hair. This produces a hopscotch pattern on the top of the head. Hair is wound in these 'squares' throughout the head giving an unstructured, tousled effect.

## TECHNICAL TIPS

The hopscotch wind can be used on the whole head or on areas which require irregular curl formation.

## Method

- Take a normal hair section.
- Thickly weave out hair and pin out of the way. Wind remaining hair on a rod.
- Wind four or five sections in this way.
- Take vertical sections and wind weaved hair so that the rods sit vertically on the previously woven section.
- Continue winding in these squares until the whole head is wound.

## Spiral wind

### Use

On medium to long hair which requires an even curl along the hair length. Use a rod one size smaller than required to allow for the weight of the hair loosening the curl.

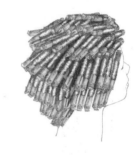

### Method

- Wind hair with lotion to ensure an even coverage and penetration.
- Start at the nape, take square sections (Fig. 3.3.4). Hold hair out from the head at right angles.
- Use an endpaper then start winding the hair at the end of the rod farthest away from the fastener.

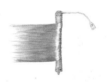

- Secure ends by winding two or three turns then wind the rest of the hair spirally down the rod.
- Continue winding round the head, up towards the front, until wind is complete.

L'Oréal

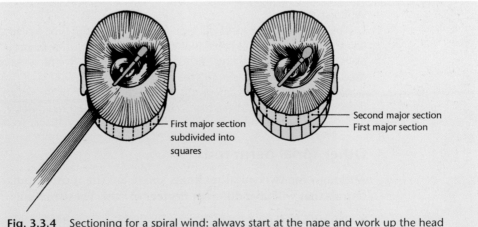

First major section subdivided into squares

Second major section
First major section

**Fig. 3.3.4**   Sectioning for a spiral wind: always start at the nape and work up the head

## Alternative spiral wind

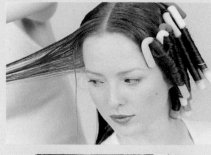

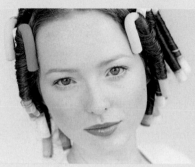

L'Oréal

Hair is wound in a similar manner to the method given in the main text, but rubber or foam rods are used instead of conventional perming rods. This gives a looser, slightly more open spiral curl. Hair can be twisted during winding to give added volume.

**POINTS TO REMEMBER**

Checking a spiral wind for development can be quite difficult as it does not always form the same type of S-shape as a conventional wind. Using a self-timing perm or placing a few **croquignole** wound rods, to use as test curls, in a position that is not obvious are ways that can resolve this problem.

Make sure that any heat used to cut down the development time is evenly applied, as the head when fully spirally wound is quite a size and difficult to place under a conventional dryer.

Rinsing this type of wind will usually require a longer time because of the amount of hair and the number of rods. Blot the rods carefully after rinsing; it is also useful to place the client under a dryer or use a hand dryer for five minutes to help remove the excess moisture before applying the neutraliser.

Again, because of the amount of hair, the application of the neutraliser must be thorough to make sure that all the hair is completely covered throughout the length of the rod.

### Other sprial perm rods

Although the two spiral methods above are the most popular, there are a variety of rods that will give different degrees of curl. These include:

- Chopsticks (Fig. 3.3.5).
- Spiral rods (Fig. 3.3.6).

**TECHNICAL TIPS**

Ensure that an endpaper is always used, and that the centre of the curl is open – this will avoid the hair becoming frizzy.

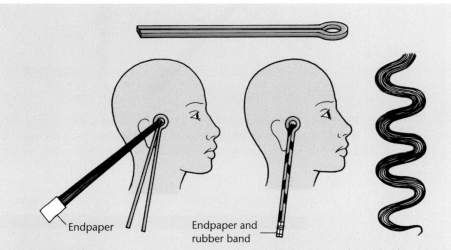

Endpaper

Endpaper and rubber band

**Fig. 3.3.5**   Spiral wind using chopsticks: hair is wound from the root, side to side down the sticks then secured with a rubber band over the end paper; finished curl is uniform and angular with lots of volume

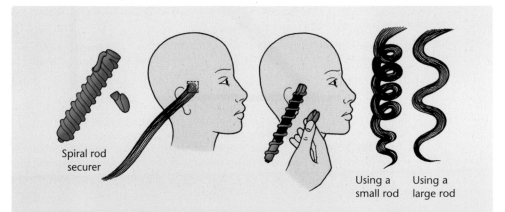

Spiral rod securer

Using a small rod

Using a large rod

**Fig. 3.3.6**   Ridged spiral rod used to wind hair down between the ridges and hold with an end securer; produces an even curl along the hair length; the larger the rod, the looser the curl

- U-stick (Fig. 3.3.7).
- Tube rods (Fig. 3.3.8).

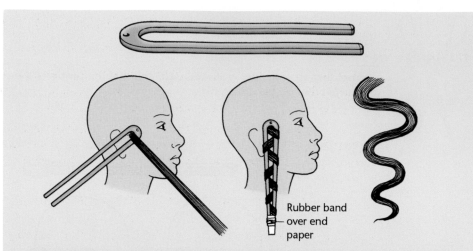

**Fig. 3.3.7**  Spiral wind using U-stick rod: hair is wound backwards and forwards between the U and secured with a rubber band over the endpapers; the two ends of the rod come together as the hair is wound producing a looser curl at the roots than at the ends

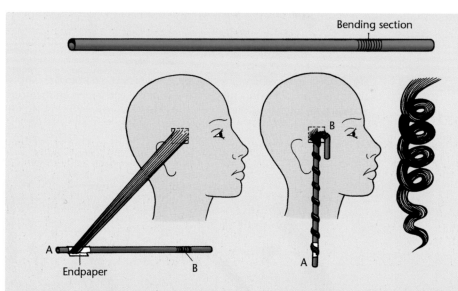

**Fig. 3.3.8**  Tube rods are shaped like straws with a corrugated section which allows them to bend: the hair is wound down the tube to the corrugated section and the tube bent over to secure; these rods produce a lot of volume with an even, tight curl along the hair length

**POINTS TO REMEMBER**    Always keep precise records of each treatment. Fashion perming offers an indivdualised service to suit the individual needs of the client, and it will therefore be extremely difficult to remember exactly the techniques and procedures used if the client requires a repeat treatment in the future.

## Considerations when chemically processing long hair

1. Remember that the ends of the hair have been there for a long time and have been subjected to physical and atmospheric influences. Therefore, the ends of the hair will be porous and will process more quickly.

2. The client must be told of the long-term implications of using potentially damaging chemicals such as perm lotion. It is very upsetting for a client who has grown their hair over a number of years to have to have it cut off because a chemical process has damaged it.

3. Always protect the hair with restructurants, pre-chemical and post-chemical treatments.

4. Use only good quality products which will do the least damage to the hair. Do not use excessively harsh lotions.

5. Do not overprocess the hair. However, when perming long hair also make sure that it is not underprocessed as it is not usually advisable to reperm on this length of hair.

6. Always advise the client on how to look after their hair by protecting it from the sun, regular conditioning, using a suitable shampoo, using oils and waxes and on the effects of overusing heated appliances such as curling tongs, hot brushes, heated rollers, etc.

## Partial combination wind

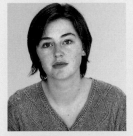 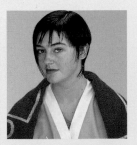 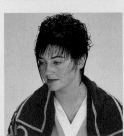 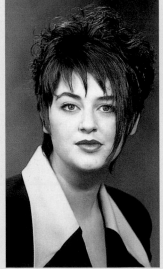

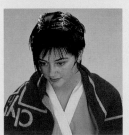 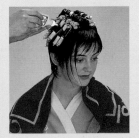 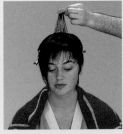

Clynol

Model's hair is restyled and combed in direction of final style. Front hair is wound first, as normal, leaving out the fringe area. Hair is woven out and permed in a hopscotch design on the top and crown area. The side hair is then wound directionally, without weaving, away from the face. Apply the perm lotion to the wound areas only. The perm has given lift and texture where it is needed for this 1970s-inspired style.

## Summary of perming faults

| Result | Cause | Remedy |
|---|---|---|
| Curl too tight | Overprocessed<br>Rod size too small | Relax if in reasonable condition |
| Curl too loose | Underprocessed<br>Lotion too weak<br>Incorrect neutralising | Reperm if condition allows<br>May need to condition or<br>restructure hair first |
| Poor condition | Overprocessed<br>Lotion too strong | Deep conditioning treatment,<br>restructurants<br>Cut off ends if necessary |
| Frizz | Overprocessed<br>Lotion too strong<br>Too much tension when<br>winding | Deep conditioning treatment,<br>restructurants<br>Cut off ends if possible |
| Uneven curl result | Uneven tension when winding<br>Incorrect sections<br>Uneven application of perm<br>or neutraliser | Use restructurant and deep<br>conditioning treatment<br>Reperm straight areas if possible |
| Band marks | Rubber bands placed on rod<br>incorrectly | Use restructurant and deep<br>conditioning treatment |

## Things to do

| Fault | Possible cause | Correction |
|---|---|---|
| Perm slow to process | | |
| Hairline and scalp irritation | | |
| Pull-burn | | |
| Straight finished result (no curl) | | |
| Hair not curly enough | | |
| Frizz (hair looks curly when wet and straight when dry) | | |
| Hair too curly | | |

1. Mistakes sometimes happen with even the most experienced stylist but this does not make the result less upsetting for the client. It is therefore extremely important that any mistakes are identified as soon as possible and remedial action taken immediately. The above table has been devised to enable you to identify some

common faults which occur if due care and attention have not been paid during the perming process. Fill in the blank spaces on the table. If you are unsure, you can check your knowledge by reading the relevant section in this unit and Unit 2.5a. You may also wish to keep the completed table to use as evidence of your knowledge for your portfolio.

2. To broaden and improve your product knowledge:

   (a) Collect information on products available for pre-perm and post-perm treatments from at least **four** different manufacturers.

   (b) Compare the uses and prices of the treatments and write a short report on each.

3. Read through Unit 2.5a then draw a diagram of the structural changes that take place in the hair during perming and neutralising. Write a summary of these changes.

4. Your responsibilities under the COSHH Regulations are to handle, use, store and dispose of products in accordance with manufacturer's instructions, salon policy and local by-laws.

   (a) Write out a fact sheet, or create a poster for the staffroom, that gives clear guidance to trainees on your salon's procedures and how they meet the requirements of manufacturers and local by-laws

   (b) If you have written a fact sheet, word process or type it out neatly then give each trainee a copy.

   (c) Present your fact sheet or poster to the trainees as a training session on health and safety.

## What do you know?

- Give the main ingredient of:
  (a) an alkaline perm
  (b) an acid perm
- Give a brief description of the softening, moulding and fixing stages of perming.
- List **four** tests that could be carried out before perming. Give their use and the adverse reaction to each of them.
- What are pre-perm treatments and why are they used?
- Explain briefly how you would carry out a pre-perm test curl.
- List **six** factors to consider before perming.
- When taking a development test curl, what would you look for, in the movement, when testing:

  (a) an acid perm?
  (b) an alkaline perm?
- Why is it sometimes better to cut the hair after perming instead of before?
- Give **nine** health and safety considerations when perming hair.
- Give **two** methods or products used to block out the ends when root perming.
- Where on the head is a candlestick wind most commonly used and what effect does it give?
- Briefly explain how you would carry out a weave wind perm.
- What is the effect of a weave-and-leave perm?
- Give the method of winding a root extension wind.

- What is the effect of a hopscotch wind and where on the head is it usually carried out?
- When would a perm and colour wind be carried out?
- Where on the head is a winding commenced for a spiral wind?

- How is the hair tested for development on spirally wound hair?
- Why is it important to keep precise, up-to-date records of all client treatments?
- List the legislation which needs to be considered when perming hair.

In this unit you will learn about:

- The principles of hair colour and colour selection.
- Preparing the hair and client for colouring.
- A variety of creative colouring techniques.
- Diagnosing and correcting colour problems.
- Bleaching hair.
- When and how to prepigment hair.
- Presoftening hair.
- Working safely, hygienically and efficiently when colouring hair.

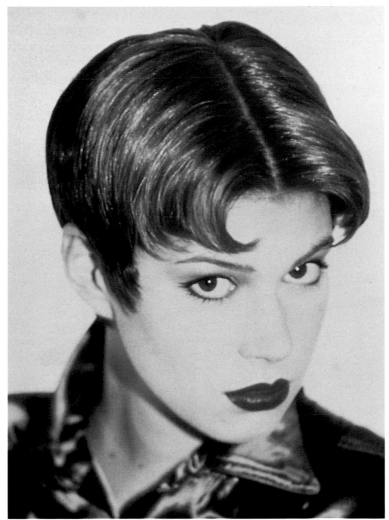

Sabre Europe

# Creative colouring

## Creative colouring

Creative colouring techniques are used to improve the look of a hairstyle by giving definition to the shape. They can give the illusion of increased weight or they can lighten 'heaviness', depending on how and where the colour is applied. Most important of all, fashion colouring techniques can be fun. The more outrageous or different the equipment and methods used, the more interest is stimulated. Clients often do not know the many effects of using colour, so it is up to you to give advice and offer new suggestions. Most clients want to improve their image and once they know of the subtle effects that can be achieved, they will be prompted to do something positive.

Creative colouring is a natural progression from basic colouring techniques. The techniques in this unit can be used on their own or in combination. You therefore need to know the principles of hair colour before you can begin to use colour to its best effect; read Unit 2.6.

**POINTS TO REMEMBER**

### Principles of hair colouring

The hair's natural colour pigment is found in the **cortex** and is produced by cells called **melanocytes**, found at the base of the hair follicle. If the hair is dark it will contain mostly **melanin** (black or brown pigments). If the hair is red or blonde, it will contain mostly **pheomelanin** (red and yellow pigments). If something goes wrong with this process, through illness or ageing, and no melanin is made then the hair will be without colour and become white. White hair is known as **canites**.

The **depth** of colour is how light or dark the colour of the hair is. The overall colour – how ash, golden or red – is determined by the combination of pigments in the hair and is known as the **tone**. Manufacturers use depth and tone to describe their colours through the International Colour Code (ICC). The ICC grades the depth of colour from 1 as the darkest colour (black) to 10 as the lightest (blonde).

## Colour selection

### First considerations

- **Hair porosity** – very porous hair will 'grab' or absorb the colour. If the hair is very porous you may have to dilute the tint, condition, or 'infill' with a restructurant to even out the porosity to help avoid an uneven result.

- **Hair texture** – fine hair will need less product and will give a more intense result; thick, coarse hair will need more product and may need presoftening or a longer development time.

- **Scalp condition** – check for cuts, abrasions or diseases. Some colours may irritate the scalp.

- **Hair condition/elasticity** – hair in poor condition or with poor elasticity could break if you use a peroxide or other product with too high a strength.

- **Fraction of white hair** – fashion shades may be too intense if there is more than 25 per cent white in the hair. Add some of the base shade if this is the case.

- **Previous treatments** – check that they will not react with the colour by carrying out an incompatibility test. Previously permed, bleached or tinted hair may be porous and absorb the colour, making it deeper than the selected shade.

- **Skin tone** – warm skin tones need warm colours. Paler, colder skin tones will need cold colours.
- **Client image** – find out if a complete revamp or a more subtle image change is needed.
- **Depth and tone of colour** – if you are lightening the hair, you will need to use a higher strength of hydrogen peroxide, bleach or tint lightener. You will also have to decide on the colour tone, whether it is to be warm or cold. (See Unit 2.6 for details of hydrogen peroxide, client preparation and mixing of colour.)

### Other critical factors

- Base colour of client's hair.
- Hair length and shape of haircut.
- Test results.
- Temperature of the salon.
- Any heat used to process the colour.

## Client preparation

Hair colour can stain clothing and skin. Make sure that you protect yourself with a tinting apron and rubber gloves. The client will also need protecting but in addition, you will also need to:

- Carry out a thorough client consultation to determine the client's needs. Use visual aids such as a shade chart, photographs and hair swatches.
- Protect the client's clothes with a tinting gown, towels and neck strip.
- Protect the client's skin with barrier cream around the hairline.
- Carry out any appropriate tests:
  - skin test
  - porosity test
  - elasticity test
  - incompatibility test
  - strand test
- Prepare the hair according to manufacturer's instructions for the products to be used.

## Creative colouring techniques

### Block colouring

Block colouring emphasises the shape of short hairstyles. Two, three or even four colours can be used, but there should be *at least* two shades difference between the colours (Fig. 3.4.1). Subtle effects are created by using similar colour tones to the client's own hair. Dramatic effects can be created by using contrasting colours, e.g. dark brown at the nape graduating to bright red-orange at the front.

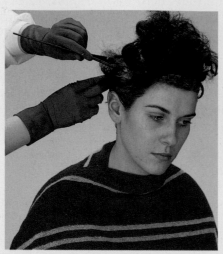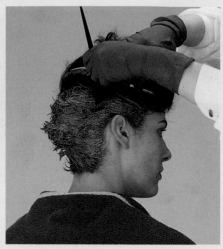

Clynol

**Fig. 3.4.1** Application for block colouring hair using two colours; a lighter colour will be used on the top and front

- Apply the darkest shade at the nape, graduating to the lighter shade at the front.
- Zigzag the partings or divisions to prevent a hard line between the shades.
- Use cotton wool/foil strips to block out each section as it is completed to stop the colours from touching each other.
- For a more subtle effect, carefully comb the tint together up from the nape to the crown when application is complete.

**POINTS TO REMEMBER**

1. When tinting lighter, allow for the effect of body heat at the scalp; the mid-lengths and ends must be tinted before the roots. When tinting darker, the tint can be applied from the roots through to the ends. It may be necessary to use both techniques on one head when block tinting.

2. The hair is naturally lighter at the front and crown area because of the effect of sunlight, etc.; by using lighter shades in these areas a more natural effect is achieved. To give a very dramatic effect, reverse the colours, i.e. darker shades at the front and lighter shades at the nape.

3. Darker shades make the hair appear more dense and therefore heavier. Lighter shades give the illusion of less weight. This is a useful fact to bear in mind when emphasising a hairstyle with colour.

**TECHNICAL TIPS**

When using two colours, mix them in a bowl before adding hydrogen peroxide or applying to the hair.

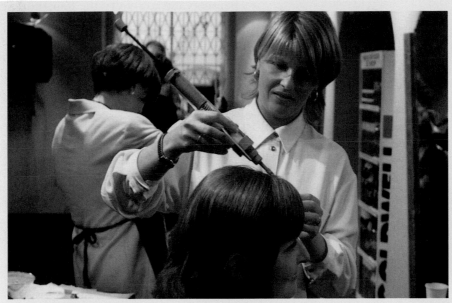

**Fig. 3.4.2** Applying painted lights using a colour gun

## Painted lights (flying colours)

Painted lights add colour and depth to a hairstyle.

- Comb the hair into shape and decide where the style needs accentuating. This may be at the nape, sides or crown.
- Paint a semi-permanent colour or permanent tint on to the hair using a vent brush, a wide-toothed comb, a fine artist's paintbrush or a colour gun.
- Apply the tint in the direction of the style (bleach can also be applied in this manner) but try not to work in straight lines as this can give a heavy effect (Fig. 3.4.2).

**POINTS TO REMEMBER**

1. A number of shades can be used throughout the head. Lighter shades at the front and darker shades at the sides and nape will give a shimmering effect.
2. This is a good method to add interest to dark hair. Paint the hair with strong red or burgundy shades of tint.
3. A tinting gun creates interest in the salon but it needs plenty of practice, so handle it with caution.
4. Painted lights are a very quick method of adding colour and are a good way of using up odd quarter tubes of tint, but remember not to get too enthusiastic. Applying too much tint (particularly tint lightener) over too great an area can give a patchy result.

## Shimmer lights

Shimmer lights have the same effect as painted lights (Fig. 3.4.3). This method can be used all over the head or just on certain areas, depending upon the effect desired.

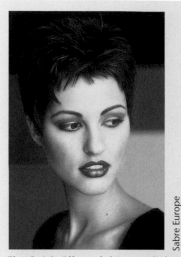

**Fig. 3.4.3** Effect of shimmer lights

Sabre Europe

- Shampoo and towel-dry the hair thoroughly then comb into the desired style with gel, using a wide-toothed comb. This will create 'tramlines' in the direction of the hairstyle.
- Choose a tint at least two shades lighter and of a brighter tone than the natural colour, then apply it carefully along the raised lines with a fine artist's brush or a tinting gun.

## Colour flashes

Colour flashes can be used on their own or with other effects. They work on hair that is long or short, curly or straight.

- Use a tint lightener to lighten a fine or thick band around the front hairline.
- For a brighter colour, the band is bleached then a permanent tint is applied to the bleached area.
- Alternatively, after banding, a semi-permanent colour can be applied over the whole head to brighten all of the hair and create a lighter tone of the same colour at the front.

**POINTS TO REMEMBER**

1. Use a zigzag parting to soften the banding line.
2. Colour flashes can be used with fine highlights of the same colour through the back of the head to give added interest or to emphasise and soften the front hairline.
3. Another use of colour flashing is to lighten the weight of a heavy forward fringe. Take out a section at the front hairline of the fringe (zigzag parting) about 10–20 mm ($\frac{3}{8}$ to $\frac{3}{4}$ in) wide, and use a tint lightener in this area. When all of the fringe is combed forward, the darker back section of the fringe will blend with the front section, creating a wispier, lighter effect.

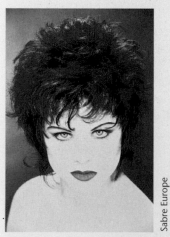

**Fig. 3.4.4** Scrunching can produce lighter roots with darker ends

Sabre Europe

## Scrunching

Scrunching gives a good effect on either long or short curly hairstyles but is not suitable for long straight styles. This quick and easy technique adds colour and depth to the ends of the hair, emphasising the outline of the hairstyle (Fig. 3.4.4).

- Shampoo the hair then rough-dry it into shape.
- Mix the desired shade of tint (usually tint lightener).
- Wear rubber gloves to spread the tint evenly onto the palms of the rubber gloves.
- Squeeze or scrunch the ends of the hair between the fingers; this places the tint on the ends of the hair only. Apply throughout the head, or wherever needed.

**POINTS TO REMEMBER**

1. If the hair is longer and tends to flop, backcomb it thoroughly at the roots then carefully lacquer the roots with a fine hairspray. This will prevent the tint from running or flopping onto the root area.

2. More than one shade of tint can be used, depending upon the result required.

3. Bleach may be used instead of tint, but care must be taken only to lighten a few shades. When bleach is developed and removed, a semi-permanent tint can be applied over the whole head to give lighter and darker tones of the same colour.

4. This technique is excellent for the client who enjoys changing their hair colour frequently or for brightening dull hair during the winter months. Because only the ends of the hair are tinted or bleached lighter, they are soon removed by cutting.

## Tortoiseshell lights

Tortoiseshell lights give a richer and more unusual effect than the usual lowlights or highlights (Fig. 3.4.5). They are suitable for any length of hair. Three to four different colours are used, ranging from one shade darker to two to three shades lighter than the natural base shade. Two different colours are applied separately to fine woven streaks of hair, usually in alternation; see Unit 2.6 for methods of highlighting using foil or packets.

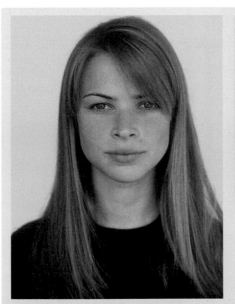
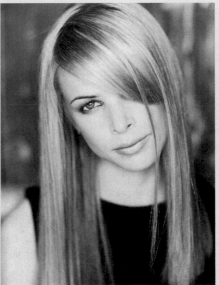

Sabre Europe

**Fig. 3.4.5** Before and after effects of tortoiseshell lights

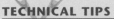

**TECHNICAL TIPS**

Always ensure there is no seepage of the tint from the easi-meche, foil or cling film, otherwise the results could be disastrous.

## Glimmering (polishing)

Glimmering is a very quick technique for any length of hair, but particularly good on very short nape hair where it is difficult to use other techniques.

- Comb the hair into style.
- Take a piece of tinfoil or cellophane and paint the surface with the chosen shade of tint.
- Hold the tinfoil or cellophane in both hands and allow it to touch the ends of the hair, then gently stroke backwards and forwards in a polishing motion in the direction of the style.
- Pull away and repeat over the whole head or just the areas that will emphasise the style.

**POINTS TO REMEMBER**

1. Do not be afraid to use bold colours as this technique gives a subtle effect.
2. Do not become too enthusiastic and cover all of the hair; it is just the ends that are tinted.
3. Polish the hair gently otherwise the tint may be inadvertently placed where it is not wanted.

## Slicing or tramming

Slicing or tramming produces a very dramatic effect (Fig. 3.4.6).

- Comb the hair into style and decide which area of the head needs emphasising (slicing usually looks more effective on the front section of the head).

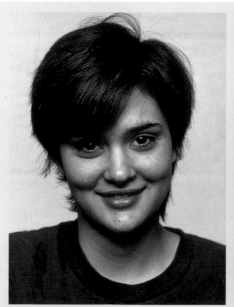
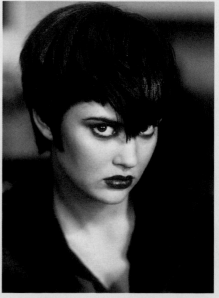

Sabre Europe

**Fig. 3.4.6** Before and after effect of colour slicing the hair using a vibrant red colour

- Section the remaining hair away from this area.
- Take a section of hair about the size of a perm rod from the area to be coloured and apply the tint to this section.
- Wrap in tinfoil, easi-meche or cling film then leave out a fine 6 mm ($\frac{1}{4}$ in) section and take the next section in the same manner as before.
- Continue across the area to be covered, tinting a section and leaving a section until completed.

**POINTS TO REMEMBER**

1. More than one colour may be used depending upon the desired result.
2. Because the hair is not woven, the colour is far more dense in certain areas and therefore more dramatic. Do not use this technique on clients who wish to have subtle coloration only.
3. The sections that do not need tinting can be kept out of the way by winding on a perm rod.
4. A vibrant effect can be achieved by bleaching the slices then colouring with a semi-permanent colour.

# Creating a new image

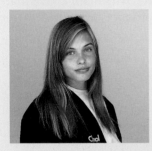
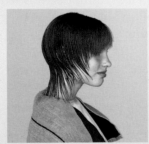
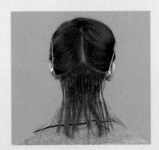

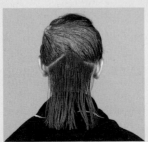
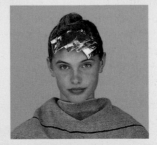
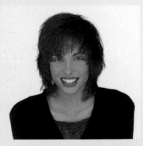

Clynol

Long hair is reshaped into a new, textured style. A V-shaped section from occipital bone to back of ears has a dark, rich brown tint applied from roots to points. Hair is parted from crown to temples and a copper tint applied to this section. Leaving out the fringe area, the crown to forehead hair has a chestnut brown colour applied to blend together all the different colour tones and create a natural effect. Finally, foil slices are used with high lift tint on the fringe area around the face to give a soft, flattering effect.

## Using a combination of techniques and equipment

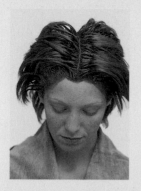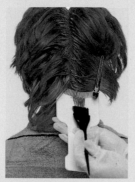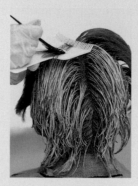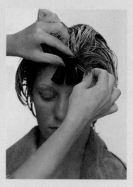

Clynol Ltd

Retouch tint is applied over whole head. Starting at the nape, a spatula is then used to apply tint to fine sections of individual slices of hair using two colours in alternation. When the front area is reached, several fine sections are left out of the fringe. Single lights are then created by pulling the hair through colour pots and applying a vibrant colour to each strand. This breaks up the fringe area to prevent a 'solid' effect.

## Bleaching

Bleaching lightens the hair by decolouring the natural colour pigments. The lightened colour is permanent and cannot be washed out. The main active ingredient is usually **hydrogen peroxide** with 'bleaching products' designed merely to make the peroxide work more efficiently.

### How bleaching works

**POINTS TO REMEMBER**

The two major colour pigments in the hair are **melanin** (dark brown to black) and **pheomelanin** (red to yellow). They can be lightened in shade by adding oxygen; melanin will lighten quite easily but pheomelanin is more resistant. The substance providing the oxygen is known as an **oxidising agent** and whatever accepts the oxygen is described as having been **oxidised**.

In hairdressing the most commonly used oxidising agent is hydrogen peroxide. It is colourless and odourless and looks like its close relative, water ($H_2O$). The difference is that hydrogen peroxide has an extra atom of oxygen ($H_2O_2$) which makes it unstable and it will easily release the extra oxygen atom to become water and oxygen gas:

$$\text{hydrogen peroxide} \rightarrow \text{water} + \text{oxygen}$$
$$H_2O_2 \rightarrow H_2O + O$$

Manufactured hydrogen peroxide is made more stable by adding some acid to it, usually **salicylic acid** or **phosphoric acid**, to give a final pH of about 5.

To help the release of oxygen, an alkali is added, usually **ammonium hydroxide**. This neutralises (cancels out) the acid stabiliser so that the oxygen can be more readily released. It also makes the bleach mixture alkaline, which swells the hair and opens the cuticle scales to allow the oxygen to penetrate into the cortex more easily. The bleaching process can be summarised in three steps (Fig. 3.4.7):

- The oxidising agent in the bleach breaks down, releasing oxygen.
- The oxygen penetrates the hair shaft and oxidises the melanin and pheomelanin to become decolourised oxymelanin.
- The oxidation process can be seen as a series of colour changes:

    black → brown → red → orange → yellow → pale yellow → white

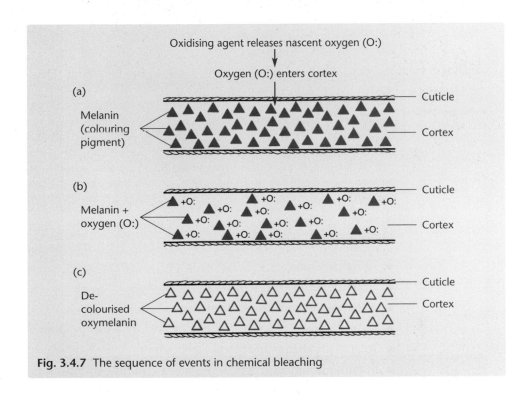

**Fig. 3.4.7** The sequence of events in chemical bleaching

## Types of bleach

- **Simple bleach** – this is 20 vol. (6 per cent) hydrogen peroxide mixed with a few drops of 0.880 ammonia solution. It will lighten the hair a few shades and does not leave behind a chemical deposit, so it does not need to be rinsed out. Simple bleach can be used to presoften resistant hair before tinting.
- **Powder bleach** – consists of magnesium carbonate powder plus ammonium carbonate powder or sodium acetate powder. The magnesium carbonate forms a paste but does not take part in the bleaching process. The ammonium carbonate or the sodium acetate makes the pH equal to 8.5, slightly alkaline, and this causes the cuticle scales to open.
- **Emulsion bleach** – this is used with boosters or activators to give a high degree of 'lift'. When mixed the emulsion bleach has a gel-like consistency, which makes it easier to apply for a full-head bleach. The emulsion itself contains an alkali, a thickening agent, conditioners and modifiers.

## Powder bleach: how it works

The powder is mixed with hydrogen peroxide to form a creamy mixture, rather like a paste. If the mixture is too thick, it will not coat the hair evenly and it will not penetrate the hair sections. Having been applied to the hair, a crust begins to form over the mixture; this slows down evaporation and allows more action of natural heat from the scalp. Powder bleaches have a high degree of lift and will usually lighten dark hair to blonde.

**POINTS TO REMEMBER**

### Boosters or activators

Boosters or activators increase the speed of the bleaching. They contain oxidising agents that release extra oxygen; this is in addition to the oxygen produced by the hydrogen peroxide. The active ingredients are usually a mixture of ammonium and potassium persulphate. Ammonium persulphate breaks down rapidly, releasing its oxygen, and is therefore fast acting. Potassium persulphate breaks down more slowly and therefore acts more slowly. Boosters or activators can only be used with hydrogen peroxide because they cannot physically break up the pigment granules in the hair. Hydrogen peroxide can do this and the boosters then speed the **decolorisation** of the pigment once the granules break up. Unit 2.6 gives full details of hydrogen peroxide.

## Uses of bleaching

- To lighten hair.
- To lighten hair before tinting.
- To lighten or remove tint from hair.
- To break down any resistant patches before a tint is applied.
- To give highlights and streaks to the hair.
- In conjunction with tint to produce extra hair colouring techniques.
- To presoften hair.

Bleach lifts the cuticle scales slightly and makes the hair more porous, so resistant hair becomes more susceptible to tinting as it can penetrate into the cortex more easily.

## Preparation for bleaching

Before starting a full-head bleach it is often safer to take a test cutting of the hair when the client books the appointment. The hair cuttings are taken from the front, crown and nape areas, as these areas can vary in porosity. If the client has been treating their own hair with chemicals, these may not have been evenly applied to the hair or may be incompatible with the bleaching agent to be used.

A skin test is not needed before bleaching unless the client has an extremely sensitive skin (strong bleach mixtures can burn sensitive skin), or in rare cases the client may have an allergy to ammonia. If in any doubt, apply a skin test as for tinting but use bleach instead of tint.

## Preparation of operator and client

Bleaching agents will remove colour from clothing, so the operator should wear rubber gloves and a tinting apron. Use a tinting gown to cover the client's clothing and preferably the chair as well. The towel should be tucked firmly into the nape to protect collars, and also to prevent the towel from slipping during the bleaching process. A cotton wool strip or neck strip placed at the nape is an added protection. A disposable plastic cape to cover the gown, towel and back of the chair prevents any bleach splashing onto these areas, removing the colour and rotting the material.

## Preparation of materials and equipment

Before the bleaching application, all materials and equipment should be assembled on the flat top of a trolley that can easily be wiped clean afterwards.

## Preparation of the bleach

Bleach is usually mixed with hydrogen peroxide in a 2:1 ratio, i.e. 2 parts hydrogen peroxide to 1 part bleach, unless otherwise stated by the manufacturer. Measure out the required amount of bleach into a non-metallic bowl then add the hydrogen peroxide slowly while mixing. Always follow the manufacturer's instructions.

## Application of a full-head bleach

1. Assemble equipment and materials.
2. Protect the client's clothing with tinting gown, towels, etc.
3. Disentangle hair and check scalp for cuts and abrasions.
4. Make sure that the client's hair is free from grease or heavy lacquer. If this is so, shampoo gently with a mild soapless (or lacquer-removing) shampoo, then dry.
5. Divide the head into six major sections.
6. Apply barrier cream around the hairline, ensuring that it is applied to the skin only.
7. Mix the bleach with the hydrogen peroxide, according to the manufacturer's instructions.
8. Start application at the nape (unless more resistant elsewhere) and apply the bleach mixture evenly to the mid-lengths and ends, if the hair is short. Mid-lengths only if the hair is long (Fig. 3.4.8). Allow approximately 10 mm ($\frac{1}{2}$ in) untreated hair at the roots to counteract the body heat which will develop the bleach more quickly. In the case of long hair, the ends are usually more porous and will therefore develop more quickly.
9. Continue applying the bleach in this manner through from sections 1 to 6 in Fig. 3.4.8. Take care to prevent the bleached areas touching the roots, otherwise the result will be patchy. To avoid this, strips of cotton wool may be placed between the subsections.

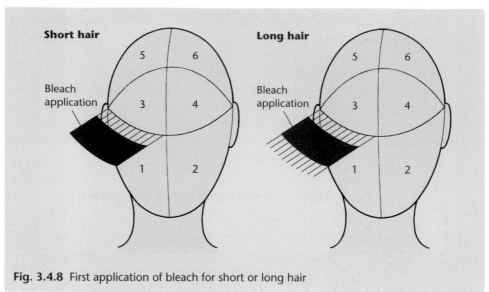

**Fig. 3.4.8** First application of bleach for short or long hair

10. When the application is complete, gently work the bleach into the hair with the fingers to ensure that the bleach has penetrated each section. In the case of long hair the bleach is now applied to the ends of the hair in the same order as before.

11. Cross-check the application to make sure that all sections are evenly and thoroughly covered.

12. Await bleach development, checking frequently by taking a strand test. If the hair is not the correct shade, reapply bleach to the strand of hair that has been checked. When the desired shade has almost been reached, mix up a fresh bleach and apply to the root areas as quickly as possible (work in the same order as previously).

13. Check that all the hair has been completely and evenly covered by cross-checking across the sections. Gently lift the hair out from the head to allow the air to circulate.

**TECHNICAL TIPS**

Remember that the scalp may be very tender at the rinsing stage and excessive massage will cause discomfort to the client.

14. Await development, checking frequently.

15. When the hair is an even shade throughout the entire length of the hair shaft, remove the bleach by rinsing thoroughly in tepid water. It is very important that all the bleach is completely removed from the hair.

16. Apply a mild acid balance or cream shampoo and massage the head gently. Rinse the hair thoroughly and repeat.

17. Apply a mild acid balance conditioner.

18. Towel-dry the hair and disentangle.
19. Apply a temporary rinse or toner to neutralise any unwanted golden or brassy tones. If a toner containing a 'para' compound is used, the client must have had a skin test 24–48 hours previously to ensure that there is no allergy to this type of tint.
20. Complete a record of work carried out and advise the client on after-care.

## Bleaching a regrowth

The bleaching of a regrowth requires far more skill and attention than the colouring of a regrowth, because of the excessive damage that can be caused to the hair by bleaching agents incorrectly applied.

- Take extra care not to overlap the bleach onto the previously treated hair. It could give a striped effect or cause breakage of the hair.
- Apply bleach quickly and evenly. It must be forced well down to the scalp to prevent the appearance of tiny black pinpricks at the roots.

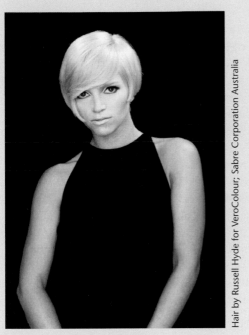

**Fig. 3.4.9** Full-head bleach

Hair by Russell Hyde for VeroColour; Sabre Corporation Australia

**SAFETY TIPS**

Treat the hair carefully because of its increased porosity and elasticity.

- Body heat has the effect of increasing the chemical activity close to the scalp, therefore the regrowth should not be allowed to exceed 1 cm ($\frac{1}{2}$ in). If the regrowth is greater than 1 cm ($\frac{1}{2}$ in), a striped effect could result and this is difficult to rectify.

## Contra-indications

Do not bleach hair in the following cases:

- If hair has been coated with a metallic substance, e.g. hair colour restorers.
- If hair is overprocessed or excessively damaged.
- If the hair is extremely fine or fragile.
- When any contagious or infectious diseases are present on the hair or scalp.
- When there are any severe cuts or abrasions on the scalp.

## Precautions and considerations

1. Always test for porosity and elasticity before bleaching.
2. Never use too high a volume strength of hydrogen peroxide on the hair, it can cause unnecessary damage.
3. Do not allow the regrowth to exceed 1 cm ($\frac{1}{2}$ in) otherwise the result could be stripy, because of the effect of body heat at the scalp.
4. Use barrier cream around the hairline.
5. Remember to allow for the effect of body heat at the roots when beginning a full-head bleach application.
6. Work quickly and methodically when bleaching the hair; the quicker the application, the more even the result.
7. Be cautious about using a steamer during processing, as it can make the bleach runny and it could run down the hair shaft on to previously bleached hair.
8. Remove all the bleach when fully developed. Any traces of the bleach left on the hair could cause creeping oxidation.
9. Bleached hair is less elastic and more porous than untreated hair. It will require more attention when conditioning, perming or tinting.
10. Give attention to the health and safety of yourself and the client at all times.

**POINTS TO REMEMBER**

Top up products and reorder stock before it gets too low. This helps to maintain an efficient and professional image of the salon by avoiding:

- Disruption to future salon services.
- Stressful situations.
- Inconvenience to the client.

## Bleach toners

Bleach toners are used to neutralise any unwanted golden tones produced by the bleaching process.

Remember that even careful bleaching will damage the cuticle scales and sometimes it creates a highly porous state. The biggest problem is that after bleaching the hair may have an *uneven* porosity, either along the hair or throughout the entire head. To avoid a patchy and uneven result, toners must therefore be applied with extra care, following the manufacturer's instructions.

### Types of toner

#### Temporary toners

Temporary toners are rinses applied to the hair after shampooing. They usually last from one shampoo to the next. However, because of the highly porous nature of bleached hair, there is often a colour build-up if these rinses are used continuously over a period of time. To correct this fault, apply the rinse to the root area only until the colour fades from the ends of the hair.

### Semi-permanent toners

Semi-permanent toners last from one bleach retouch to the next, although when applied to bleached hair they can fade more quickly. Application should be made with a brush to the roots first as they are not as porous as the points of the hair. The manufacturer's instructions should be carefully followed (some manufacturers produce semi-permanent tints specifically designed for bleached hair).

Check the development of the application carefully. Because of the damage to the cuticle scales by the bleach, the toner is absorbed quickly but is also easily removed; therefore development may appear complete, but on rinsing the colour may almost disappear. Alternatively, the development may be rapid and if the toner is left in contact with the hair too long, the finished result will be too dark.

**SAFETY TIPS**

Protect the skin with barrier cream; this also prevents staining.

A semi-permanent toner used regularly after each bleach retouch may create a colour build-up on the ends of the hair after a period of time. To rectify this, apply the toner to the root area only, then comb through to the ends of the hair, if and when necessary.

### Permanent toners

No toner used on bleached hair can be truly permanent. The degree of porosity of bleached hair causes any toner to fade quite quickly. A permanent toner is usually a para dye, which is mixed with 10 vol. (3 per cent) hydrogen peroxide. If this type of toner is used, a skin test is necessary because the client might have a reaction to the para compound. Care must be taken not to damage the hair still further by the use of too high a volume strength of hydrogen peroxide with the tint.

## Toning after highlighting with a cap

When toning the hair after highlighting with a toner that is mixed with hydrogen peroxide, remember that the hydrogen peroxide could alter the natural base shade of the client. To prevent this, apply the toner to the highlights before the highlighting cap is removed, thus colouring only the highlights. If using a semi-permanent toner without hydrogen peroxide, apply it in the same manner as above or remove the highlighting cap and apply the toner to the whole head.

POINTS TO
REMEMBER

## Returning bleached hair to a natural colour

It is more difficult to return bleached hair to its natural colour than to return tinted hair to its natural colour. During the bleaching process, the chemical action of the oxygen from the hydrogen peroxide causes the hair to progress through several colour changes, from the base shade of the hair to pale yellow or white. However, the red shade of pigment is the most difficult colour to convert and there is usually a lot of this colour pigment present in the hair shaft. If brown pigment, which is a mixture of red, blue and yellow, is added to the bleached hair, the hair absorbs the red from the brown pigment, leaving a green (blue + yellow) discoloration of the hair.

To avoid this discoloration, **prepigmentation** of the hair is necessary, using red colour particles. The red tint can be temporary, semi-permanent or permanent; the choice depends on the porosity of the hair and the needs of the client.

## How to prepigment hair

1. Take a test cutting of the hair.
2. Ensure that the client has had a skin test if using a 'para' dye.
3. Assemble materials and equipment. Protect client's and your own clothing.
4. Disentangle the hair and check for cuts and abrasions on the scalp.
5. Section hair into six major sections as for permanent tinting.
6. Apply a red semi-permanent tint using a brush, sponge or nozzle, to the bleached areas only. To damage the hair as little as possible, it is preferable to use a semi-permanent tint that does not require the addition of hydrogen peroxide.
7. Check the application.
8. Leave to develop according to the manufacturer's instructions but check frequently with a swab of damp cotton wool.
9. When the development is complete, rinse hair with warm water until the water runs clear.
10. Dry the hair and resection into six as before.
11. Proceed as for a normal full-head tint, using the shade of tint required but applying to the prepigmented areas only.
12. Complete a record of work carried out.
13. Advise the client on the after-care of the hair.

## After-care advice

- The hair will need deep conditioning and restructurants as it will be in a highly porous state due to all the chemicals it has been subjected to.
- It will take 6–12 months for the treated hair to grow out, depending on how short the client wears their hair.
- Cover the hair and protect it from the sun and the atmosphere. The hair may look a natural colour but it has bleach underneath.
- The hair must be carefully tested if it needs perming before the bleached ends have grown out.
- The hair may need recolouring after a few weeks. The increased porosity may cause the new colour to fade.

**Table 3.4.1** Bleaching faults and how to correct them

| Fault | Cause | Remedies |
|---|---|---|
| Hair breakage | Use of too strong a bleach mixture<br>Overlapping when retouching the roots<br>Incompatible chemicals present on the hair<br>prior to bleaching, e.g. metallic dyes<br>Bleaching of hair that is already in a porous and<br>weakened state<br>Overprocessing<br>Use of other strong chemicals over the bleached<br>hair, e.g. permanent wave lotion<br>Unnecessary application of heat during processing | Condition the hair<br>and apply restructurant |
| Scalp irritation or inflammation | Sensitive skin<br>Use of too strong a bleach mixture<br>Cuts and abrasions present on the scalp prior to<br>bleaching | Seek medical aid |
| Hair feels slimy and slippery<br>when wet and takes a long<br>time to dry | Hair in a highly porous state<br>Use of too strong a bleach mixture<br>Overprocessing<br>Use of other strong chemicals over the bleached hair | Condition the hair and use restructurant |
| Tiny dark pinpricks<br>at the root of the hair | Bleach not pressed into the root area firmly enough | Leave, but the client will require a<br>retouch application sooner than normal |
| Uneven colour along the<br>length of the hair shaft | Underprocessed retouch<br>Overprocessed retouch<br>No allowance made for the effect of body heat<br>on a full-head application<br>Uneven application<br>Overlapping<br>Regrowth allowed to exceed 1.25 cm ($\frac{1}{2}$ in) | Spot bleach darker areas. Rebleach if<br>underprocessed. Tone lighter areas if<br>overprocessed |
| Uneven colour throughout the<br>whole head | Commencing application at the most porous<br>area instead of the most resistant (this causes hair<br>to be lighter in some areas than others)<br>Uneven application<br>Application too slow<br>Sections too large | Spot bleach or rebleach darker areas |
| Finished result has an<br>orangey-red cast | Base colour too dark for strength of bleach<br>mixture used<br>Excessive amount of red pigment present in the<br>hair shaft<br>Use of too weak a bleach mixture<br>Too much ammonia present in the bleach mixture | Test hair for strength and porosity. If<br>satisfactory, rebleach; if unsatisfactory,<br>apply a green or matt toner |
| Hair too yellow or brassy | Underprocessed<br>Incorrect bleach for the base shade<br>Incorrect volume strength of the hydrogen peroxide | Apply a violet/mauve corrective toner |

## Hair discoloration and unwanted colour tones

An unwanted discoloration of the hair can often be masked by adding another colour. This is because brown hair colour is made up of three primary colours (blue, yellow and red). By mixing the primary colours blue, yellow and red it is possible to produce the secondary colours green, orange and purple:

    green   = blue + yellow
    orange = yellow + red
    purple = red + blue

If all three primary colours are mixed together, they produce brown, which is a neutral or tertiary colour:

    brown = blue + yellow + red

Any discoloration of the hair can be masked and brought to a neutral brown colour by adding the missing colour. For example, a green discoloration can be brought to brown by the addition of red:

    green        = blue + yellow
    green + red = blue + yellow + red   (add red)
             = brown

Thus, the colours opposite each other on the colour star will cancel each other out and bring the hair back to a neutral brown or beige colour depending on the depth of the original colour (Fig. 3.4.10):

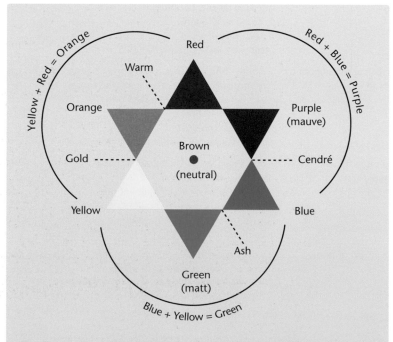

**Fig. 3.4.10** The colour star showing primary colours (blue, yellow and red) and secondary colours (green, orange and purple)

- Orange discoloration is masked by blue.
- Yellow discoloration is masked by purple (mauve).
- Red discoloration is masked by green (matt).
- Gold discoloration is masked by cendré.
- Warm tones are masked by ash.

Manufacturers take the characters from around the colour star and add them to various depths to create a range of shades.

## TECHNICAL TIPS

When masking unwanted colour tones by adding a contrasting colour, remember that the depth of both colours must be the same, e.g. pale yellow can be masked by pale purple (mauve) to produce pale brown (beige).

## Removing unwanted colour

If the unwanted colour cannot be masked by another colour, it may have to be removed by reduction or oxidation. Colour removal should always be carried out methodically and with extreme care. Every head is particular to each individual and so creates different problems; therefore, test cuttings *must* be taken to ensure that the colour can be successfully removed. The results of the tests should be shown to the client so they will know in advance what to expect.

Thorough consultation is very important in order to find out what products have been used on the hair and what the client expects from the treatment. Using shade charts and pictures helps to identify the exact requirements and whether they may be attainable. If the client has practised home tinting, an incompatibility test will be needed as the product they have used may contain metallic salts. If the client has had their hair tinted by another hairdresser, try to find out the manufacturer of the previous tint; most colouring manufacturers have an advisory service and can give valuable assistance to the hairdresser.

Do not take details of a previous treatment at face value. Clients are often reluctant to admit what they have actually used on their hair, particularly when the results have been unsatisfactory. They also do not realise that a permanent product applied to the hair several months previously could still be on the ends of the hair; therefore, always check all the facts thoroughly before deciding upon the best method of colour correction to use.

Before starting any form of colour removal, try to find out these details:

- Condition of the hair and the scalp.
- Porosity of the hair.
- History of any skin troubles.
- Make and type of any previous treatments.
- Shade of any previous tints.

- General colour state, e.g. patchy, dull, multicoloured.
- Final colour shade required.

**TECHNICAL TIPS**

Take test cuttings from various parts of the head, particularly if the unwanted colour is patchy.

**POINTS TO REMEMBER**

### Reduction is an acid removal

The oxygen is removed from the converted colour molecules which are then converted into colourless **leuco-compounds**. This means that only the artificial colour pigment is removed and the natural colour pigment is left unlightened; it also means that the lightening power of the reducers is limited.

Colour reducers, or reducters as they are sometimes known, are usually in liquid or powder form and may be mixed with either water or peroxide. They must be used in strict accordance with the manufacturer's instructions.

For simple cases the reducer is mixed with water and this will take the hair colour down by approximately one shade. If the hair is dark through colour build-up and requires more lightening, the reducer is mixed with 10 or 20 vol. (3 or 6 per cent) hydrogen peroxide. Occasionally, for very dark shades and dramatic removal, 30 vol. (9 per cent) hydrogen peroxide may be used, but never stronger than this.

It is not possible to obtain cold or flat shades when reducing as some of the red pigment will stay in the hair. A toning shade of matt will therefore be necessary to mask any unwanted warm shades.

Colour reducers make the hair more porous; therefore a tint applied after reducing is likely to process more quickly or produce a deeper shade than expected. To counteract this, it is advisable to use a tint that is one shade lighter than the tint required to achieve the best results.

The condition of the hair is also affected by colour reducers. It is important to condition the hair thoroughly after the treatment and extra care should be taken when perming decoloured hair.

### How to remove colour by reduction

1. Check all tests are satisfactory.
2. Protect the client's clothing with dark gown, towels, etc.
3. Check the scalp for cuts and abrasions.
4. Divide the hair into four major sections (forehead to nape and ear to ear across the top of the head).
5. Mix the reducer in a non-metallic bowl (do not allow the mixture to come into contact with metal comb or clips).
6. Start application with a sponge or tinting brush, taking intersecting partings across the crown.

7. Application must be done speedily and thoroughly. Apply the mixture to the tinted hair only, and avoid the root section if there is a natural colour regrowth. The natural regrowth can be blocked out with cotton wool strips if necessary.

8. When the application is complete, comb through but do not allow the reducer to come into contact with the root area. Pay particular attention to the front hairline and the ends of the hair as this usually has the highest concentration of tint.

9. Leave to develop, usually up to 50 minutes but check with the manufacturer's instructions.

10. When the development time is up, check that the hair has sufficiently lightened then rinse thoroughly and shampoo.

11. Rinse hair with a stabilising solution of 10 vol. (3 per cent) hydrogen peroxide and comb through gently. This will show whether all the colour pigment has been removed from the hair.

12. If the hair redarkens after combing through, it means that the pigment has not been successfully removed and it will be necessary to repeat the application.

13. Dry the hair to check the colour. If patchy, reapply the reducer to the patches. If the colour is even but the shade is too orange, red or brassy, tone out with a semi-permanent or permanent tint.

14. Condition the hair well.

15. Complete a record of work carried out.

16. Advise on after-care conditioning treatments.

**TECHNICAL TIPS**

Never apply the reducer to the untreated (virgin) parts of the hair.

## How to remove colour by oxidation

Oxidation is an alkaline method of removal done with bleaching preparations. It will lighten both the artificial and natural colour pigments. The bleach mixture is applied to the tinted area of the hair only, in the same way as a reducer, It may, however, be necessary to bleach the hair a shade or two lighter than the required colour to allow for corrective tinting afterwards. When an even, bleached base has been achieved, a permanent tint can then be applied to obtain the colour that is required.

It is very important when carrying out colour removal to test the hair for breakage and tensile strength during the processing. Remember that the hair is probably in a very porous state before colour removal and the addition of still more chemicals to the hair can be very damaging. The importance of test cutting before the application cannot be stressed too strongly nor too often. The client will also require advice on after-care conditioning treatments to counteract the damaging effect of the chemicals.

## Contra-indications

Do not proceed with colour removal in any of the following cases:

- Contagious or infectious disease of the hair and/or scalp.
- Excessively weak and porous hair.
- Incompatible chemicals present on the hair shaft.
- Adverse reaction to the test cuttings.
- Adverse reaction to the skin test (if using para after the decolouring).
- Highly sensitive scalp.
- Build-up of very dark products that are impossible to remove.

## Precautions and considerations

1. Always check the client's final requirements thoroughly. It may not be possible to achieve the exact colour they desire, due to the previous treatments, and the client should be made aware of this.
2. Always test the hair before starting a decolouring process.
3. Make sure the hair is in reasonable condition before strong colour removal.
4. Be aware of the health and safety of yourself and the client at all times.

## Health and safety

- Carry out all necessary tests before beginning any treatment.
- Protect yourself with a tinting apron and rubber gloves and protect the client with a gown and towels.
- Make sure that tools and equipment are assembled and positioned, before starting, for ease of use and efficient working.
- Make sure the client is comfortable and in the correct position at all times.
- Mop up any spillage immediately.
- Make sure the water temperature and flow are correct when removing products.
- Keep alert for any potential hazards.
- Dispose of waste products and materials safely in the correct place.
- Clean and sterilise tools and equipment after use.

## Things to do

1. (a) Take an old hair block and practise the following creative colouring techniques on different parts of the head:
   - painted lights
   - colour flashes
   - scrunching
   - glimmering
   - slicing

   (b) Write a short report on each technique in part (a). Use the following headings in each report:
   - what was easy about this technique
   - what was difficult about this technique
   - the type of client this technique could be used on
   - time taken

2. Read through Unit 2.6 to make sure you understand the basic theories and principles of hair colouring.

3. The following case study is a means of testing your understanding of colour correction principles by asking you to apply them to a problem which could occur in the salon.

   A member of staff asks you to look discreetly at a client's hair after having woven highlights. The product has swollen over the packet and has left lines of colour on the roots.

   Describe how you would handle this situation with reference to:
   (a) the interpersonal skills necessary to prevent losing the client
   (b) the interpersonal skills needed and the discussion you would have with the staff member
   (c) correction of the colouring mistake
   (d) any advice needed for the client and staff member

4. (a) Carry out a risk assessment on the chemicals, tools and equipment that you need to use for creative colouring.
   (b) Write a short report then place it in your file for future reference.

## What do you know?

- What is the difference between melanin and pheomelanin?
- What is meant by colour tone?
- What is the International Colour Code?
- How can creative colouring improve the look of a hairstyle?
- List **ten** factors that you need to consider when choosing a colour.
- Give a brief description of how you would prepare the client before colouring or bleaching.
- Name **five** creative colouring techniques.
- Give a brief description of what happens to the hair during the bleaching process.
- Which type of bleach are boosters used with?
- List **five** contra-indications when bleaching.
- Why is it necessary to reorder before stock levels become too low?
- What is meant by the term prepigmentation?
- How would you mask a green discoloration?
- List the primary colours.
- List the secondary colours.
- List the **three** types of bleach toners and give the use of each.
- What information is needed before beginning a colour removal?
- List the contra-indications for colour removal.
- What is the difference between removing colour by oxidation (bleach) and removing colour by a reducer?
- List **nine** health and safety considerations when colouring or decolouring hair.

# 5

In this unit you will learn about:

- Types of salon resources.
- Management of stock.
- Productivity levels and how to improve performance.
- Setting targets.

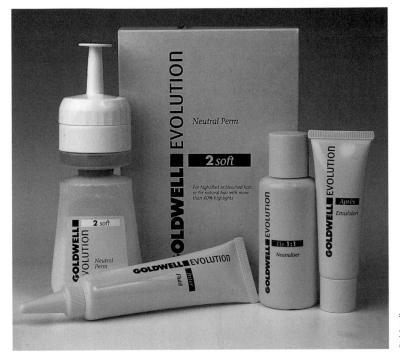

Goldwell

# Financial effectiveness

## Profit

Many places in this book emphasise the business aspects of the salon. A successful salon business is one that cares about its staff and clients and makes a profit. Profit is what keeps a salon in business and it is easy to define:

Profit = total income – total cost to operate business

From this it follows that there are two key areas in the profitability of a business:

- Maximising income.
- Minimising costs.

## Resources

A resource is something that can be used and has a value. The use of resources is governed by legal and organisational factors. Here are some of the resources for a hairdressing salon:

- **People** – the staff and clients.
- **Finance** – the income generated by salon sales and services.
- **Information systems** – these may be paper-based or more usually computerised.
- **Utilities** – electricity, gas, water, telephone, fax.
- **Tools and equipment** – instruments used to cut and style hair.
- **Time** – there is the old saying 'time is money'.
- **Space** – use it effectively for displays, secure storage, etc.

The health and safety requirements of using tools and equipment are considered in detail in Unit 3.6, but here is a summary:

- The Health and Safety at Work Act makes everyone responsible for their own safety and the safety of others (both clients and colleagues).
- The COSHH Regulations cover the storage, use and disposal of products in the salon.
- The Electrical Equipment Regulations cover the safe use of this equipment and arrangements for competent maintenance.

Working without the appropriate resources can be dangerous; it can lead to lower income for the salon and lower earnings for the staff; it can even lead to disciplinary action. All three reasons make it very important to monitor resources properly.

### Documentation

Documentation does not have to be complicated but it does have to be accurate. Indeed, if the system is too complex, staff will be less likely to complete the documentation and keep it up to date.

All stock that is for use or sale within the salon, including tools, equipment and products containing chemicals, should be entered in some type of **stock book** or **computerised system**. It is usually convenient to divide the stock into broad categories which make the checking of stock levels far easier. If anyone needs to know the current stock level of a certain shampoo type, they have to be able to find it easily and quickly. Wasted time is expensive for any business.

The documentation should be designed to accommodate the monitoring of day-to-day usage and also the retail sales of stock within the salon. However, the system is only as good as those who use it, therefore to be effective all staff must be made aware, both verbally and in writing, of how the system operates and why it is important to keep regular and accurate records.

## Security and safe handling

Part of the reason for having a well-controlled stock system is to help prevent pilfering. It is a sad fact that some people will be tempted to take what is not theirs given the opportunity. Although a tight stock control system will not totally prevent this from happening, it will act as a strong deterrent; if a stock check is carried out daily it gives some indication of when the stock went missing and may therefore help to identify what has happened to it.

Staff should also be made aware of the need for correct and safe handling of stock in accordance with the Health and Safety at Work Act and the COSHH Regulations to ensure the protection of themselves and others at work.

## Stocktaking procedures

The purpose of stocktaking is twofold: as an **internal audit** to ensure that stock levels are maintained and to aid the internal security system, and to provide documentation for **external audit** requirements.

It is up to each organisation to determine how often they will require the stock to be checked. However, it is of the utmost importance to keep an up-to-date record of stock levels; when an item of stock is removed, it should be entered in the records. Taking regular, random stock checks is usually a means of ensuring that this is the case. A full stocktake of *all* stock and equipment must be carried out at least once a year to comply with external audit requirements and the specifications of the Inland Revenue when completing year-end account books for audit.

## Stock rotation, replacement and safety

Good stockkeeping involves checking that the products are in supply when needed and that they are easily located in the stockroom. Running out of stock is unprofessional and gives a very bad impression of the salon. There is nothing more irritating to a client than to arrive for a treatment only to find that the colour or perm is out of stock. To help prevent this happening, it is important to have a system of stock control which carefully monitors stock levels so that materials can be ordered in plenty of time. Remember that when stock is ordered through the post it may be several days before the order is received. If stock is required immediately then it has to be obtained from a cash and carry.

Unforeseen circumstances and abnormal situations can arise from time to time. For example, the salon could have a sudden surge of clients requiring perms or the suppliers themselves could be out of the particular stock item that the salon needs. These problems, although unforeseen, still reflect badly on the organisation of the salon if they cause inconvenience to the client. Planning ahead and having a system of stock control which has back-up supplies, particularly of popular items, can prevent a crisis occurring.

Hairdressers work with many hazardous substances and it is therefore extremely important that all staff members are aware of the ingredients and potential dangers of all substances used in the salon. They should be given training in what to do in an emergency and, indeed, it is now a requirement of law that all salons carry out an assessment of the substances used in the workplace. This legislation is known as the **COSHH Regulations** and is intended as a safety measure to protect both staff and clients.

To ensure that stock is maintained in optimum condition and is safely stored away to avoid risking the health and safety of both staff and clients, check the storage instructions and shelf life of all stock *each* time it is delivered. These instructions should include specific guidance and will influence safe storage and stock rotation.

## Safe storage

Stock should be stored with due regard to product size and accessibility. For safety reasons, large, heavy items such as gallon containers must be stored at ground level whereas smaller, lighter items such as cotton wool should be stored at higher levels. Products which have a quick turnover, such as tints and perms, should be placed at eye level for easy access and to help prevent back strain.

Follow the manufacturer's storage instructions exactly. If they stipulate a cool, dark place then do not store the product on a window ledge or over a radiator, else it will deteriorate very rapidly or perhaps become unstable. Hydrogen peroxide can explode if stored incorrectly.

When staff are dealing with stock and equipment, there are certain laws of the land (legislation) which ought to be noted. **The Health and Safety at Work Act 1974** gives guidance regarding the safe handling of tools, equipment and substances; it is very important. All staff members should be aware of the content of this act and there are many leaflets produced by a variety of organisations for this purpose. Relevant literature should be available for staff perusal at all times and can usually be obtained from the local environmental health officer or the regional office of the Health and Safety Executive. Both are listed in the phone book.

## Rotation

Products with a limited shelf life should be sold or used in rotation to ensure that they do not go over their sell-by date and become ineffective. To alleviate this problem, always place new stock behind or underneath the old stock.

Stock that has been stored incorrectly (e.g. in the wrong place or with the cap left off) can become useless before the stated sell-by date. Items which have been dropped or where the packaging has become damaged may affect the product's effectiveness when used. For this reason it is advisable to conduct regular spot checks of the storage arrangements and the condition of the products. Products for retail also need to be regularly checked to ensure that clients are not sold goods which are damaged or have an exhausted shelf life.

## Product deterioration

Product deterioration can be the fault of the salon or the supplier. If a product has deteriorated through bad salon practices, such as incorrect storage or non-rotation of products, then it should be disposed of in an appropriate manner with the consent of the employer. A note must be made in the stock documents regarding any stock which has to be discarded, to ensure that records are correct and stock is not just presumed to be missing. Hairdressing products are expensive and if any have to be discarded in this way, perhaps new methods of stock organisation and staff training need to be considered.

Always check the soundness of stock when it is received. If goods purchased from the supplier are damaged or faulty, they should be returned immediately with a letter stating why they are being returned. No payment should be made until you are entirely satisfied with the standard of the product. Remember that the ineffectiveness of any item used or sold in the salon reflects on you as the practitioner or retailer.

## Incoming deliveries

All stock must be carefully checked as soon as it is received to ensure that any shortages, discrepancies, damaged or inferior goods within the order are quickly identified and dealt with. All goods used or sold by the salon must be of high quality as there is legislation which protects the client (consumer). They are entitled by law to receive what they have paid for. If a particular permanent wave claims to have certain properties or give a certain result then this is what the client is entitled to, and if the salon fails to supply this then they are obliged by law to reimburse the client. All staff should be aware of their responsibilities regarding the relevant sections of the **Consumer Protection Act** so that any problems are dealt with professionally and within the requirements of the law.

When stock is ordered and delivered through the post, the following overall system usually operates:

1. New stock is ordered. A copy of this order must be kept for future reference.
2. The new stock is delivered. It is usual for the driver of the delivery van to ask for a signature to prove that the stock has been delivered safely. Before signing make sure that the merchandise is in good condition with no breakages. If there are any defects, send the whole order back and refuse to sign.
3. A **delivery note** will be found with the order when it is delivered. The contents of this must be checked against the **original order** and the **actual** stock delivered. This is to check that what was originally ordered has in fact been delivered.

4. An **invoice** may also be included inside the order or it may be sent through the post separately. This document lists the various products contained in the order, gives their prices and also shows the amount of value added tax (VAT) payable. The invoice should be checked against the delivery note to make sure that the correct products are being charged for. Once checked the invoice must be kept in a safe place as it will be required when paying for the goods and also as proof of purchase within the yearly business accounts.

5. A **statement** will be received separately and does not itemise the stock delivered; it simply gives the date and number of the invoices.

Once a statement has been received and there are no discrepancies between the stock ordered and the stock received, then the stock must be paid for.

The cross-checking of the order in this manner is very important as mistakes can often be made somewhere between the placing of the order and its actual delivery. If such a mistake should occur, immediately notify the supplier (and employer if appropriate) else problems can arise.

## Activity

Carry out research into the different methods of computerised and manual stock control systems. Trade journals will usually have contact addresses to enable you to obtain information regarding the different computer programs which can be used for controlling and monitoring stock. Write a short summary of your findings under the following headings: methods, advantages and disadvantages, comparison and evaluation.

## Types of resources

### Human resources

Unit 2.8 covers the development and maintenance of effective teamwork in the salon. It is important not to overload staff with too much work, responsibility or both. They need to be clear about:

- Levels of responsibility and limits to authority of themselves and other salon staff. This needs to be made clear in all job descriptions.
- The rungs on the ladder of salon communications.
- Effective communication by means of memos, staff meetings, training sessions and notices.

Some hairdressers overload themselves by taking on extra work outside their job at the salon. Perhaps they travel to meet these extra clients or perhaps they work from home. It is probably wise to discourage too much of this extra work and some salons have a policy which forbids it altogether.

## Financial resources

It is quite common for salons to have problems with financial resources. Examples include the accidental giving of wrong change or mishandling of non-cash payments and the deliberate theft of money or stock. Here are two pieces of good practice for cash payments:

- Put any banknotes on the cash register until the change has been given.
- Look at any banknote the customer has given you and say its value out loud, e.g. £20.

Commission is another aspect of financial resources. Some salons work on a commission-only basis. Others use a basic wage with commission earned on top. The commission is an incentive and may be calculated on the actual income generated or a fixed payment for particular services.

Whenever commission is involved it is in everyone's interests to ensure it is accurately worked out. Most salons use a validation system which checks services against the appointments made. Stock control is important as commission is often paid on retail goods as well as on salon services.

## Information

Information is a resource; it should be kept **confidential**. Commercial confidentiality covers areas such as pay, pay structure and pricing of goods and services. Client details may be of a sensitive nature or, more usually, they are important to give the client a feeling of being valued. Make an effort to record details that may help with later appointments. People like to be remembered and made to feel important. Salons have strict rules about confidentiality of client details and, in many salons, failure to keep to the rules results in dismissal. The Data Protection Act means that a breach of confidence in computer records can be prosecuted.

## Utilities

Salons use a lot of water and electricity, and they may also use gas. The main factor is misuse by wasting energy or water, particularly hot water. Minimising waste should be a matter of routine and the relevant procedures should be followed automatically. Misuse of the salon phone can also be included here. The phone should only be used for salon business, not just because of the cost but due to creating difficulties for clients and potential clients when phoning in.

## Spillages and waste

Spillages occur even in the best-run salons. Remembering to put the caps back on containers minimises the risk, but what if a spill does occur? The best advice is to wash it off and clean it up using lots of water. Avoid skin contact. If the spill is onto someone, wash clothes and skin under the tap. Report the spill to your supervisor.

Breakages do not happen often in the salon. Very few hairdressing products are supplied in breakable containers – most are in plastic which does not break easily. Some pieces of hairdressing equipment are more vulnerable – blow-dryers for example can break if dropped. All salon lotions should be stored in well-labelled containers and not put on high shelves, as they may be dropped when people reach up to get them. Particular care needs to be taken with stored hydrogen peroxide and pressurised aerosol sprays. Both can explode if heated, so they should never be stored near heaters or in direct sunlight.

If a container has lost its label or the contents cannot be identified then dispose of it. Empty pressurised cans should be disposed of carefully. They should not be punctured or burned (incinerated) as the pressure left inside could cause an explosion. Warnings about this are printed on the container.

Waste is expensive. The usual cause of waste in the salon is using too much of something, such as using too much shampoo on a client's scalp, or too much hot water which has cost money to heat up. In addition bad planning and technique can waste people's time and effort, both of which cost money, cause frustration and reduce morale. Encourage staff to report spillages and breakages to their supervisor, along with any ideas for improving resource use.

## Tools and equipment

Ensure that tools and equipment are:

● Properly looked after and maintained.

● Used only for hairdressing in the salon.

## Time

People's time is an important resource and should not be wasted. This has a lot to do with self-motivation of staff. Staff sitting about gives a very poor impression. The 'find something to do' rule is important here. There are always things that need doing in the salon.

## Space

The careful use of space is important in the salon. Space is often at a premium and things can go wrong:

● **At reception** – too much clutter on chairs, surfaces, untidy displays which get in the way.

● **In the salon** – staff bags, coats and personal possessions.

The salon layout needs to be planned to give working room, waiting room, display areas, reception and storage areas. Badly planned space can be a constant problem and good communication systems, such as staff meetings, can help develop better practice and suggestions for better space utilisation.

## Salon productivity

Salon productivity is the amount of work carried out (and so the amount of turnover) in a given length of time. Many salons use incentives, particularly commission payments to staff, in order to enhance productivity. Some salons operate a 'commission only' payment system to staff, whereas others operate a basic payment with commission added on. In some salons the commission is based on the numbers of operations, whereas in others it is on the income generated by the services provided. In any event it is important for all salon staff to be aware that their own work and how they do it (their work performance) are important to the success of the salon business. This can be encouraged by:

● Providing opportunities to review salon services in terms of improving productivity. This gets people to think about what they are doing.

● Promotion of self and salon by workshops, training sessions, marketing, retailing and shows. This helps staff to identify commercial opportunities and new products as well as encouraging team building.

### Setting productivity levels

Setting realistic targets for performance is a key aspect of salon management. This can be through one-to-one discussions (including formal appraisal in larger salons), staff meetings or setting general expected levels of activity. This helps to prevent the abuse sometimes encountered in salons where too few clients are deliberately booked in (or even non-existent bogus clients are put down) to give an easy time to a stylist. Another problem (mostly by accident) is the failure to pass on in the client's bill the proper cost of the resources used, e.g. payment for a cheaper alkaline perm when in fact a more expensive acid perm has been used.

Setting targets also helps to clarify how long a service or process should take and then helps to identify if problems in working speeds are present. In many salons staff keep a work log as an independent method of recording (in addition to the appointment record) what they have done over a period of time. This is often used in calculations for commission or bonus payments for exceeding targets.

It is important to maintain the motivation and enthusiasm of staff and key aspects of this are:

● Clear and realistic target setting.

● Good, effective, two-way communication.

● Staff see that appropriate action is taken.

● Appropriate action may be to ensure implementation of salon and legal requirements of operations, e.g. dismissal for breach of confidentiality, misappropriation of stock, etc.

## Things to do

1. The following case study has been devised to give you an opportunity to formulate 'proposals' which could improve the effectiveness of the organisation. If a proposal is well researched and produced in a logical and coherent manner, the senior manager is more likely to take your suggestions seriously.

   Read the case study carefully then carry out the tasks indicated. Evaluating and discussing your ideas with others is a useful exercise as it will enable you to identify any perceived difficulties and will also allow you to see another viewpoint.

   *The manager of your salon is very concerned that junior staff are not exercising enough care and attention when they are dealing with stock and equipment. The manager discusses the problem with you and asks if you will come up with some ideas for the next meeting.*

   (a) Draft out a list of simple and realistic guidelines regarding security and safe handling of stock.

   (b) List any other additional ideas you may have.

   (c) Present your proposals to your manager (or other members of your group).

   (d) Discuss and evaluate the proposals. Are they realistic? Would they be easily implemented? Are they cost-effective?

   (e) Amend your proposals, if necessary.

   (f) Keep a copy of your amended proposals in an evidence file or your portfolio.

2. (a) Complete the resource, income and cost lists for an actual salon (opposite).

   (b) Carry out a study of the use of resources in a salon. Suggest **improvements** that could realistically be made.

   (c) What is meant by salon productivity? Make a list of factors which influence productivity for an actual salon. From your list select some areas where improvements could be made and explain how they could realistically be achieved.

**Resources used**

- 
- 
- 
- 
- 
- 
- 

↓

**Income from**

- 
- 
- 
- 
- 
- 
- 

↓

**Example costs**

- 
- 
- 
- 
- 
- 
- 

↓

**PROFIT**

## What do you know?

- List **seven** types of resources used in salons.
- Explain the **legal** and **organisational** factors which influence resource use.
- What are the potential consequences of **misusing** resources?
- How does **waste** affect profit?
- Identify who is responsible for **resource allocation** and use in the salon.
- List some **effective** types of communication.
- Why is **effective** communication important?
- What is **productivity**?
- How might you encourage contributions to improving salon productivity?
- What should be taken into account to ensure a **satisfactory** stock control system?

- What is the **difference** between an external audit and an internal audit?
- Why is it necessary to keep accurate and up-to-date **records** of stock levels
- How can you ease the problem of **unforeseen** circumstances with regard to stock?
- What are the **COSHH** Regulations?
- Why should stock be used in **rotation**?
- Why is it necessary to store the stock with **due regard** for product size and accessibility?
- Why should new stock be checked **immediately** that it is received?
- What is the **purpose** of an invoice?
- Give a brief summary of the procedure for the **receipt** of incoming stock deliveries at your salon.

# 6

In this unit you will learn about:

- Health and safety hazards.
- The legal requirements with regard to salon health and safety.
- How to maintain a safe and healthy salon environment.
- First-aid procedures.
- Salon security.

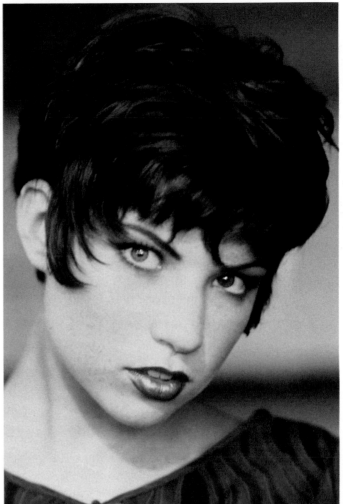

Sabre Europe

# Salon health, safety and security

## Health and safety hazards

A large hairdressing salon on a busy day may have over one hundred clients using the premises. Most of those people will be concerned only with the finished style and few, if any, will give any thought to the possible hazards in the salon. The hairdresser needs to be much more aware of these health and safety issues so that possible accidents or infections can be prevented. The hairdresser and the client can be put at risk from several possible sources:

- **Physical hazards** – these include physical injury (e.g. cuts and knocks), fire and heat burns, electricity (e.g. electric shock).
- **Chemical hazards** – these include chemical burns (including chemicals on the skin and the eyes), storage and disposal of chemicals (e.g. hydrogen peroxide and aerosol containers), dermatitis or eczema (e.g. from hair dyes).
- **Biological hazards** – these include infections caused by micro-organisms (germs), e.g. impetigo, and infestations caused by animal parasites, e.g. head lice.

Hairdressers have a responsibility to protect themselves and their clients. This is a moral responsibility, in that it is wrong to cause pain or discomfort, and a practical responsibility due to:

- The legal responsibilities placed on the salon owner and worker.
- The bad publicity from accidents or infections in the salon.

This unit develops the areas covered in Levels 1 and 2 and the relevant health and safety legislation required for Level 3.

## Legal requirements for salon health and safety

The legislation, regulations and guidance advice in this area are under constant review and change. What follows is a brief outline of the legislation and regulations of particular importance to hairdressing. These are correct at the time of writing but it is strongly advised that current information be sought if significant time has passed.

Information can be obtained from a variety of sources:

- Trade publications.
- Manufacturers and wholesalers.
- Local environmental health officers.
- Community health organisations.
- Health and Safety Executive.

The Health and Safety Executive (HSE) have regional offices (in the phone book) and are an extremely good source of up-to-date information. They produce a range of leaflets and pamphlets on legislation and regulations along with practical guides to implementation. Here are some examples:

- How to use hair preparations safely in the salon.
- Guidelines on Aids and hepatitis B for hairdressers.
- Five steps for completing a COSHH assessment.

The HSE has information and publication centres; more details on these centres can be obtained from regional offices.

## Some important health and safety legislation

- Management of Health and Safety at Work Regulations 1992.
- Health and Safety at Work Act 1974.
- Workplace (Health, Safety and Welfare) Regulations 1992.
- Manual Handling Operations Regulations 1992.
- Personal Protective Equipment at Work Regulations 1992.
- Control of Substances Hazardous to Health Regulations 1988 (COSHH).
- Health and Safety (Training for Employment) Regulations 1988.
- Reporting of Injuries, Diseases and Dangerous Occurrences Regulations 1985.
- Health and Safety Information to Employees Regulations 1989.
- Health and Safety (First Aid) Regulations 1981.
- Electricity at Work Regulations 1989.

The Management of Health and Safety at Work Regulations 1992 requires salons to set up codes of practice to carry out aspects of the Health and Safety at Work Act and the COSHH Regulations. Here are some examples:

- Risk assessment.
- Keeping records.
- Preventive measures.
- Training.

The Health and Safety Information to Employees Regulations 1989 place a duty on employers to inform employees on exposure and risk as well as policies and procedures on health and safety.

- **The Electricity at Work Regulations 1989** state that electrical equipment must be used safely and must be checked every year by a 'competent person'.
- **The Provision and Use of Work Equipment Regulations 1992** have a very wide scope and will eventually cover both new and old equipment. They regulate areas such as the use, repair, maintenance and cleaning of equipment and they place a duty on the employer to protect the employee. The regulations cover equipment used in hairdressing and extend to lighting.
- **The Workplace (Health, Safety and Welfare) Regulations 1992** replace large parts of the older Factories Act 1961 and the Offices, Shops and Railway Premises Act 1963. They contain large numbers of areas relevant to hairdressing.

The regulations cover areas such as:

- Equipment maintenance – 'good working order and in good repair'.
- Ventilation – 'sufficient' fresh air or purified air.
- Workplace, temperature – at least 16°C.
- Lighting – 'suitable and sufficient'.
- Cleanliness – of the workplace, furniture and fittings.

The regulations cover floors and indoor traffic routes which should be cleaned 'at least once a week' and should be 'non-slip' and not cause a person to drop anything.

Workstations and seating need to be 'suitable' for the stylist and client, and there should be places to put a person's own clothing and overalls, and facilities for changing. There should also be facilities for rest and meals, including protecting non-smokers from the discomfort caused by smokers. Toilets and wash facilities must also be provided.

## Health and Safety at Work Act 1974

The Health and Safety at Work Act 1974 extends to all working situations and sets out the responsibilities of both the employer and the employee in terms of:

- General health and safety.
- First-aid arrangements and reporting of accidents.
- Enforcement of the act.

### General health and safety

The duties of the *employer* include:

- Care and maintenance of equipment.
- Prevention of risk in the storage and use of materials.
- Instruction and training employees in safe practices.
- Maintaining the place of work so it is safe.
- With five or more employees, the employer needs to produce a written policy statement in terms of the general policy operated concerning health and safety.

For the *employee* the duties are:

- To take reasonable care for the health and safety of themselves and others who may be affected by their actions.
- To cooperate with the employer and others to ensure health and safety at work.

The act also lists 'dangerous occurrences' and recommends that they must be reported and a record kept. This is taken further in the Notification of Accidents and Dangerous Occurrences Regulations 1980, which stipulate that 'dangerous occurrences' must be noted whether a person is injured or not.

### Enforcement of the act

Enforcement is carried out by area offices of the Health and Safety Executive by means of health and safety inspectors. These inspectors have the right of entry to premises and the power to:

- Order improvements to be made.
- Prohibit the use of apparatus or premises.
- Seize, render harmless or destroy dangerous equipment.

The Health and Safety (Training for Employment) Regulations 1988 extended health and safety legislation to cover trainees and those on work experience.

## COSHH Regulations

The COSHH Regulations are concerned with chemical hazards. The main principles of these regulations are:

- Assessment of risk from substances – much of this depends on information supplied by manufacturer.
- Provision, use and upkeep of adequate control measure for chemicals – the main point is to prevent exposure if practicable or have adequate control.
- Monitoring exposure of employees to potential hazards.
- Health surveillance of employees – this means monitoring the health of people exposed to potential hazards.
- Education and training of employees in terms of:
  - purpose of personal protective clothing
  - how to avoid endangering themselves and others
  - storage and disposal
  - emergency procedures

## Maintaining a healthy and safe working environment

The working environment includes the salon, access to and from the salon, the stockroom, toilets, wash areas and restrooms, and offices. Having covered the underpinning legislation and regulations on salon health and safety, here is an outline of practical health, safety and hygiene theory and practice. Other information is given in Unit 1.5 and Unit 2.9.

## Maintaining equipment for long and reliable service

- Every client should have a clean brush and comb used on their hair. Combs should be kept in antiseptic and brushes in a sterilising cabinet.

- Chairs should be kept clean and free from hair. A vinyl covering makes cleaning easier. They should be wiped down every day, including the backs of the chairs and the legs, which tend to get splashed with lotions. Any splitting or tearing of the material must be attended to immediately so it does not get worse.

- Light fittings should be kept clean. It is important that the salon is well lit from all angles.

- Dryers do long duty hours. If kept clean and dust free, the wear and tear on them is kept to a minimum. Regularly unscrew the top and remove dust and fluff from the fan, otherwise there is a real risk of fire. Arrange a yearly contract for servicing; there are firms that specialise in this service.

- Steamers and infrared lamps should be cleaned after use. Always ensure that the water bottle on the steamer has enough water in it before use (distilled water should be used) and give the steamer a regular clean out. Infrared bulbs should be checked before use and any faulty bulbs replaced. Servicing once a year will prolong the life of this equipment and maintain its safety of use.

- Make sure that the vapour steriliser cabinet is checked each day and refilled with sterilising solution. Keep vapour and ultraviolet cabinets clean inside and out.

**POINTS TO REMEMBER**    Routine hygiene practices and procedures should always be followed by all staff.

## Safe use of electricity

People can be at risk for two different reasons: from overheating of electrical appliances or from receiving an electric shock. The amount of electricity and hence the severity of the electric shock depend on the **voltage** and **current** of the electrical supply involved, and the **electrical resistance** between the person and the item from which they receive the shock.

The electricity supplied to and used in most salons has a voltage of 240 volts and a current of 13 amps. This is sufficient to produce a severe shock, especially if the electrical resistance between the person's body and the item causing the shock is low. A good example of this is when wet hands are used to plug in, switch on, or handle electrical apparatus. Water is a conductor of electricity and this lowers the resistance between a person and whatever they are touching. The water could also get inside plugs, sockets, switches and equipment and conduct (carry) the electricity into a person. Therefore, always use dry hands to plug in, switch on or handle electrical equipment.

A further factor in the amount of electricity received by the body is the **earthing** of equipment. In outline, the function of the earth (E) cable is to carry electricity from metal parts of electrical equipment into the earth (or ground). This provides an easy route for electricity to flow and it will take this path rather than pass through the person's body and produce an electric shock. Regular and expert checking is important to detect faults likely to cause electric shocks and to ensure that the earthing circuit is functioning properly.

In the UK electricity is supplied to consumers, including hairdressing salons, in quantities which can be very dangerous, either directly by electric shock or indirectly by fire. Fuses (or circuit breakers) are deliberately placed in circuits for reasons of safety. The fuses help to prevent fires and earthing helps to prevent electric shock. Many of the accidents that occur when using electricity are simply due to thoughtlessness, carelessness or downright bad practice.

## Bad ventilation in the salon

Routine activities in the hairdressing salon produce damp, warm, contaminated (stale) air, which tends to rise to the ceiling as warm air is lighter than cooler air. The aim of a good ventilation system is to provide fresh air (i.e. less humid, cooler and with fewer micro-organisms) but without producing any draughts or low temperatures in the salon and therefore making conditions uncomfortable.

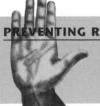

**PREVENTING RSI**

Arrange your station and your client so that you are not looking into the light, at a white wall or at a mirror which shows their reflection. The glare can be very tiring and irritating to your eyes.

### Effects on comfort

The body cooling system depends on the evaporation of sweat from the skin. In conditions of high humidity (i.e. moist air) the evaporation process is reduced so the body tends to overheat very slightly. This produces feelings of drowsiness in clients and staff, or even feelings of being uncomfortably hot, if combined with warmth.

### Effects on hygiene

One type of micro-organism (germ) is a virus, some of which attack humans and are described as **pathogenic**, e.g. cold and influenza (flu). These are mostly spread in tiny droplets of moisture which shoot out of a person's mouth and nose when they cough or sneeze. The more humid the air, the slower these droplets evaporate and the longer the viruses survive, increasing the chance of them being breathed in by other clients and staff. Bacteria also thrive in damp conditions; they are another type of micro-organism.

## Effects on hair

The major influence is due to the hair's ability to absorb water from the atmosphere – its tendency to be **hygroscopic**. The more humid the air, the more quickly this happens, so it is more difficult to carry out both wet and dry setting and blow-drying in conditions where the hair is continually reabsorbing water from humid air.

## Chemical hazards in the salon

Hairdressing operations very often involve the use of chemicals on the hair and some of them are sprayed onto the hair using pressurised containers, e.g. hair lacquers. The chemical hazards in the salon come from three main sources: chemicals getting onto the skin or into the eyes, storage and disposal, or dermatitis (eczema).

### Contact with eyes or skin

The main prevention here is to be aware of the risk involved in carrying out any hairdressing operation (even shampooing) that involves chemicals and to handle chemicals with care. Chemicals can be swallowed, especially by children, so care should be taken to put them out of reach.

Accidental spills can be avoided by replacing caps and stoppers on containers immediately after use.

Do not use **caustic soda** (sodium hydroxide) to clear blocked drains, get a plumber instead to clear the blockage. Caustic soda can cause severe skin burns.

### Storage and disposal

All salon products should be stored in well-labelled containers and not put onto high shelves; there is always a risk they will be dropped when taken down. Particular care needs to be taken with stored hydrogen peroxide and pressurised aerosol sprays. Both can explode if heated, so they should never be stored near heaters or in direct sunlight.

If a container has lost its label or the contents cannot be identified with certainty for any other reason, then dispose of it. Careful disposal of empty pressurised cans is important.

### Dermatitis (eczema)

Dermatitis involves the body overreacting to a substance to which it has been exposed. Many of the chemicals used in hairdressing may cause dermatitis, but **paraphenylenediamine** used in some tints is strongly linked to people developing dermatitis. Both the hairdresser and the client are at risk, with the hairdresser at greatest risk due to their repeated and long-term exposure to hairdressing chemicals. The client can be protected against para dye dermatitis by carrying out a skin test before going ahead with the tint. The hairdresser can be protected by using rubber gloves for any hairdressing operation that involves chemicals, including shampooing.

## Biological hazards in the salon

### Infections by micro-organisms

Infections are caused by harmful germs or, more properly, **pathogenic micro-organisms**. They can be passed between people or transmitted in the salon. Here are some common examples in the salon:

- Impetigo.
- Boils.
- Eye infections, e.g. conjunctivitis.
- Ringworm.
- Cold sores (herpes).
- Some types of wart.

It is important to be able to recognise these conditions and distinguish between the infectious or contagious complaints and the non-infectious or non-contagious conditions. Also you should know which of them prohibit hairdressing operations. Impetigo, eye infections and ringworm *definitely* mean that hairdressing operations should not start (or should stop if already started).

#### Aids and hepatitis B

Aids and hepatitis B are both very serious infections which can be transmitted by small amounts of blood or serum (clear liquid in blisters) from one person to another. The risk to hairdressers is slight. There is a useful pamphlet produced by the government's Health Department with notes for guidance. Transmission of both diseases can be avoided by using simple and routine hygiene practices, sterilisation of tools and equipment, and prevention of infection or infestation.

### Infestations by animal parasites

Infestations occur when larger animal parasites live on the body. They can be passed between people or transmitted in the salon. Here are some examples:

- Head and body lice.
- Fleas.
- Itchmites (which cause scabies).

With head lice particularly, the hairdresser can be the first person to definitely detect the presence of these parasites. In all the examples above, hairdressing operations should not start (or should stop if already begun).

## Preventing infection or infestation

1. Be able to recognise which scalp conditions are infectious or contagious and know what to do if they are.
2. Carry out routine hygiene procedures in the salon, coupled with design considerations, like the choice of wall and floor coverings, upholstery, ventilation and temperature control. Here are some examples:
   - **Between clients:** washing your hands; sterilising personal tools and equipment; cleaning shampoo basins.
   - **For each client:** preparing a clean towel (or towels) and neck strip; sterilising any tools accidentally dropped onto the floor; not keeping tools and equipment in pockets.
   - **Regular:** washing down of walls, floors, work surfaces with an alcohol-based disinfectant; sweeping up hair clippings and putting waste into a closed container.
   - **Personal routine:** not putting hairpins and clips in the mouth; wearing closed-in shoes with low heels.
   - **General:** not allowing animals in the salon; ensuring an adequate ventilation and heating system.

## Some basic first-aid procedures

First aid can be defined as 'the skilled application of accepted principles of treatment on the occurrence of any injury or sudden illness, using facilities available at the time. It is the approved method of treating a casualty until placed, if necessary, in the care of a doctor or removed to hospital' (authorised manual of St John Ambulance, St Andrews Ambulance Association, British Red Cross Society).

The best thing to do with accidents is to prevent them. However, even in the best-run salons, accidents will sometimes happen. There are also cases where events occur which are not under the control of anyone in the salon, a client suffering a heart attack for example. It is important to know what to do and the best method of learning this is to complete a first aid course. There are a number of these organised by the St John Ambulance, Red Cross, or at your local college of further education. It is an extremely good idea to have at least one trained first aider in the salon. Table 3.6.1 suggests how to put together a **first-aid kit**.

There is no real substitute for completing a proper first-aid course, but here are a few guidelines.

## Cuts

- **Minor wounds** – cover the wound as soon as possible with a sterile dressing.
- **Major wounds** – send for expert help immediately. Try to control the bleeding by pulling the sides of the wound together and hold firmly until the bleeding

**Table 3.6.1** How to put together a first-aid kit

| Item | Number of employees | | |
|---|---|---|---|
| | 1–5 | 6–10 | 11–50 |
| Card giving general first-aid guidance | 1 | 1 | 1 |
| Individually wrapped sterile, adhesive dressings | 10 | 20 | 40 |
| Sterile eye pads, with attachment | 1 | 2 | 4 |
| Triangular bandage | 1 | 2 | 4 |
| Sterile dressing for serious wounds* | 1 | 2 | 4 |
| Safety pins | 6 | 6 | 12 |
| Sterile, unmedicated wound dressings | | | |
| Medium | 3 | 6 | 8 |
| Large | 1 | 2 | 4 |
| Extra large | 1 | 2 | 4 |

*These should be provided if the triangular bandages are not sterile.

stops. Apply a pad of sterile dressings and hold in place (use disposable plastic gloves if possible). If they become soaked with blood, add more dressings.

- **Blood spills** – pour neat bleach onto the blood. Leave for a few minutes. Put on disposable plastic gloves. Wash off with a large amount of hot water containing some washing-up liquid or shampoo.

## Burns

- **Heat burns** – cool immediately under cold water. If the person is seriously burnt, send for expert medical help. If the burn is widespread, cover it with loose dressings. Do not attempt to remove clothing sticking to the burnt area.
- **Chemical burns** – wash off with plenty of cold water. Remove any clothing which may have chemical on it. Apply a sterile dressing. Refer the person to expert medical help if necessary.

## Eye injuries

- **Object in the eye** – attempt to remove the object with the moistened corner of a sterile dressing. If it cannot be removed or the eye is still painful after the object has been removed, cover with an eyepatch and quickly send the person to a hospital or a doctor.
- **Chemical in the eye** – if a chemical has run into the eye, wash it out with a large amount of cold water. Force the eye open if necessary. Cover it with an eyepad then send the person to a hospital or a doctor, or summon expert help.

## Collapse

A person may collapse from electric shock, heart attack, epileptic fit, fainting, etc. They may be partly conscious or completely unconscious. Whatever their state of consciousness, talk reassuringly to the collapsed person. They may also have knocked or cut themselves while falling.

### Electric shock

Switch off the supply. If this is not possible then use an insulator (rug, clothing, paper or plastic) to pull the person away from the source of the shock. Decide whether the shocked person is conscious or unconscious. If they are partly **conscious** then keep talking and reassuring them. Keep them warm and if they do not recover within a few minutes, send for expert medical help. If they are **unconscious** then follow these steps:

- Send immediately for expert help.
- Check their heartbeat by trying to find the pulse in the neck.
- Check their breathing by watching for breathing movements or by holding a mirror, e.g. compact lid mirror or watch glass, over their mouth and looking for misting.
- If the heart has stopped, start external cardiac massage and/or if breathing has stopped, start mouth-to-mouth resuscitation (the kiss of life).
- Continue cardiac massage and/or mouth-to-mouth resuscitation until help arrives.
- Keep talking in a reassuring manner, even if the person is unconscious.

### Heart attack

- If the person is **partly conscious** they will probably complain of chest pains (often severe). They may have some medication with them. Loosen their clothes and talk reassuringly to them. Send for expert medical help.
- If the person is **unconscious** then treat them as for electric shock.

### Epileptic fit

Epileptic fits can vary from a mild attack with only a brief loss of consciousness (much like fainting) to severe attacks involving the person becoming unconscious, going stiff and having convulsions, e.g. arms and legs twitching violently. Try to prevent them hurting themselves by protecting the head. The attack will pass. Keep talking reassuringly.

**SAFETY TIPS**

Complete a first-aid course to learn how to find the pulse and how to carry out cardiac massage and mouth-to-mouth resuscitation.

**Fainting**

Fainting can be partial or complete. If **partial**, the person will feel faint but will not be unconscious. Put their head between their knees or lie them down with their feet raised above their head. Loosen tight clothing. Keep them warm and supply fresh air. If they have fainted fully and are **unconscious**, lie them down with their feet raised above their head. Loosen their clothing and keep them warm. They should recover rapidly, but if not then summon expert medical help.

## Security in the salon

The key is to prevent theft of money, stock and people's belongings. Salons will have their own security arrangements and policies on, for example, what to do if a member of staff is caught pilfering. Crime prevention officers can give valuable help on the physical security and the management of security for people and premises.

### Security audits

Security audits are regular reviews of the security of the salon, open and closed. Team involvement is important as team members can:

- See security being taken seriously.
- Contribute a variety of views and ideas.

When staff can see that security is being taken seriously, it may reassure the honest and deter the dishonest. A good approach is to consider how the premises could be broken into, and how stock and money could be stolen. When can someone steal unobserved? Put yourself in the place of someone intending to steal.

### Stock control procedures

Stock control procedures (Unit 3.5) are very important in the prevention of security problems. They are needed to cross-check what has been used, how much money has been taken and by whom.

## Things to do

Good hygiene and safety practices are essential in any working environment and great care must always be taken when dealing with any potentially hazardous tools, chemicals or equipment. The following tasks have been devised to help you become aware of any potential dangers and the precautions that can be taken to ensure your salon is a safe place for you and your clients.

1. (a) Use your workplace or training salon to identify any items or situations which could be a safety hazard.

   (b) Make a chart listing the potentially hazardous items or situations together with any precautions which could minimise the risk to health and safety. Use the following layout for your chart:

   | Item/situation | Precautions |
   | --- | --- |
   | Frayed electrical wires | Check all wires before using any electrical equipment. Rewire if necessary |

2. Find out from your salon employment or work placement the procedure in case of fire on the premises. Design a bright, noticeable poster for display in the salon staffroom which illustrates the risks of fire and your own salon's procedure should a fire occur. The poster should be on A4 paper of any colour using whatever medium or combination of mediums you consider suitable, e.g. paint, pastels, ink, collage.

3. Carry out a case study on the security arrangements of a salon. Include stock, money, people's possessions, prevention of break-ins when the salon is closed. Suggest where improvements could be made.

## What do you know?

- List the **three** major groups of hazards to which a client or hairdresser may be exposed.

- Give **two** reasons for regularly cleaning the salon.

- List the **regulations** of particular importance to the salon.

- Why is it necessary to **unplug** electrical apparatus before cleaning?

- What **two** types of accident are particularly linked to using electrical apparatus?

- What is the **first** action if a chemical has run onto the skin or into the eyes?

- What **precautions** need to be taken in the use, storage and disposal of aerosol spray cans?

- What is the **difference** between infection and infestation?

- How in particular can a **hairdresser** avoid dermatitis?

- Name **three** dangers linked to trailing electrical flexes.

# Unit

# 7

In this unit you will learn about:

- Planning commercial, avant-garde and fantasy hairstyles and images.
- How to carry out research into your chosen area or image.
- Combining different techniques to create a total look.
- Making use of additional materials such as added hair, make-up, ornamentation and clothes.
- Presenting your final images.
- The importance of effective communication skills.
- Styling hair for special occasions.
- Planning a photographic session and hair show.

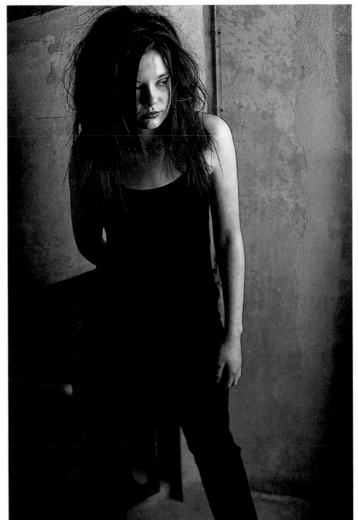

Plassey Hair Studio, Wrexham

# Creating images

## Creating images

One of the most exciting aspects of hairdressing is being able to express yourself creatively. Unfortunately, unless you work in an avant-garde salon, a lot of the day-to-day styling will be of a more mundane, commercial nature and it is only the occasional client who will allow experimentation or alternative styling on their hair.

However, creativity is the lifeblood of the hairdressing industry; without creativity, fashions would never change and new techniques would never be born. Keeping your own creativity alive and actively encouraging staff members to work imaginatively promotes an enthusiastic team spirit and is also good for business. Most of the images fall into three broad categories:

- **Commercial** – popular styles that form most of a stylist's work.
- **Avant-garde** – styles that exaggerate a commercial style or are genuine innovations that will set a fashion trend.
- **Fantasy** – totally outlandish and imaginative, these styles would seldom be worn by a client under normal circumstances. They are often based on a theme and may be used to promote the salon image.

There are various opportunities that allow stylists and junior staff to practise and use their creative skills, including photographic work, staging a hair show, styling hair for special occasions and competition work.

## Created images

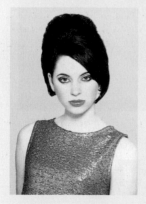 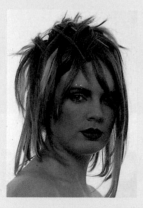 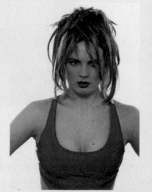 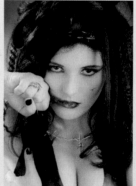

Examples of a 1960s style, avant-garde looks (also used as a promotional image) and a fantasy image
Goldwell (left), Plassey Hair Studio, Wrexham (centre images), hair by Steve Johnson, make-up by Katherine for Peter West (right)

## Photographic work

Photography for promotional purposes is a specialist skill, so unless you are a very keen amateur photographer it is much better to engage an expert. Organising a photographic shoot takes careful planning and many hours of preparation, therefore it is very upsetting, and indeed too late, if after the event the pictures taken do not turn out or are not what you wanted.

Styling hair for photographic work requires imagination and often problem-solving skills too. The idea is to create an image, and besides the commercial styles, the image can be fantasy, avant-garde or for a special occasion such as a wedding. It all depends on the type of salon image you want to portray and what you are trying to achieve through the publicity it will generate.

## Doing the planning

**A design plan helps you organise**

- Think of a theme.
- Research your ideas.
- Check for any budgetary constraints.
- Write up your ideas and include photographs or sketches.
- Talk over your ideas and show your plan to colleagues.
- Amend your plan if necessary.

**Carry out some research**

Look for ideas on your ideas. Use libraries, trade journals, magazines, television and film. If you have access to a computer, try looking on the Web for information. Talk to friends and colleagues about your ideas; this can easily spark off even more ideas.

**Plan a session checklist**

1. Decide on the look and the purpose of the photographs. Remember that any photographs can also be used as a training aid for other staff members.
2. Sketch out your ideas and make notes; this will give you your **design plan**. Looking at other photographs in fashion magazines often generates ideas. Note the angle and background of the shots, it will help you decide which may be the most effective for your own work.
3. Decide on the model to use. It is a good idea to use other staff members, particularly junior members if possible, as this generates a team spirit and is also a good learning experience for them. It is surprising how much they will learn through helping or just being there.
4. Practise the styles beforehand. Use gels, waxes, lacquers or even sugar and water to create the look you want; remember that it is an illusion you are creating and the style does not have to last. If it is only a front view then it does not matter what the back of the head looks like.

5. Make sure that the model's clothes and make-up create a total look with the hairstyle.
6. Make a list of who is responsible for what and discuss it with them.
7. Work out a schedule for the photographic shoot. Be organised; a photographer's time costs money, so have everything prepared and ready when they arrive. And finally, always allow for the session taking much longer than you thought.

## Carrying out a photo session

### Choosing the model

The model, Fleur, was chosen first and her slight build inspired a fairy theme. The whole look – hair, make-up, clothes and background props – was then built around this theme.

## Created images

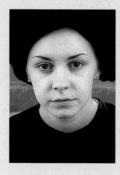 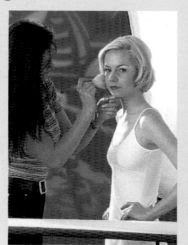 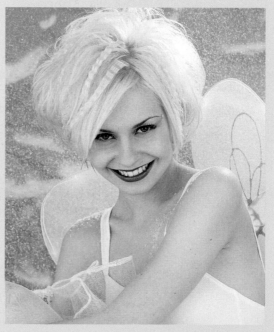

At the beginning of the session the model's hair is bleached very light blonde to go with the snowy, fairy look to be achieved. Make-up is applied before dressing the hair. Pale foundation and very blue eye make-up are used to complement the 'white and blue' colour scheme and a small silver star is placed at the corner of the eyebrow to mirror the illusion of ice and snow. The hair is then dressed with plenty of volume with random sections of hair crimped with the crimping irons to give added volume and interest. The tips of the hair around the face have been lightly tipped with blue mascara paints. Artificial snow is sprinkled onto the shoulders and wings of the fairy just before the shoot.

Hair by Steve Johnson, make-up by Katherine for Peter West

**Session checklist**

1. Arrive early to set everything up and get the model organised and ready.
2. Make sure that the background for the photographs is suitable. Does it contrast with the hair colour? A dark background does not work with a black-haired model.
3. Make sure the lighting is adequate and make sure there is additional lighting in case you should need it.
4. Always take lots of photographs (Fig. 3.7.1). When they are developed, you will find that many shots will be unsuitable for one reason or another.
5. For future reference, keep a record of how the shoot was planned and carried out. Evaluate what went well and what did not work; this will help you to improve future sessions.

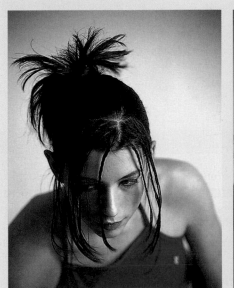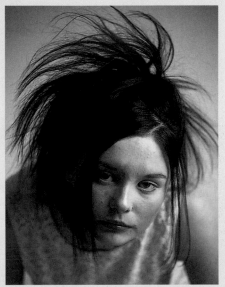

Plassey Hair Studio, Wrexham

**Fig. 3.7.1** These avant-garde shots can be used on promotional materials or as framed photographs in the salon.

**After the session**

If the shoot has gone well, you will have lots of photographs to choose from. Which ones you choose will depend on the image you want to project to the public.

## After the photo shoot

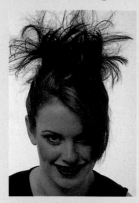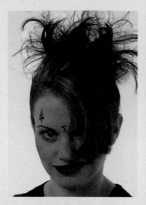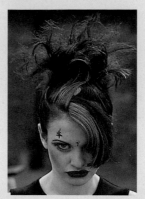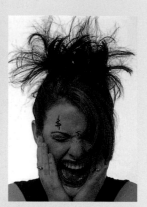

If the shoot has gone well, you will have lots of photographs to choose from. Which ones you choose will depend on the image you want to project to the public. You can choose a demure look, be sultry, bad, or add face paint and scream!

Plassey Hair Studio, Wrexham

## Staging a hair show

A hair show is a very useful team-building and staff development exercise. It is also a very efficient method of promoting the salon and gaining additional clients. Even those clients satisfied with the work of their present salon will be more likely to consider your salon should they ever wish a change. Unit 3.10 gives more detail on the organisation and planning for a hair show.

### Effective communication skills

#### Communication with colleagues

Talk to your colleagues and actively listen to what they say; this can generate more ideas and create a team spirit.

#### Communication with your audience

Pay attention to what you say and how you say it. Photographs are a form of non-verbal communication that tell the client what type of salon you are. How you present your hair show, both verbally and visually, can increase your business, enhance your salon's image and show your professionalism.

### Using themes within a hair show

You can use a theme within a hair show to give a dramatic effect and act as a contrast to the more commercial styles you may be showing. The following ideas show how other materials such as props, make-up, clothes, ornamentation and added hair are used to give a total look.

### The devil

The simplest props can be very effective to create an avant-garde look. Black leather jacket, red horns and pitchfork are enough to suggest the devil (Fig. 3.7.2).

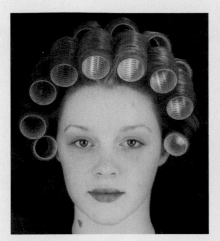
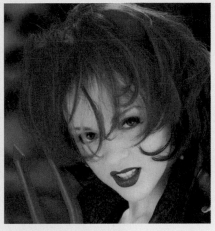

Hair by Steve Johnson, make-up by Katherine for Peter West

**Fig. 3.7.2** The model's hair is dry set on large rollers. The finished effect shows that a fine fringe section has been bleached yellow. The red flame effects on the front of the hair have been painted on with washout hair mascara.

### Vampire

The model for 'the devil' has now been given a vampire look (Fig. 3.7.3). The set is built from trees with an old papier mâché cross borrowed from a local school together with a gravestone. The teeth were specially made to create the right effect.

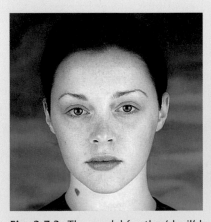
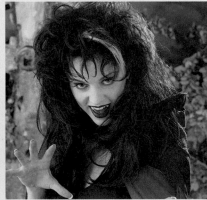

Hair by Steve Johnson, make-up by Katherine for Peter West

**Fig. 3.7.3** The model for the 'devil' has now been given a vampire look. A long, dark hairpiece has been added with an extra piece of white hair at the front as a streak. A black and red cloak is worn and the make-up is very dramatic, particularly the eyes and the blood-red mouth.

### Soldier Girl

The soldier idea came from the film *GI Jane*. It took almost four hours to paint the body. The hair is simple to give focus to the body paint (Fig. 3.7.4).

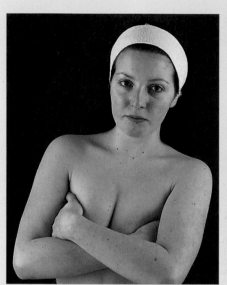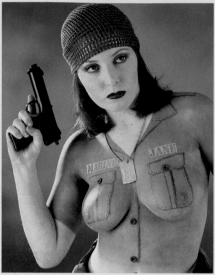

Hair by Steve Johnson, make-up by Katherine for Peter West

**Fig. 3.7.4** The model's upper body has been realistically painted; the neck tag and gun reinforce the soldier image. The net scarf makes a suitable hair ornamentation.

## Styling hair for special occasions

Special occasions allow the stylist to be creative. Very often ornamentation will also be used to allow more creativity and enhance the final dressing. The most common special occasion is a wedding.

### Bridal hairstyling

Because a wedding day is considered so important, it is essential that any ornamentation forms part of the client's total look, together with the hairstyle and the dress. This applies to all the members of the wedding party but in particular the bride and the bridesmaids. It is also important to plan carefully beforehand to ensure the ornamentation is suitable and to the client's liking. When creating the bride's hairstyle, consider:

- Hair type and length.
- Style of dress.
- Other accessories.
- Client personality.

**Checklist**

- Ask about all other accessories: headdress, type of veil, flowers, etc.
- Find out the style of the wedding dress: Victorian, Edwardian, Pre-Raphàelite, modern, etc.
- Research styles that are in keeping with the dress.
- Encourage a practice run.
- Organise any cutting, perming or tinting of the hair *before* the big day.
- Leave plenty of time when scheduling the appointment.
- If styling the hair in the bride's home, leave plenty of time as the house is usually chaotic.

## Competition work

Competition work stretches practical ability, giving more confidence to try out new techniques and ideas. Local colleges and the National Hairdressing Federation (NHF) usually hold local hairdressing competitions which have different events for all levels of experience. Encouraging junior staff members to enter these competitions helps to foster a culture of creativity within the salon right from the beginning.

Competition styling is often quite different from commercial styling, particularly at a more experienced level. It is the opportunity to show off artistic ability and therefore may have little to do with commercial wearability.

### Planning competition work

Planning, preparation and practice, then even more practice, is the secret of successful competition work. The following suggestions are by no means complete but they could help the novice competition worker:

1. Attend some competitions before entering them. This will give an insight into what is expected. Look carefully at the winning heads, and take photographs to give you ideas of the types of hairstyles.
2. Choose a suitable model. They should have good bone structure and an oval face shape as this suits most hairstyles. The texture of the hair should be manageable, neither too thick nor too thin. But most importantly of all, the model must have the time for practice sessions and be willing to be adventurous with their hair colour and shape.
3. Decide on the competition to be entered; look through trade magazines then sketch out various ideas to try out.
4. Make out a time schedule for practice sessions and preparing the hair. Work back from the competition date. You will need time to practise the style, colour the hair and cut it. Hair for competition work should not be soft and silky as this is more difficult to work on, therefore it will need time to settle after the tint or bleach, but if tinted too soon there will be a regrowth.

5. Decide on the type of clothes and make-up to be worn by the model. The clothing should be suitable for the occasion and must also complement the colour and style of the hair. Do not choose an outfit with a collar or high neckline as this could disturb the hair at the nape of the neck.

## Designing and producing the style

1. Wet the hair then mould it in different directions until the style evolves. Shorter hair is easier to manage unless the competition stipulates that it must be long hair. Draw the style in detail, on paper, how it was done, otherwise you may forget how you did it.
2. Set or blow-dry the hair, depending on the type of competition, in the direction of the final dressing. Make a note on the drawing of any alterations you have made.
3. Once the style is decided upon, cut the hair to accentuate the shape. This may mean razor cutting or thinning out any unwanted bulk in the hair, but remember that the model must be able to wear it commercially afterwards.
4. Redo the hair and take a note of how long it takes. The competition will have a time limit, so time yourself when practising.
5. Keep practising the style until you know exactly where each hair is going and until you are able to keep within the time limit. This stage will usually take weeks not days.
6. Decide on how the hair is to be coloured or bleached. Bleached hair is often easier to work on for competitions. The colours used should emphasise the movements of the style and it is worth noting that lighter, brighter colours show the hair off to its best advantage on the competition floor.
7. Have a final dress rehearsal the day before the competition to make sure there is time to carry out any alterations to clothing or make-up. On the day, leave plenty of time to reach the venue, take lots of photos of your work and enjoy yourself.

## Using added hair

Using additional hair and hairpieces can make natural hair appear longer, thicker, or almost instantly different depending on how, why and when they are used (see page 435).

Hair extensions are a popular type of added hair. Made from synthetic fibre or real hair, they are woven onto the client's natural hair either throughout the head or just where they are needed. For example, on extremely short hair which is clipper cut at the back, the client may only require the extensions at the front.

### Hair extensions

Hair extensions are a specialised service and they are very time-consuming. Small sections of hair are sectioned off and long strands of synthetic fibre are woven into them. The extension is then sealed onto the hair with heat. This is one of the reasons why synthetic fibres are used in preference to human hair; they can be melted with heat and fused together, so the hairpiece can be attached more securely. If the hairpiece is made of real hair, it is woven into the natural hair; no heat is used.

Extensions should remain in the hair until they grow out. Harsh brushing or tugging on the hair will loosen the fibre, so the client must be given the correct after-care advice to look after their extensions properly. An extension for Afro-Caribbean hair is shown in Fig. 3.7.5.

## Hairpieces

Hairpieces were at their most popular during the 1960s and the 1970s but they are still useful today for special occasions, photographic work or show work.

They are available in various hair lengths and sizes. Their base can be hand woven or machine woven, or it can be hand knotted. Most types of hairpiece can be obtained in synthetic hair or human hair and the price will depend on the quality.

When using hairpieces, remember to select the most suitable type of hairpiece for the effect you wish to achieve (Fig. 3.7.6). Postiche is like natural hair in that you can only work within the confines of what you have. Thus, if the client requires a plait then the hairpiece must have enough length to achieve this effect.

Set or blow-dry the hairpiece on a headform or malleable block. If the piece is made of synthetic fibre then follow the manufacturer's instructions as the fibres will usually melt if any kind of heat is used.

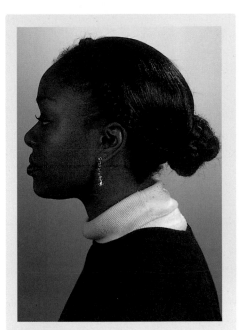

**Fig. 3.7.5** Extension enables hair to appear longer than it is

### Attaching a hairpiece

- Brush or comb the hair in the direction of the style.
- Decide on the position of the hairpiece on the head then section off a square section of hair in the centre of this position, curl it round in a pincurl and secure it with two crossed hairgrips.
- If the base of the hairpiece has a comb, push it under the grips to hold it firm.
- Use hairgrips to attach the hairpiece to the scalp, taking care not to harm the base.
- Backcomb or backbrush the client's hair if needed then blend the hair with the hairpiece, making sure its base is camouflaged.
- Advise the client on the care of the hairpiece and demonstrate how it is attached and removed.

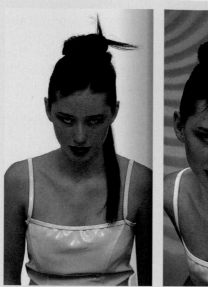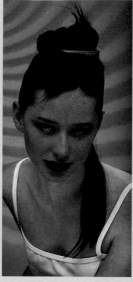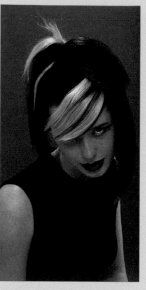

Plassey Hair Studio, Wrexham

**Fig. 3.7.6** Take one model and three hairpieces to create three different looks in no time at all!

## Things to do

1. Collect pictures and photographs of creative styles.

   Separate them under three headings, commercial, avant-garde and fantasy. Mount them on plain paper under those headings. Keep them for future reference and as a teaching aid for junior staff.

2. You are asked by your salon manager to organise a photographic shoot. The purpose of the event is to market your salon's new range of hair products. The manager wishes to see a layout of your plan and your ideas before it is implemented. The following stages may help you to organise the shoot:

   (a) Identify a suitable time and venue which will cause the minimum inconvenience and disruption to normal working practice. Decide who is to take the photographs.

   (b) Make a list of objectives – what you are hoping to achieve from the event.

   (c) Write out a memo to inform the staff involved; give them enough time to organise their schedules and to practise any hairstyles they need to.

   (d) Contact all models who may be required and have a back-up in case of emergencies.

   (e) Make sure all resources and equipment are available and in working order on the date required.

   (f) Discuss with other staff members what incentives, if any, can be used to bring additional trade to the salon through the event.

   (g) Plan how you will evaluate the effectiveness of the event.

## What do you know?

- Explain what is meant by an **avant-garde** hairstyle.
- Briefly describe how you would create a **design plan** for a photographic session.
- List **three** sources of information where you could research ideas and themes.
- Give **five** points you could include on a checklist before a photographic shoot.
- What additional materials (media) can you use to create a **total** look?

- Why is it beneficial to include **junior** staff members in promotional activities?
- Why is it important to **plan** any event?
- How do good **communication** skills help the salon?
- What considerations are necessary when **choosing a model** for competition styling?
- What **four** points should you consider when styling hair for a bride?

In this unit you will learn about:

- Differences between Caucasian and Afro-Caribbean hair.
- Styling hair using thermal (heat) techniques.
- The tools and equipment needed to thermally style the hair.
- Testing and preparing hair.
- Identifying possible problems and their solutions.
- Corrective relaxing treatments.
- Working safely and efficiently.

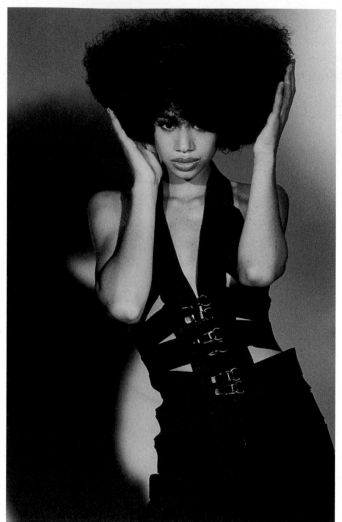

Sabre Europe

# Afro-Caribbean styling

## Straightening Afro-Caribbean hair

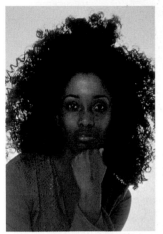

Goldwell

Straightening can be either permanent or temporary. Permanent straightening is known as relaxing and is covered in detail in Unit 2.5b. Temporary straightening can be carried out on wet or dry hair but it needs some form of heat to be successful. The two main methods of temporarily straightening hair are:

- Wet setting: blow-drying, roller setting, etc.
- Dry setting.

Dry setting means pulling the hair straighter using pressing combs and then curling with heated curling tongs, marcel waving irons, hot brushes or heated rollers.

**POINTS TO REMEMBER**

### Afro-Caribbean hair

The main difference between Afro-Caribbean hair and European (Caucasian) hair is that while European hair is either fine, medium or coarse textured, the texture of Afro-Caribbean hair varies along the actual hair shaft (Fig. 3.8.1). This results in an uneven porosity along the length of each individual hair, which creates special problems when chemicals are applied. Extra care and thought are essential before and during the treatment of Afro-Caribbean hair to prevent damage and/or breakage to the weaker and more porous areas.

The degree of curl in this type of hair also differs from that of most European hair. Afro-Caribbean hair has a very diffuse hair growth direction pattern which makes it difficult to manage as it does not fall in uniform waves. It is usually extremely dry and brittle, which means it can easily be broken during combing or when using heated appliances. Both the hair and the scalp should be kept well oiled and supple through the use of conditioners, oils and waxes. Because of the excess dryness, specialised products containing ingredients such as protein, lanolin, natural and mineral oils are more effective than the conditioning agents formulated for European hair.

The anagen stage of Afro-Caribbean hair growth may last only nine to ten months and the growth rate is also often slower, therefore Afro-Caribbean hair is considered to be long if it is 18–20 cm (7–8 in). However, because of its tightly coiled nature the hair usually appears shorter than it actually is. The amount of curl present in the hair will depend on hereditary factors, e.g. African hair is very curly whereas Guyanese hair is merely curly.

When permanently changing the shape of Afro-Caribbean hair (curling or straightening), the same structural alteration takes place as in European hair, i.e. breaking sufficient chemical bonds within the hair and rejoining them in a new shape. However, specialised Afro-Caribbean straighteners are very strong and could easily dissolve the hair if not used correctly.

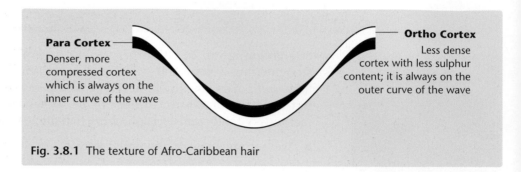

**Para Cortex** — Denser, more compressed cortex which is always on the inner curve of the wave

**Ortho Cortex** — Less dense cortex with less sulphur content; it is always on the outer curve of the wave

**Fig. 3.8.1** The texture of Afro-Caribbean hair

## Thermal styling

Thermal styling is the term used for styling the hair using heat. Unless the hair has been permanently straightened, this usually involves straightening the hair before curling it into style. Afro-Caribbean hair can be temporarily straightened by blow-drying using a wide-toothed comb attachment fitted to the nozzle of the hair dryer or by using a pressing comb (Fig. 3.8.2).

### How it works

Some of the water found naturally in the cortex is turned into steam by the heat of the dryer or pressing comb. This steam breaks some of the weaker hydrogen cross-linkages. The cross-linkages reform themselves in their new, straightened positions as the hair cools. The greater the heat used on the hair, the more bonds are broken. If the equipment is too cool then the straightening will not last, but if it is too hot then the hair may be burned or singed. Chemically treated hair has bonds

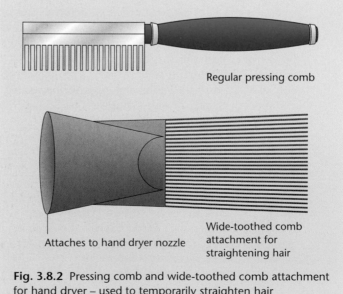

Regular pressing comb

Attaches to hand dryer nozzle

Wide-toothed comb attachment for straightening hair

**Fig. 3.8.2** Pressing comb and wide-toothed comb attachment for hand dryer – used to temporarily straighten hair

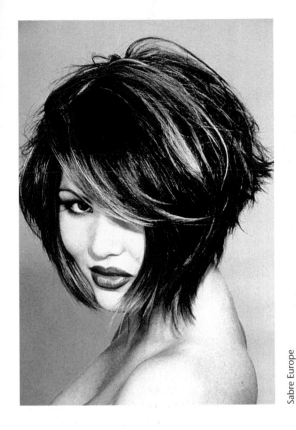

Sabre Europe

which will break more easily, so extra care must be taken when dealing with this type of hair.

There are two main ways of temporarily straightening Afro-Caribbean hair using heat:

- **Soft pressing** – sometimes referred to as single-comb pressing, this is straightening the hair with the pressing comb once all over the head. It will remove 70 per cent of the curl.

- **Hard pressing** – this is straightening the hair twice with the pressing comb. Compared with soft pressing, twice the amount of heat is applied and this makes it unsuitable for more fragile hair. Hard pressing is sometimes known as double-comb pressing.

## Tools and equipment

- Pressing combs of various sizes.
- Electric or gas heater (unless the pressing combs are electrically heated).
- Vulcanite comb.
- Protective pressing cream or oil.
- Finishing oils or waxes.
- Heated curling tongs.
- Hot brushes.
- Heated rollers.

## Preparation

- Carry out a client consultation to determine their needs and the final effect.
- Protect the client with gown and towels.
- Carry out a thorough hair and scalp analysis. Note the hair texture, condition and curl pattern.
- Check the hair and scalp for contra-indications.
- Carry out porosity and elasticity tests on the hair.
- If the hair is in poor condition, recommend a course of deep conditioning treatments and postpone pressing until the hair is stronger and more supple.
- Assemble any tools and equipment.
- Shampoo the hair with a suitable shampoo then dry.

## Contra-indications

Do not straighten the hair by pressing if:

- There are any infectious or contagious conditions present.
- There are major cuts and scratches or sores on the scalp.
- The hair is in a fragile state or hair breakage is present.
- The hair is excessively porous or highly bleached.
- The client has a headache, as the pulling action when tension is applied could be unbearable for the client.

**SAFETY TIPS**

Excessive heat on the hair can cause scorching and loss of colour or maybe discoloration.

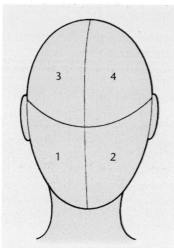

**Fig. 3.8.3** Sectioning hair for soft pressing

## Soft pressing

1. Prepare the client as above.
2. Divide the hair into four sections (Fig. 3.8.3).
3. Starting at the nape, take a 1.25 cm ($\frac{1}{2}$ in) section of hair and apply oil or conditioning cream to the section. Lift the hair away from the scalp at 90° using index finger and thumb.
4. Check the heat of the pressing comb on some tissue paper then insert the pressing comb teeth into the hair section 1.25 cm ($\frac{1}{2}$ in) away from the scalp.
5. Slide the comb down the hair mesh, turning it so the back of the comb is positioned on top of the hair section. The angle of the comb is very important as it is the back of the comb which creates the tension and actually straightens the hair (Fig. 3.8.4).
6. Comb each section two or three times in this manner until the hair is straight.
7. Continue towards the front of the head taking 1.25 cm ($\frac{1}{2}$ in) sections until the whole head has been completed.
8. Apply dressing cream or oil to the hair and brush thoroughly.
9. Style the hair with curling tongs, hot brush or heated rollers (Fig. 3.8.5).
10. Complete a record of work and advise the client on the care of their hairstyle, including any preparations that would help the condition of the hair and maintain the style for longer.

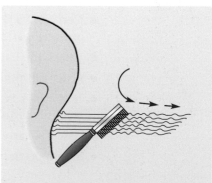

**Fig. 3.8.4** Straightening hair with the pressing comb

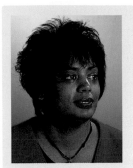

**Fig. 3.8.5** Soft pressed and thermally styled hair

## Hard pressing

Hard pressing will remove almost all the curl but will also weaken the hair, so great caution is needed when carrying out this service. Proceed as for soft pressing then either repeat the process or restraighten using heated curling tongs.

## Touching up

Hair is hygroscopic, and because the heat from the pressing comb has removed most of the hair's natural moisture from the cortex, any water or dampness in the atmosphere will make the hair revert back to its previous curly state. What is known as touch-up pressing of the unwanted curly parts of the hairstyle is done if this occurs.

Touching up is carried out, between shampoos, to prolong the life of the pressing by restraightening any part of the hair which has reverted back to its curly state through water or atmospheric moisture. Sometimes it is only the roots, or a small area, which will require touching up, in which case a spot touch-up is all that is required. If a larger area requires restraightening, then the same procedure as for soft pressing is followed but the shampooing stage is omitted.

## Effects on hair

- Has a drying effect on the hair as the heat from the equipment evaporates the moisture in the hair.

## POINTS TO REMEMBER

The oil based products used before pressing or applying heat to the hair contain **silicones** and **long-chain hydrocarbons**.

- Provides the client with looser movement in the hair.
- The protective oils give a coating to the hair and add shine (Fig. 3.8.6).

## Initial considerations

- Check that the hair is strong enough to withstand the tension and heat needed during the process.
- Coarse hair is often the most difficult to press and will need the most heat, medium textured hair responds well to pressing, and fine hair requires less pressure and a lower heat as it could break or burn more easily.
- Bleached, tinted or porous hair needs special attention. Use a lower heat and less pressure on this type of hair. It may be necessary to condition and moisturise the hair beforehand.

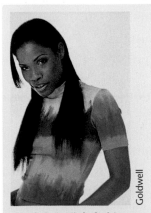

Goldwell

**Fig. 3.8.6** High-fashion, avant-garde styling

- Take care not to discolour grey or white hair. Use a lower heat if necessary.
- Always use oil-based products on the hair before pressing. This will lubricate the hair, make it more pliable and help to prevent burning and scorching.
- During the process, make sure that the back of the comb is pulled along the top of the hair section as it is this part of the comb which smooths and straightens the hair.
- Make sure that enough tension is used on the hair to make it straight.
- Advise the client that pressing is a temporary means of straightening hair and will only last between seven and ten days. Any dampness in the atmosphere will cause the hair to revert back to its curly state.
- Always use a dressing cream or oil after the process to replace some of the natural oils and give the hair shine.
- Advise the client on the after-care of their hair. Hairsprays, oils and gloss will all help to protect the hair from the effect of atmospheric moisture, prolonging the life of the pressing.

**POINTS TO REMEMBER**    If the hair is burnt or singed during the thermal styling process, nothing can repair it.

## Health and safety

- Make sure the client is well protected.
- All tools and equipment should be in good working order and only used for their intended purpose.
- Before using any electrical equipment, check the date when it was last tested and do a visual examination for any damage, loose wires or loose connections.
- Use protective products on the hair to help prevent burning.
- Test hot, non-electrical equipment such as tongs and pressing combs on tissue paper before using on the hair.
- Always assess the hair and scalp thoroughly before pressing the hair; carry out any necessary tests before starting the treatment.
- Take all necessary precautions to avoid burning the client's skin, particularly if the hair is short. Be aware of health and safety at all times.
- Clean all tools and equipment after use. The oils used on the hair tend to burn onto the pressing comb and other electrical equipment. This causes a build-up if they are not removed after each service and it makes the equipment less efficient.

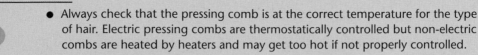

**SAFETY TIPS**

- Always check that the pressing comb is at the correct temperature for the type of hair. Electric pressing combs are thermostatically controlled but non-electric combs are heated by heaters and may get too hot if not properly controlled.
- Great care must be taken not to touch the scalp or skin with the hot comb or burning will occur.
- Do not attempt to straighten very short hair as there is a danger of burning the scalp and skin.

## Relaxing hair

Relaxing is permanently straightening hair through chemical processes (Fig. 3.8.7). What happens to hair and the methods used are covered in detail in Unit 2.5b. Relaxing is done to remove curl or to reduce the degree of curl. If a relaxing process needs to be corrected, the following factors must be taken into consideration:

- Hair condition and strength.
- Scalp sensitivity.
- Sequence of application.
- Temperature and time.

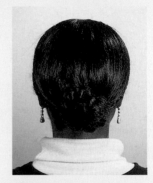

**Fig. 3.8.7** Relaxed hair, styled with hair extension

**POINTS TO REMEMBER**

### The relaxing process

Calcium hydroxide, potassium hydroxide or sodium hydroxide are the chemicals used to relax hair; sodium hydroxide is the one most commonly used. They are extremely alkaline with a pH of between 10 and 14 and can therefore cause a great deal of damage to the hair if not used correctly and in strict accordance with the manufacturer's instructions. It is also important to use the correct neutralising shampoo for the relaxing agent otherwise there could be an adverse reaction between the chemicals used. Unlike perming, which is a reduction followed by an oxidation, relaxing occurs through **hydrolysis.** This is a complicated process and is detailed in Unit 2.5b.

Because of the damage that can be caused by relaxing agents, it is very important that a porosity test, elasticity test and pre-perm test are carried out before starting the treatment to make sure that the hair can withstand the chemicals. The tests will also give some idea of the development time and the strength of relaxer to use. An incompatibility test may also need to be carried out if the client has been treating their own hair with unknown chemicals. These unknown chemicals could contain metallic salts which might react with the relaxing agent. If there is any doubt, do not proceed with the relaxing treatment. A selection of possible problems, their causes and their remedies is given in Table 3.8.1.

## Protecting the client

Relaxer creams are extremely strong chemicals so it is very important to protect the client and their clothing (Fig. 3.8.8). Here are some guidelines:

- Protect the client's clothing with a gown and towel tucked well down at the neck.
- Pin a piece of polythene to hair at the nape; the polythene covers the neck and gives extra protection.
- Protect the skin with petroleum jelly, known as **base cream**.
- Read the manufacturer's instructions regarding **basing** and **development** times.
- Take elasticity, porosity and test cuttings of the hair before treatment.
- Condition the hair before and after treatment.
- Work safely with an awareness of your responsibilities under health and safety legislation and the COSHH Regulations.

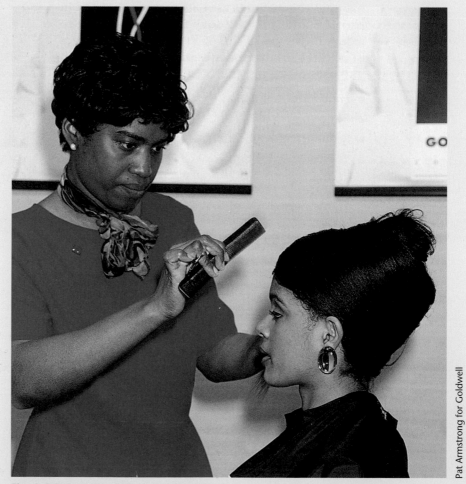

**Fig. 3.8.8** Dressing African Caribbean hair

Pat Armstrong for Goldwell

## Basing method

Section the hair into four, forehead to nape then ear to ear across the back. Take small sections of hair and press the cream onto the scalp; be careful not to rub or spread the cream else it could coat the hair and form a barrier. The client's body heat melts the cream, enabling it to cover all the scalp.

**Table 3.8.1** Some problems

| Problem | Cause and remedy |
|---|---|
| Hair reverts back to curly | • Oily barrier on the hair<br>• Relaxer too weak<br>• Product is off, not correctly sealed after use<br>*Remedy: Condition and test hair for elasticity and strength. Re-relax if the hair is strong enough* |
| Hair breakage | • Too much tension while developing<br>• Relaxer too strong<br>• Development too long<br>• Hair in poor condition<br>*Remedy: Condition and moisturise hair thoroughly with specialised products. Hair may need cutting* |
| Appearance of orange bands on the hair | • Overlapping of relaxer onto previously relaxed hair – hair will break<br>*Remedy: Condition and moisturise thoroughly with specialised products* |
| Skin irritation or burns | • Not enough basing cream applied to skin<br>• Relaxer in contact with skin<br>*Remedy: Rinse thoroughly in plenty of water. Apply neutralising shampoo to counteract alkalinity. Seek medical aid* |
| Hair very dry and brittle | • No pre-perm treatment used<br>• Relaxer too strong<br>• Not conditioned enough after treatment<br>*Remedy: Condition and moisturise thoroughly using specialised products* |
| Relaxer enters eye | • Not rinsing at backwash<br>• Sloppy application<br>*Remedy: Rinse thoroughly in plenty of water. Seek medical aid* |
| Trying to perm relaxed hair | • The perm will not take<br>• The hair gets badly damaged<br>*Remedy: Don't do it!* |

## Partial and corrective relaxing

Partial relaxing is often done on shorter hair, particularly men's hair, when only the longer top layers of the hair need to be straightened (Fig. 3.8.9). However, you may also have to carry out partial relaxing as a corrective treatment. For a corrective treatment, always follow these guidelines:

- Carry out a full hair and scalp analysis.
- Test, test and test the hair to make sure it has enough strength for the treatment.
- Use deep conditioning treatments and protective products before the treatment.
- Find out exactly what has been used on the hair and everything you can about the previous treatment.
- Postpone the treatment if you have any doubts.

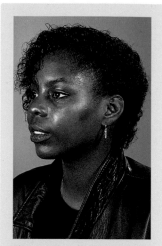

**Fig. 3.8.9** Following partial or corrective relaxing the hair still retains some curl

### Method

1. Carry out a hair and scalp analysis and any necessary tests. Consult with the client to determine their requirements.
2. If all tests are satisfactory, proceed with the relaxing treatment.
3. Protect the client with gown and towels. Protect yourself with rubber gloves and plastic or tinting apron. Apply protective cream around the hairline and scalp if necessary (follow manufacturer's instructions).
4. Apply barrier cream or conditioner to the hair that is to be left untreated as this will protect it from the relaxer. A strip of cotton wool may also be placed over this hair as an added barrier.
5. Do not shampoo the hair unless heavily coated in oils and waxes. Apply pre-perm treatment if necessary to the hair to be relaxed. Cut the hair after the treatment when it will be more manageable.
6. Starting with the underneath hair, take sections of 1.25 cm ($\frac{1}{2}$ in). Place relaxing cream on the back of the gloved hand for ease of access. Apply relaxer to the hair section, 1.25 cm ($\frac{1}{2}$ in) from the scalp with either a tinting brush or tail comb.
7. When application is complete, cross-check the hair to ensure an even coverage. Leave it to develop according to the manufacturer's instructions. Do not be tempted to leave the relaxer in contact with the hair longer than the recommended time or it could be irreparably damaged.
8. When processed, comb through the hair gently. Then rinse thoroughly, at a back wash, in warm water using the force of the water to remove the relaxer. Handle the hair as little as possible at this point as it is in a fragile state.
9. Apply the correct acidic neutralising shampoo to neutralise the alkalinity of the relaxer. Follow manufacturer's instructions as it may be necessary to shampoo the hair two or three times. Do not rub the hair, use effleurage stroking movements to minimise any tangling or damage. Rinse thoroughly.
10. Apply conditioning or moisturising agent. This may need to be left in contact with the hair for five to ten minutes. Remove and blot the hair gently; it is important not to rub the hair at any stage of the process.
11. Cut and style into shape as required. Advise the client on the after-care of their hair. Complete a record card.

## Health and safety

- Carry out all relevant tests before beginning the relaxing.
- Wait at least 72 hours after tinting to relax the hair.
- Leave braided hair unbraided for at least a week before relaxing.
- Do not relax the hair if there are cuts and abrasions on the scalp.
- If hair needs re-relaxing, do not carry out the second application within one week of the first and always test the hair to make sure it can withstand a further treatment.
- Do not relax the hair if there is any breakage present. Once you agree to treat the hair, any breakage (including the previous breakage) becomes your salon's responsibility.

- Do not shampoo the hair before relaxing; it will remove the protective layer of sebum from the scalp.
- Always wear protective rubber gloves when carrying out the treatment.
- Never use heat to quicken the development time.
- Always use the weakest product possible for the hair. If development is slow, reapply with a stronger product.
- Use the complementary neutralising shampoo for the relaxing product used.
- Always replace the lid firmly on the relaxer cream to prevent it going off.
- Different products do vary slightly; always follow the manufacturer's instructions very strictly together with all safety guidelines.
- Afro-Caribbean hair requires a higher level of moisture than Caucasian hair. Always use specialised Afro-Caribbean products as they are specifically designed to moisturise thoroughly.
- Keep a precise record of all work carried out for future reference and in case of any future problems.

## Things to do

1. Knowing your products and what they can do helps to prevent mistakes. Here is a task to help you increase your knowledge.
   (a) Collect information on different ranges of Afro-Caribbean products. Carry out a comparison of what the manufacturers are offering (range) and prices.
   (b) Organise a demonstration where a manufacturer's technical representative shows their products to other staff members.
   (c) Write a report on the demonstration under the following headings:
      - strengths of the presentation
      - how the demonstration could be improved
      - most effective products and their benefits to your organisation

2. Health and safety is particularly important when thermal styling and relaxing because of the potential damage that could be done to the hair. Obtain a copy of the following regulations. Copies can be obtained from the Stationery Office, bookshops, the Hairdressing Manufacturers and Wholesalers Association, individual manufacturers.
   (a) COSHH
   (b) Cosmetic Products (Safety) Regulations 1989
   (c) Health and Safety at Work Act
   Summarise the main points of each. Keep the information and your summaries in a file for future reference.

3. (a) Collect pictures of Afro-Caribbean hairstyles.
   (b) Mount them on plain paper then divide them under these headings: short hairstyles, medium-length hairstyles, long hairstyles.
   (c) Produce an Afro-Caribbean style book for use in your salon. You can also use it for training sessions with junior staff members.

## What do you know?

- List the tools and equipment needed to **thermally** style hair.
- Give **eight** steps for preparing the client before pressing and thermal styling.
- Give **three** effects of thermal styling.
- Briefly explain what is meant by **touching up** Afro-Caribbean hair.
- What are the ingredients of **oil-based** products for use before pressing?
- What are the **two** main purposes of relaxing hair?
- State as many **health and safety** precautions as you can when soft and hard pressing the hair.
- List **six** contra-indications when soft and hard pressing hair.

- Which type of hair is **most difficult** to press?
- Describe what happens to the **internal** structure of the hair when pressing the hair.
- Give a **brief** summary of the advice you would give to a client regarding the after-care of a pressing treatment
- List the guidelines for protecting the **client** when relaxing hair.
- What is the **main** active ingredient in relaxing creams?
- What happens to the **internal** structure of the hair during the relaxing process?
- List any possible **problems** that could occur when relaxing the hair. Give possible **solutions** to the problems you have listed.

# 9

In this unit you will learn about:

- The effect of humidity on the internal structure of the hair.
- Setting hair using a variety of techniques.
- Dressing hair into a variety of styles.
- Dealing with long hair.
- Working safely and efficiently.

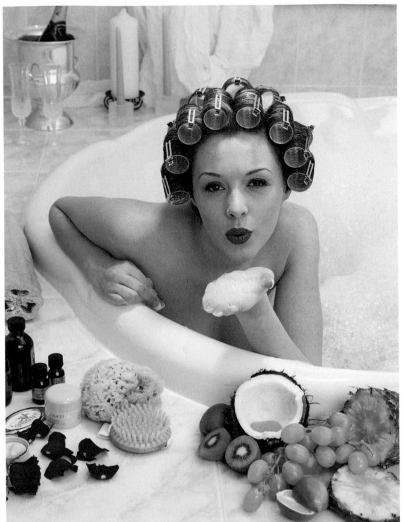

Peter West

# Setting and dressing hair creatively

## Creative setting

Creative setting is using your imagination to create the look you want. You may need to use rollers, rods, pincurls, fingers or even clothes pegs to get the right effect and you may have to use blow-drying, waving, finger drying and setting all on one head. The effects created can be:

- **Conventional** – classical looks that stand the test of time. They usually only need to be updated slightly to remain fashionable. The bob of the 1960s is a good example of this.
- **Alternative** – avant-garde styles that are striking and often unusual. But even the most outlandish looks are often adapted to become more conventional (Fig. 3.9.1).

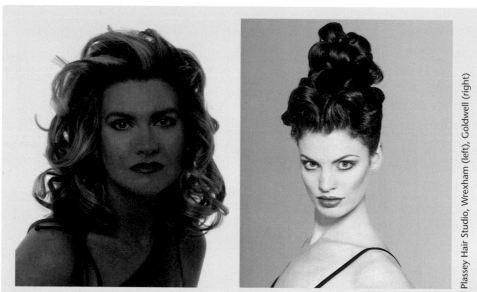

Plassey Hair Studio, Wrexham (left), Goldwell (right)

**Fig. 3.9.1** Conventional and more alternative looks achieved on longer hair

## How setting works

Setting is covered in Unit 2.3; here is a summary. In the cortex of the hair are long, buckled chains of keratin called **polypeptide** chains. These chains are held together by **cystine linkages**. When the hair is wet, stretched, and dried the buckled polypeptide chains straighten out slightly and the hair will stay in this position until it is wet again. This is known as going from **alpha** keratin to **beta** keratin.

Unfortunately, hair is **hygroscopic** – it can absorb moisture. As they absorb moisture from the atmosphere, the polypeptide chains revert back to their buckled state (alpha keratin) and the set drops. To help prevent this happening, setting agents, gels, lacquers and waxes are used to coat the hair, forming a barrier and protecting it from the moisture. This helps the set to last longer.

## Hairstyling aids

- **Mousse, setting and blow-styling lotions** – various holding power, for general use to prolong the life of the set.
- **Gel** – in tub or spray form; stronger than mousse or lotions, used to mould or strand wet or dry hair.
- **Volumising lotion** – builds texture and volume into the style.
- **Moisturiser** – restores the strength, elasticity and shine to damaged and dehydrated hair.
- **Leave-in reconditioning spray** – restores moisture balance in the hair; helps to repair cuticle damage and increases strength and shine; good for fine hair.
- **Reconstructor** – penetrates areas of extreme damage and dehydration; good for chemically treated and damaged or dry hair.
- **Holding spray** – used on finished dressing to hold the style and protect from atmospheric moisture.
- **Spray shine/gloss** – used on finished dressing to add shine and give UV protection.

## Creative setting techniques

Basic setting techniques are usually combined and adapted to create the look you are trying to achieve, but here are some other styling aids you can use:

- Curling tongs.
- Crimping irons
- Straightening irons.
- Molton Brown bendy curlers.
- Pincurl clips.
- Pipe cleaners.

The effects you can achieve by combining them on wet or dry hair are limitless. Here are some examples of how basic techniques can be adapted.

### Spiral set

A spiral set is similar to a spiral perm but the hair should be damp, not wet, and the sections should be larger than those taken when perming, otherwise there will be too much curl. Rectangular-shaped rods can be used to create angular-shaped curls.

#### Method

- Comb hair in the direction of the final hair position with any partings or fringes.
- Apply a suitable setting aid.
- Wind hair spirally on the rods, taking square sections from the nape up towards the front of the head.

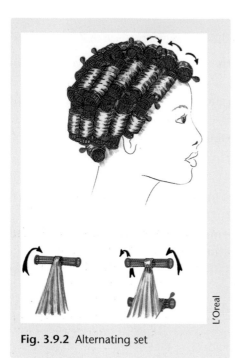

**Fig. 3.9.2** Alternating set

L'Oreal

- Place the client under a suitable drying appliance. Spirally wound hair is very bulky and may not fit under a conventional dryer; therefore a climazone, octopus or rollerball machine may have to be used.
- When the hair is dry, dress it into style using your fingers; combing spirally wound hair can often produce too much curl.
- Use wax, gel, mousse or lacquer as appropriate to achieve the desired effect.

## Alternating set

This set will produce volume in the hair. The rollers are placed in the direction of the finished dressing but where the additional volume is needed, one roller is wound up then the next down so that the curls or movements are pushed against each other, creating volume in the hair. This type of set is normally used with other methods (Fig. 3.9.2).

## Pincurl set

Square sections of hair are moulded into a circle (Fig. 3.9.3). The smaller the curl, the curlier the result. Hair can be just moulded and placed if it is very short.

## Directional set

- Comb the hair in the direction and shape of the finished dressing.
- Decide how much curl or movement you need; identify where the hair needs to be lifted and where flat.
- Select your tools and equipment and set the hair in the direction it has been combed.

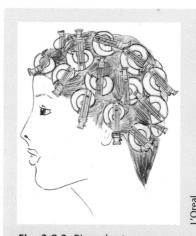

**Fig. 3.9.3** Pincurl set

L'Oreal

### TECHNICAL TIPS

Remember that any rollers placed in the hair will give lift. Controlled overdirecting or dragging of the hair at the root will give various types of lift depending on the position of the rollers. Experimenting with placing the rollers at different angles and base positions can create endless possibilities.

Before you begin any set, think about the things that will influence you:

- Talk to the client to find out their needs and the total look you are aiming for.
- Look at the length of the hair and the shape of the haircut.
- Feel the hair texture.
- Determine any strong hair growth patterns or abnormalities.
- Look at the client's features, their face and head shape.

## Dealing with long hair

Long hair is often believed to be the most difficult to deal with, and this frightens many stylists. It is certainly true that long hair usually takes more time to style than shorter hair, but long hair opens up a whole new world of creativity and, as with any other skill, the more you practise, the better you will become.

Long-haired blocks are ideal for practising on as they can be used whenever there is a free or quiet moment in the salon or they can be taken home to try out any new ideas. To look its best, long hair must be shiny with no breakage or split ends; therefore, the **condition** of the hair is always of the utmost importance. There are many differences between dealing with short and long hair, and the following checklist outlines the main areas to consider.

### Dealing with long hair

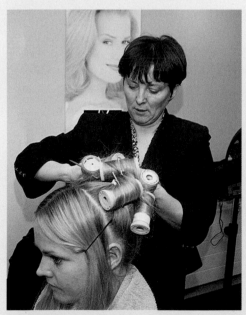
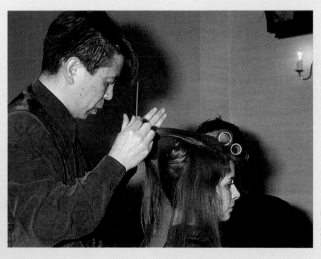

Goldwell

The stylist uses manageable sections to dry set her model's hair. Dressing the top hair over a 'pad' creates height without having to backcomb the hair.

## Considerations when setting and drying long hair

- For a better result, set the hair when it is damp as the finished result tends to be too curly if it is set from wet. Use a good, suitable setting agent such as mousse to give the hair body and protection.
- Choose the roller size carefully. Unless a lot of curl is needed, use a large roller to achieve most effects.
- Because of its length, long hair takes a long time to dry. Therefore, before styling, near-dry the hair first to remove the excess moisture.
- When drying the hair it is often more efficient to use the fingers instead of a brush. Aim the airstream down the hair shaft alternating between hot and cold air to smooth the hair.
- Do not overdry the hair. Leave it slightly damp before using heated rollers, tongs or hot sticks. The heat from these appliances will finish the drying process.
- Use a diffuser attachment on the blow-dryer when drying long, curly hair which needs curl in the finished style. It helps to prevent frizzing.
- Wind the front tendrils of hair around your finger to give a less frizzy result around the face.
- Do not use a heat that is too high, as it can damage the hair and dry out its moisture content.

## Considerations when dressing long hair

- Use a dressing cream, moisturiser, oil or wax, particularly on the ends of the hair, to replace the natural oil and give the hair shine.
- Try to restrict backcombing to the root area only, to minimise the risk of breakage or damage to the hair.

## Dressing long hair

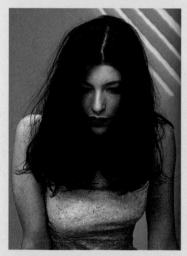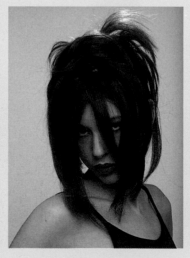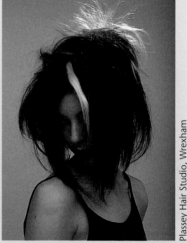

Plassey Hair Studio, Wrexham

Long hair, worn loose, is then dressed in an alternative style which can be instantly changed using added hair.

- Make sure that smooth styles are thoroughly brushed before dressing. However, styles which are very curly are usually dressed using only the fingers or an Afro-type comb to prevent hair frizzing.
- Use bands which are covered and grips which have covered ends; this will prevent damage to the hair.
- Trying to cope with a large amount of hair can be overwhelming. Decide on the overall effect to be achieved before starting, then break down the task into small stages.
- Work methodically. Don't panic!
- Keep the head in the correct position or it could alter the balance of the style.
- Because of its weight, very long hair, e.g. waist length, is difficult to secure. It is usually easier, quicker and firmer to tie the hair itself into an ordinary knot then secure in position with hairgrips. By sectioning the hair and knotting it in different places, many different and unusual effects can be achieved.
- When you have finished, check the shape from all angles, particularly if the hair has been put up or drawn away from the face.
- Aim for a natural look when dressing long hair down or in a combination of up and down.

## Dressing long hair into a classic knot on the crown

1. Position the client's head at the appropriate angle. Brush the hair thoroughly away from the hairline and up towards the crown (Fig. 3.9.4). Secure in a ponytail with a covered band.
2. Twist the hair in an anticlockwise direction and secure with hairgrips.
3. Tuck the ends of the hair underneath the previously wound hair and make firm with hairgrips.
4. Variations to the style include creating a knot at the nape or side; see Unit 2.3 for other classical dressings.

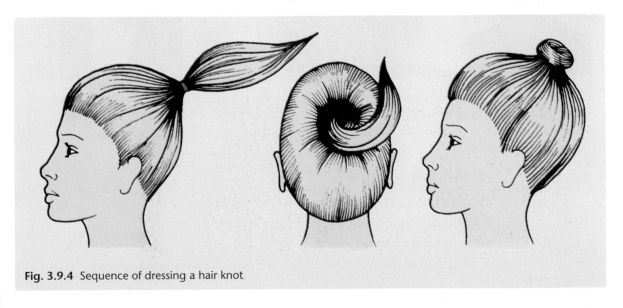

**Fig. 3.9.4** Sequence of dressing a hair knot

## Styling long hair down

The preparation of the hair before setting will determine the amount and crispness of any curl or movement. Here are some of the options.

### Wet set

Not recommended for very long hair as the drying time would be too long. Moulding hair from wet will usually make it more crisp with a longer-lasting curl. However, it can often be difficult to dress because of the amount of bounce that is produced.

### Damp dried then set

This is usually the most suitable preparation for long hair as it cuts down drying time and the hair tends to be more manageable to dress.

### Completely dried then curled or straightened

This method is often used in conjunction with heated curling tongs, hot brush or straightening irons, depending on the required result. It is possible to produce very effective results with this method, and the hair can be made as curly or as straight as necessary, depending on the equipment used.

## Creative long hair work

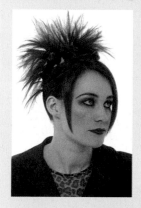 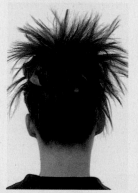 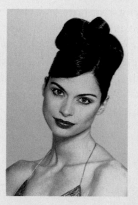 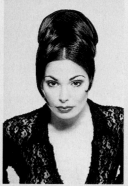

Plassey Hair Studio, Wrexham (left and centre left), Goldwell (centre right, right)

Front view of an alternative, avant-garde style created by gelling the hair and straightening the front sections with straightening irons. The back view shows how a twisted scarf gives support. Classical styles have been adapted creatively to create two stunning long hair looks.

## Health and safety

- Protect your client's clothing and skin at all times.
- Check all electrical appliances before you use them.
- Do not leave trailing wires.
- Switch off at the socket when you have finished and store safely.

- Keep your workstation and all tools and equipment tidy, clean and sterile.
- Use only a medium heat on the hair otherwise it may burn and its moisture content may be removed.
- Do not let heated electrical appliances touch the skin.
- Take care when removing rollers from long hair; they could tangle or tear the hair.
- Use backcombing sparing; it could tear the hair when you try to remove it.
- Use covered elastic bands and hairgrips on long hair.
- Be aware and understand your responsibilities under the COSHH Regulations and the Electricity at Work Regulations.

## Things to do

1. (a) Read about the structure of the hair in Unit 2.3.
   (b) Make notes then try to answer the questions at the end of the chapter.

2. Write a short summary of your responsibilities for:
   (a) COSHH when using styling aids
   (b) Electricity at Work Regulations

3. A junior member of staff accidentally leaves curling tongs switched on, with trailing wires, on a plastic tray of a trolley. As a client walks past, she knocks the hot tongs onto the floor but also burns her hand. Write a brief description of:
   (a) how you cope with the client
   (b) how you cope with the junior staff member
   (c) the future action you will take

## What do you know?

- What **two** main effects can be created when setting hair?
- What are **chains** of keratin called?
- What does **hygroscopic** mean?
- List **six** styling tools you could use.
- Give a brief description of how you would carry out a **directional** set.
- List **five** influencing factors before beginning a set.

- Why is it important not to use **too high** a heat on the hair and skin?
- Give a **brief** description of what dressing creams, moisturisers, oils and waxes are used for.
- Give **five** health and safety considerations when dressing long hair.
- What are **your** responsibilities under the Electricity at Work Regulations?

In this unit you will learn about:

- Types of salon promotion.
- Planning a promotional event.
- Setting and achieving objectives.
- Organising and staging a promotional show.
- Using incentives.
- Promotional materials and their uses.

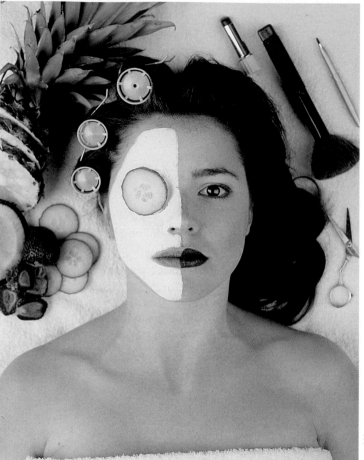

Peter West

# Promotional activities

## Promotional events

Promotional events are an important part of marketing the salon's goods and services. Here are some options:

- Demonstrations to staff and the public.
- Staging displays.
- Taking part in shows.
- Use of incentives.
- Use of promotional materials.

Demonstrations, displays and shows are very similar and they are considered together in the next section.

## Demonstrating

### Demonstrating practical skills to staff

Demonstrations to staff must be carefully planned to ensure they clearly illustrate the key points you wish to emphasise and the practical skills involved. Remember that an audience has an attention span of about 20 minutes, so the demonstration should vary in pace and allow time for the trainee to experiment or practise themselves. Learning is more efficient if the trainee is allowed to use as many of the senses as possible, including touch and smell.

Good preparation is the key to success when demonstrating and planning specific areas (Fig. 3.10.1). Unit 3.11 gives more information on demonstrating to

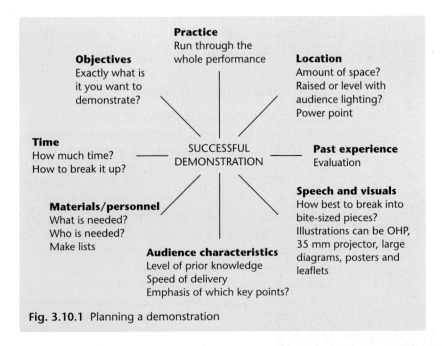

**Fig. 3.10.1** Planning a demonstration

staff. There are several ways of laying out plans for demonstrations and training; Fig. 3.10.2 shows an example.

| Title _____ | | Time allowed _____ | |
| --- | --- | --- | --- |
| Objective | Time | Method | Materials |
| | | | |

**Fig. 3.10.2** Example of a session plan

## Feedback from a public audience

Feedback is the information you receive from the audience during (and after) your demonstration. During the performance look at the audience, to determine what signals they are sending. Are the signals negative, with shifting around, talking or staring into space, or are they positive, with people giving their full attention, everyone sitting still and smiling when you make eye contact? There may be a mixture of negative and positive signals and it is important to assess the reasons for the differences.

At the end of the demonstration, the level of questions and the length of time people linger are signs of their attitudes. Individuals may say flattering (or unflattering) things to you. However, be aware that these are probably people who feel much more strongly than the average audience member. Formal feedback can be obtained using a short questionnaire on a postcard or small sheet of paper. Keep them short and clear. Try to use tick boxes for speed but allow some space for written reactions and comments.

## Evaluating a demonstration

Evaluation is the important stage of reflecting on how the demonstration has gone. It should be very thorough and needs to be taken into consideration when planning the next demonstration. In addition to staff and audience feedback, the model and your own evaluation of the session will help you to assess the level of success. When demonstrating to trainees, their feedback allows you to define success in terms of whether you have reached the training goals with those trainees.

Always find the time to write down a summary of what went well or what did not and any lessons for the future. It may be some time before you do the same thing again and you will then be able to learn from any mistakes as well as the parts of the session which went well.

One final point is that it is essential to stress the importance of safety to both the client and the operator during any demonstrated process. Good hygiene procedures and practices should also be emphasised.

## Staging and taking part in promotional shows

Shows are an extremely effective means of improving public relations and promoting the salon. They are also a good way to motivate the entire staff as everyone from the top stylist to the shampooist can be involved. Staging a show is a stimulating experience which reinforces working together as a team and encourages the stylists to give full vent to their creativity.

Hair shows can be linked up with talks on different aspects of hair care or can be used as a showcase to present a specific look which the salon is promoting. They can be staged by the salon on its own or as a joint venture with another organisation. For example, boutiques or in-store fashion shows need hairdressers and make-up artists to make the most of their models and show off their fashion clothes to best effect.

The best way to get involved with this type of work is to write to or go to see the store or boutique in question, usually in your client catchment area, taking photographs of the salon's work to give an indication of the standard and variety of work the salon can achieve. Invite relevant managers or the public relations officer (PRO) along to your salon to see the work you are doing and offer very competitive rates or, better still, do the show free of charge at first.

The type of audience you wish to attract will make a difference to the type of show you present. Organising a hairdressing demonstration for younger people at a youth club will obviously be approached differently from staging a high-profile show to a mixed audience in a top-class hotel. If the audience has paid a high price for a ticket to attend a top-class venue, then their expectations will differ from the audience that is attending a free demonstration. For this reason, it is important to decide at the beginning what type of event you wish to present and what the target audience will be.

**POINTS TO REMEMBER**
Every hair and fashion event must be organised to the very last detail and timing needs to be split-second. If not, there can be embarrassing gaps in the programme, misleading information given about the hairstyles and clothes, or the wrong clothes may be worn for that part of the programme.

## Delegating tasks: some roles to allocate

### Coordinator

This is the key role as the coordinator has overall responsibility for organising and liaising with management on the venue, music, lighting, seating, advertising, and printing and distribution of any necessary tickets. They must also make out a schedule of work and timetable both for the countdown and the actual day of the event to ensure that everyone knows exactly what they are doing and when.

## Backstage reality?

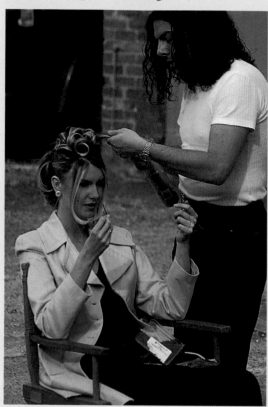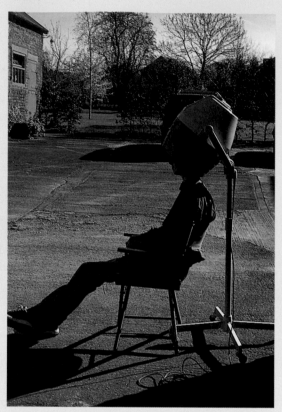

Plassey Hair Studio, Wrexham

Not all venues have ideal facilities! Check in advance that they meet your requirements.

### Compère

This is also an important role, as the person selected will have to speak through a microphone in front of the audience. Therefore, they must have good communication skills and the self-confidence to speak in public.

They must be able to handle interruptions from the audience. Sometimes questions asked during the show can be a useful means of explaining certain processes being carried out on stage, but this really depends on the type of event. Too many questions may sidetrack the commentary and then become an intrusion. It may be necessary to insist that all questions be saved until the end of the session.

The compère must be sensitive at all times to the atmosphere conveyed by the audience and must be able to pitch the commentary at the correct level for the type of audience. Making the commentary too technical may bore the audience; pitching it at too low a level is embarrassing and will make them feel uncomfortable.

If people appear restless or uninterested, then the compère must be able to regain their attention by various strategies, e.g. humour, increasing the pace of the show adding anecdotes.

For shows, linked to haircare it may be possible to contact leading manufacturers to see if any of their senior sales staff would be willing to take on this role.

### Hairstylists

They must be quick and efficient. If dressing the hair in public they must be confident working in front of an audience. When styling the hair for a fashion show, they often have to work in very cramped backstage quarters. They must be able to create and convert hairstyles on long or short hair quickly, using temporary methods of curling, such as heated rollers, hot sticks or curling tongs, as it may not be possible to wet the hair.

### Trainees and juniors

They are needed to carry out any of the preliminary tasks on the hair or to help the stylists before, during and after the performance. They must make sure that everywhere is cleaned and tidied after use and check that all equipment is cleaned and returned to the salon. Often it is useful to allow the trainees to help the stylist at the show, as it gives them valuable experience of working in front of an audience, boosts their confidence and makes them feel important members of the team.

### Make-up artist

They must be fully briefed about the clothes and hairstyles that the models will be wearing and should be given a full list of who is wearing what, so they can make sure the hair, clothes, colours and make-up styles all match.

If you do not know a freelance beautician, try the local press, Yellow Pages or final-year students on a beauty therapy course at a local college. However, always check the standard of the make-up artist's work first before engaging them, and remember that stage make-up needs to be slightly darker and heavier than normal, to counteract the strong lighting.

### Wardrobe mistress or dresser

A person is needed to take charge of the clothing and accessories and to make sure they are coordinated with the hair and make-up. Before a hair and fashion show, the clothing must be clean, pressed and placed in the correct order, usually on a rail in the changing room. The wardrobe mistress must then make sure the correct outfit is worn by the correct person during the show. All clothing should be checked and then safely returned after the event. A useful tip when having a lot of costume changes is to list (or sketch) all clothes, accessories and shoes on a piece of paper and pin this to the outside of a black plastic bag which contains all the parts of the particular outfit.

### Disc jockey

The DJ must be carefully briefed on the format of the show and should be given a list with the order of any scenes, e.g. sports, bridal, together with who will be appearing and what music is required for each particular part. Very specific instructions should also be given as to the volume of the music, and when it needs to be faded out completely, perhaps while the compère is talking.

The music should not be an intrusion but should complement the looks that are being portrayed. It must also be on cue, as any unwanted silent gaps are embarrassing to both the audience and the people involved. Always go through the music carefully with the DJ and rectify any misunderstandings or problems at the rehearsal stage.

### Models

Depending on the type of show, the models should be chosen to display the hair and clothes to best effect. If all they will be doing is sitting to have their hair styled onstage then standing at the end, it will probably be sufficient to employ attractive clients from the salon. However, many girls are shy and find it difficult to walk down a catwalk correctly to music; therefore, it is often better to use professional models. If this is too expensive ask at the local college, university or private modelling school to see if any of their final-year modelling or fashion students would be willing to model. Often they are delighted to gain the experience, and the photographs of them in action are very useful when they are creating their portfolios.

### Photographer

Local newspapers can be contacted to cover the event. For added marketing impact, the event could be linked to an advertisement that give discounts to clients who attend the show. Always have your own photographer, as news photographers do not always take the shots you would like and sometimes do not even attend.

Decide on the general effect you want from the finished photographs and then, if possible, give the photographer a list of the shots you require. Remember that any good pictures can be blown up and displayed in the salon or sent to various newspapers and magazines with a short report of the event as an interest story. If it is published, this is an excellent way of promoting the salon.

A video of the event is a good training and evaluation aid for present and future staff, as it can show any mistakes and where improvements can be made. If it is edited, it can be used as a marketing tool to show the standard and variety of work that can be achieved by the salon.

## Planning the event: some checklist items

### Legal requirements

In addition to the general health and safety legislation (Health and Safety at Work Act and the COSHH Regulations) the use of many locations outside the salon will involve other regulations governing:

- Fire safety.
- Electrical equipment.
- Public liability.

There may also be local by-laws to observe. The venue chosen will usually be able to give information on all of these aspects; another source of information is the local authority.

## Venue

The venue will depend on the type of event and the funds available. If the salon is servicing an in-store fashion show, then obviously there will be no charge. If the venue is a hotel or community centre, there may be a fee. Before committing yourself, compare the prices and facilities of several venues.

Consider carefully the lighting, seating space, staging, access to water, electric sockets, changing area and fire precautions. Check what car parking facilities are available and whether the venue is easily accessible by public transport.

These issues are important as they will affect your final choice of venue. They will determine the size of your audience (fire precautions also often limit numbers) and the type of event it is possible to stage. For example, a big fund-raising event will require a central location, good car parking facilities, enough seating space, and adequate lighting to give good visual impact to the whole audience.

### TECHNICAL TIPS

Sometimes it is necessary to bring additional spot lighting. If this is the case, always make sure the electrical systems can withstand the additional load.

## Date

The date may depend on the venue; perhaps only certain dates are available. If there is a free choice, decide on the type of audience you wish to target and check local newspapers, libraries, etc., to make sure the date you have chosen will not clash with any other events.

Consider any holidays, such as annual or bank holidays, and the time of year. During busy summer months will your staff have time to put in the necessary preparation before the show? In winter will the weather be too bad for people to attend?

## Printing and publicity

If tickets and programmes are required, enquire into sponsorship by manufacturers or local businesses. They may be willing to print the tickets and/or programmes free of charge in return for publicity. Asking local businesses to advertise in the programme for a small fee will often offset the printing costs. Always acknowledge any sponsorship, advertising or other help received.

Publicise the event well in advance in the local press and place posters in local shops (including your own salon), local colleges, libraries and community centres. Remember that people can only attend if they know all about it well in advance. It may also be worthwhile sending free tickets to local dignitaries and VIPs, as this gives added interest to the press. After the event send photographs and a short report to your local newspaper and trade journals.

## Costings

Make a list of all the outgoings for the show. This list could include hire of venue; printing, publicity, flowers; materials used on the hair such as mousse, lacquer and gels; laundering of gowns and towels; refreshments; helpers' fees (e.g. make-up artist); and any other sundry expenses. Add together the outgoings and then divide this figure by the number of people you expect to attend. This will give you the minimum price required for each ticket. Remember that there may not be a full attendance and therefore it may be necessary to charge more, and donate any profit to charity. Some salons prefer to stage a show free of charge and offset the expenses as advertising or promotion of the salon.

### Refreshments

Refreshments can be anything from coffee or cheese and wine to a full buffet, depending on the type of event, the budget allowance and when it is to be held, i.e. during the day or in the evening. Refreshments can be served in the middle of the presentation as an interval, or at the end so that staff and models can mingle with the audience to answer any questions and talk about the hair salon. This part of the event can be especially good for the salon's public relations.

### Schedule of work

Make out a list of the people needed to help with the show and then write a detailed timetable for practice sessions and rehearsals, ensuring that everyone attends.

Work out a countdown timesheet and then a timetable for the actual day of the show. Everyone involved in the show must know not only their own role but also where they fit into the programme as a whole. So, to keep the event under control, write down each production number in order, together with the following information:

- Music for the scene.
- Names of models.
- What clothes they will be wearing.
- What accessories, e.g. shoes, hair ornaments.
- What hairstyle for each model.
- Prices, if necessary.

Give a copy of this information to the compère, DJ, hairstylists, make-up artist, wardrobe mistress and models. Pin another copy next to the door in the changing room for communal reference so that everyone knows the schedule and exactly what is going on.

**PREVENTING RSI**

If the event has been carefully prepared beforehand, there will be less chance of excessive stress on the day.

## Evaluation and feedback

Evaluation and feedback can take place during and after the event. During the show the audience will express either positive or negative reactions. Positive reactions can be determined by the way in which the audience listens attentively, asks relevant questions when appropriate, and can also be felt in the general atmosphere. Negative reactions can be very noticeable if people fidget in their seats, lack concentration and attention, talk together or walk out either during the show or at the interval.

Walking among the audience after the show will also give a good indication as to whether it has been successful or not. If the audience is enthusiastic and wanting to know more about the hairstyles, the clothes and the salon, then this is usually an indication of a successful event. If the audience is non-committal, unwilling to give an opinion or avoids eye contact, this could be an indication that they have not enjoyed themselves.

It is very important to have a debriefing session with the entire staff as soon as possible after the event to find out what worked well and what problems there were. Write down all the important points to use for future reference and give an indication of how to improve future performance. Keep a record of all transactions and costings to evaluate whether your predictions were accurate. Make notes on any improvements or savings that could be made.

Feedback from clients may take a period of time. Regular clients are usually delighted that their salon has a high profile. However, other members of the audience may be perfectly happy with their current salon, but may become a new client much later. Staff should be encouraged to ask any new clients whether they attended the event, in order to determine its impact on the local community.

## Sample timesheet for a hair show

### Night before

Collect clothes, accessories and any props. Check that all equipment, tools and materials needed for the hair are clean and ready.

### 8.00 am

Arrive at venue. Divide clothes into production numbers or looks and place in order on the rail. Pin up the schedule on the wall.

### 8.30 am

Models, hairstylists and make-up artist arrive.

### 9.00–10.45 am

Rehearsals. Make sure that everything is in the correct order and that the compère and DJ have been fully briefed. Anything that goes wrong or missing can be rectified at this stage.

**10.45–12.00 noon**

Dress models. Do hair and make-up. Check that programmes are laid out on the audience's seats. Make sure the photographer and local press are positioned where they can see. Also check that the compère's script has the details about any VIPs or sponsorship and all credits for make-up artists, boutique or fashion house, and hair salon.

**12.00–12.45 pm**

The presentation.

**12.45 pm onwards**

Refreshments. Models and stylists mingle with the audience, answering any questions on the hair and salon. Make a note of all comments made by the audience for the future debriefing session.

**3.00 pm**

Collect all clothes and equipment and check that nothing is missing.

## Using incentives

Incentives are designed to get people to try something. They can be anything – the only limits are imagination, appropriateness and finance. Staff can also be offered incentives through commission. Many salons offer incentives to clients through:

● Reduced prices.
● Reduced rates to particular groups.
● Providing extras in a set price.

The basic idea is to tempt clients into the salon and so impress them that they will not only return but publicise the salon's goods and services to their friends.

## Promotional materials

There are lots of promotional materials to choose from; they range from inserts in local newspapers to leaflets under car windscreen wipers. Promotions often include a money-off or free trial voucher but to be effective they must be carefully planned and professionally carried out, otherwise they will lose prospective clients instead of attracting them. There are many methods of advertising, and some are more appropriate for a salon than others. Factors which will influence this choice are cost, target population and product.

### Cost

Any type of advertising must be cost-effective and the overall price of the advertising campaign must be measured against the potential profit from selling the goods. A large organisation may have more funds at their disposal than a smaller salon. They may also have a certain amount set aside for advertising which has been built into their yearly budget.

## Target population

The target population is the category of client that is most likely to be attracted to the product. They may be within a local area or a national area. The type of potential client and where they live will greatly influence where and how the goods are advertised.

## Product

The type of product will also influence the type of advertising necessary. For example, demonstrating toupees at an all-women WI meeting would not be particularly effective as the target population for toupees is usually men.

## Methods of advertising

Once the factors of cost, target population and product have been decided then it is possible to consider the most appropriate method of advertising to give the best results. Here are some of the options.

### Newspapers and magazines

Four types of newspaper are available: nationals, regional dailies, local weeklies and free newspapers. The cost of advertising in these papers will vary but usually the national press is the most expensive. Any newspaper advertisement should be noticeable but easy to read and understand. The price of the advertisement will depend on the number of words, so keep it brief, snappy and to the point. The following points should be considered when selecting which newspaper to use:

- A local paper would be the most suitable for a local target population as a national newspaper would not be selective enough.
- Local weekly papers have a reading life of one week or more, so the advertisement will have more chance of being seen.
- Advertisers have to pay to advertise in the free papers but research indicates that they are read by a high percentage of the population in each delivery area.

National magazine advertising is usually well out of the price range of most salons, but other magazines such as parish magazines, carnival programmes and cinema, theatre or bingo programmes are worth considering if the target population is local. An advertisement placed in any of these magazines should have visual appeal as this type of literature is usually hastily read.

### Direct mail and leaflets

Direct mail and leaflets can be a good way of informing local people of the services that the salon offers. The literature must be well produced and visually interesting so it is noticeable and creates a good impression. Care should be taken with the wording to ensure all the information is clearly stated and precise without being too long-winded. If too much information is crammed onto the sheet, no one will bother to read it.

There are sometimes offers available for salons using direct mailing for the first time (e.g. free postage on first mailshot). A specialist mailing house will provide a mailing list and will also produce and mail the publicity material for the salon. However, some salons prefer to produce their own material, particularly those with access to word processing or desktop publishing facilities, in which case the electoral register may be used for the mailing list.

Leaflets can be delivered locally by hand and there are various organisations who are willing to carry out this task for a donation. Sometimes, for a fee, a local newsagent (or local newspaper itself) will slip a leaflet inside each newspaper before it is delivered.

### Posters

Posters are used to attract local trade and can be displayed at local halls, bus stops, and businesses including the salon. They must look professional and be designed to attract attention. It is often worth enlisting the help of a graphic artist or art student from a local college. Desktop publishing can also produce professional posters which can be enlarged on a photocopier.

### Business directories

Business directories list businesses together under their specialist areas to enable consumers to easily find the service they require (e.g. Yellow Pages). They are good for long-term publicity as they are delivered to all homes within the locality that have a telephone. However, the salon will be listed with other competing salons, so the entry has to be carefully worded.

### Local radio and cinema

Advertising on local radio has the advantage that audiences vary throughout the day, so it is possible to target potential customers. However, it is cost-effective only in areas of high population such as cities or large towns. Advertisements in local cinemas last approximately 15 seconds and the commercial itself is usually a generalised, pre-recorded item on hairdressing which is then personalised with the salon's name, address and services offered. The salon has to enter into a contract with the cinema so this is more of a long-term commitment and, unless the cinema is situated near the salon, it could have little effect.

### Internet

There is rapid growth in the commercial use of the Internet (e-commerce) and a wide variety of companies now provide Internet access as well as help with designing a website. A website can be used to market a range of products and services, and email allows customers to give their feedback.

### Transport advertising

Advertisements can be displayed on the inside or outside of buses, trains, taxis, tubes or cars. Commuters do tend to read display advertising while they are sitting immobile during transit. Advertisements appearing on the outside of transport must be visually exciting with a simple message so they are easy to see and read. However, to be effective, the transport must travel through the salon's area so it can be easily identified by potential clients.

### Demonstrations

Demonstrations are an extremely effective way to promote the salon's services and image. They give potential clients a very clear indication, at first hand, of what the salon can achieve. They also allow the consumer the opportunity to see what is on offer without any obligation or commitment to buy the goods. However, to be successful and to attain the desired result, demonstrations must be carefully planned and professionally executed irrespective of the size of audience or venue.

### Window display

Window displays are also known as 'point-of-sale advertising' and can be carried through to the reception area with displays and special offers. Local events, national incidents and seasonal displays (e.g. Christmas) can all be used as a vehicle for the display or promotion. All displays should be changed regularly otherwise they lose their impact and prospective clients fail to notice them. Large stores are extremely conscious of the power of an effective window display and use various devices to entice the consumer into the shop. Next time you walk down the high street, notice how many people are looking in the shop windows and try to see what has attracted them. See Unit 2.11 for a more detailed explanation.

### Personal selling

Personal selling is one of the most important forms of advertising but it relies heavily on the expertise of the stylist, receptionist and other staff members as salespeople. The whole process is far more personal and allows the client to find out more about the product or service by being able to ask questions. However, to be effective, the staff must be aware of the importance of their role and must also have adequate product or service knowledge to give informed advice to the client. The staff should be encouraged to wear different forms of false hair themselves if this is the salon's speciality, e.g. hair extensions; that will enable the client to see a finished product and also enable the staff to discuss and advise the client from first-hand experience.

**POINTS TO REMEMBER**

Marketing is a highly professional and expensive area. It is very easy to produce materials or use incentives which are not particularly good or effective. People are constantly bombarded with marketing ploys of all kinds. Many of these ploys have involved very large expenditure which a salon could not hope to match. Remember that the most effective marketing is word of mouth – personal recommendation. Making sure each client is satisfied with the service and treatment they have received repays all the effort put into ensuring a highly professional and top quality experience for the client.

## Review and evaluation

Review and evaluate any promotions soon after they have ended. Follow these guidelines for a successful review that helps to generate improvements:

- Be honest but not overly critical.
- Evaluate the promotion against the planned objectives.
- Use feedback from the participants as a major source of information.
- Make notes on how to improve things for next time.

### Things to do

You are asked by your salon manager to organise a day or evening of staff development, to take place within the salon, in conjunction with a manufacturing firm's technical services team. The purpose of the event is to acquaint all staff with a new range of products. The manager wishes to see a layout of your plan and your ideas before it is implemented. The following stages may help you to organise your session:

(a) Identify a suitable time and date which will cause the minimum of inconvenience and disruption to the normal working week.

(b) Make a list of objectives, i.e. what you hope to achieve through the session.

(c) Contact the manufacturer to determine availability of a technician on the chosen date and time.

(d) Write out a memo to all staff informing them of the event and allowing enough time to organise their schedules.

(e) Contact any models who may be required and have a back-up in case of emergencies.

(f) Ensure all resources and equipment are available and in working order on the date required.

(g) Plan how you will evaluate the effectiveness of the session.

(h) Plan how you can motivate the staff to provide ideas for incentives to market the new products to their clients.

## What do you know?

- What is meant by marketing a salon's services?
- What can be used as incentives in marketing?
- Why is personal recommendation so important in publicising a salon?
- What is evaluation?
- What is feedback?
- List **four** ways of obtaining feedback from a training programme.
- What is the best way to get involved in outside hair demonstrations?

- What can happen if a hair demonstration is not organised down to the very last detail?
- List the tasks and roles that should be delegated to people when organising an outside demonstration.
- List **seven** areas that need to be carefully considered when planning a demonstration of the salon's hairdressing skills to an outside audience.
- Outline **five** features of an effective review and evaluation of a promotional event.

# 11

In this unit you will learn about:

- Demonstration techniques for individuals and groups.
- Organising training.
- Instructing learners.
- Evaluating training sessions.
- Key areas for training.
- Developing training plans for individual learners.

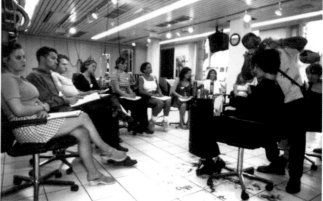

L'Oreal

# Instructing learners

## Demonstrating

Demonstrating is a technique which combines oral explanation with the handling or operation of equipment to teach or show a skill. It can be carried out on a one-to-one basis or in a group. Instructional demonstrations to trainees fall into three main types:

● **Familiarisation** – showing a trainee how to carry out a conditioning treatment.

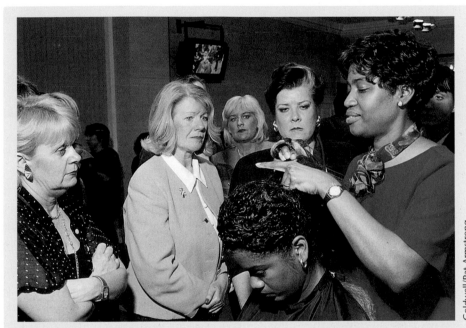

**Fig. 3.11.1** Demonstration of Afro-Caribbean styling

Goldwell/Pat Armstrong

● **Concepts and principles** – showing a trainee, on a hair cutting, what happens to the hair if it is overprocessed.

● **Skills** – used as instruction to trainees or for promotional purposes, as when putting on a hair show (Fig. 3.11.1).

There are three stages to providing a demonstration for trainees, and indeed when any kind of formal instruction takes place. These three stages are preparation, delivery and evaluation.

### Preparing for the demonstration

Any instructional technique is always more effective if it is well planned in advance with clear objectives or outcomes. These should be written down in simple terms, stating exactly what you want the trainee to know, or be able to do, at the end of the demonstration. The following guidelines may be useful when planning a demonstration for trainees.

- Decide on the specific outcomes (objectives) for the trainee.
- Explain the purpose of the demonstration to the trainee. They need to fully understand exactly what is expected of them and why.
- Plan the most effective and efficient time to carry out the demonstration.
- Carefully plan the content of the demonstration to have a clear introduction with each stage of the process logically sequenced. List the key points you wish to make to prevent them being missed out during the demonstration by mistake.
- Estimate the time needed for the demonstration. Remember that additional time should be included to allow the trainee practice time for the skill afterwards.
- Consider the room or the surroundings where the demonstration will take place.
- Familiarise yourself with the equipment you will use, making sure it complies with health and safety and is in good working order.
- Make sure any additional visual aids, such as posters, videos, shade charts, etc., are up to date and available.
- Have completed examples of the finished result, or product, so the trainee can see exactly what they are aiming for. They need not be too complex, a magazine picture or completed practice head would be sufficient.

## Delivering the demonstration

Demonstrating is more complex than it seems. Experienced stylists often assume that their trainees know more than they actually do. Think back to learning a new skill yourself; driving a car is a particularly good example, not enough hands and too much to remember is usually the first reaction. To learn effectively the trainee needs to be taken through the skill they are learning stage by stage, in small steps. To help their understanding, it is important to be very clear and precise about what you are doing and why. Encourage lots of questions and stress any key points, including health and safety, throughout the demonstration. Here are some other points to consider:

- Make sure the trainee can see and hear (Fig. 3.11.2).
- Talk to the trainee not the equipment.
- Explain fully any new or unfamiliar terms or processes.
- Clarify in simple terms any difficult or complicated areas.
- Relate facts to the trainee's own experiences wherever possible.
- Move at the correct pace for the skill demonstrated.
- Ask the trainee to predict outcomes and give solutions to hypothetical questions.
- Watch out for signs of confusion or inattention.
- Summarise key points and health and safety at the end.
- Provide opportunity for practice.

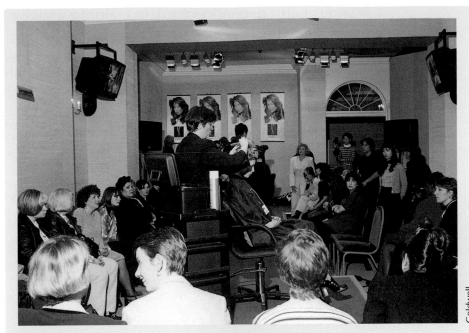

**Fig. 3.11.2** Make sure everyone can see what is being demonstrated

## Evaluation after the demonstration

Check whether the outcomes and objectives set for the trainee have been met. To improve future demonstrations, it is also necessary to evaluate your own performance and ask yourself whether your delivery has helped the trainee learn in the way you had hoped. At the end of the demonstration remember to:

- Encourage the trainee to practise the skills immediately afterwards (and during the demonstration too if possible).
- Ask questions.
- Allow the trainee to demonstrate the procedure.
- Test understanding and knowledge, particularly of key points, health and safety and any legislative requirements.

## Organising the training

Training is a skill and, like all skills, a good performance is smooth, polished and looks easy. Try to remember occasions when you thought something was really good. Reflect on why this was, in terms of the technique and delivery. You will probably find that it involved careful preparation, good delivery and assessment then critical evaluation. Experienced trainers often do much of this automatically (almost unconsciously), but beginners will need to plan.

## Planning and preparing for the training activity

Planning and preparation are extremely important to the success of a training programme. Care and attention to detail at this stage is very worthwhile. The place to start planning is with the **specific objectives**. In other words, what is it exactly that the trainee should be able to do at the end of the session that they could not do at the start?

The more precise you are about this, the easier the planning of the stages to achieve objectives will be. BEEP is a useful aid in planning to reach a training objective; it can be used for whole programmes, individual sessions or parts of sessions.

**B** *Before the training*

What is the level of existing competence? Are the trainees starting from nothing or do they have previous experience?

**E** *Experience*

Practice and experimentation must be built into the training programme to enable the trainee to achieve the desired level of competence.

**E** *Environment*

Where is the training to take place? What equipment and other resources will be needed from within the salon and/or from outside?

**P** *Performance*

What are they to be able to do and to what standard, using which procedure and in what length of time?

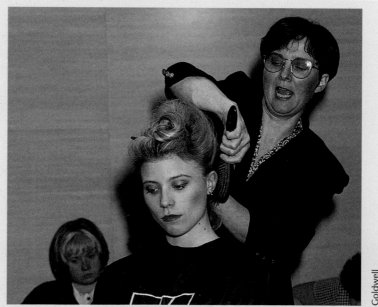

**Fig. 3.11.3** Training session

The following notes should help you in planning and preparing better training sessions (Fig. 3.11.3):

- Specific descriptions of competency levels and how to measure them are given in the Hairdressing Training Board's publication on the National Vocational Qualifications (NVQs) in hairdressing. The NVQ is based on competence statements and includes very useful analyses of what is needed to be competent in the major hairdressing operations.

- Having identified what you want to achieve, this clarifies and informs you on what to do. Your planning should identify the key stages in the learning; concentrate on these. Exactly what these are will depend on the level of previous experience of the trainee.

- Having planned what you want to achieve and the steps needed to get there, you need to decide how you are going to achieve it. What facilities will you need? While the essential facilities and equipment will be those always available in a salon, basic visual aids could be included such as videos, colour slides, wallcharts, training manuals, articles cut from magazines and trade journals. Help can also be obtained from outside the salon from manufacturers' training schools, short courses at your local further education college, textbooks, video games, demonstrations by manufacturers' technicians, day seminars, and workshops held by leading stylists and private hairdressing schools.

- Does the trainee receive training from another organisation, such as off-the-job training at college? If so, make sure you are fully aware of the content of the programme. There may be flexibility in these programmes to meet your trainee's needs and it will be worthwhile finding out if their analysis of the training needs of the trainee agrees with yours. In general, it is very useful to make contact and cooperate with others who provide hairdressing training for your trainees.

- Will the material you have selected for your training be suitable for a wide range of trainees: male as well as female; older people; people from various ethnic groups? It is very easy to see hairdressers as stereotypes – young, white and female. Always bear this in mind, not just because of the desirability (even legal requirement) of equal opportunities but so that your time and effort in planning and preparing the session materials can be used as widely as possible.

## Carrying out the training: instructing the learner

Having set clear objectives then carefully planned and organised your delivery in terms of content, pace and resources, you are ready to run the session (Fig. 3.11.3). The best training sessions involve:

- Learning by doing (activity learning).
- Tolerance of mistakes or errors.
- Responding positively to individuals.

Plan your session to involve as little showing and as much doing as possible. Use as much time as possible on one-to-one discussions if working with a group. Be active and vigilant and respond positively to any request for help or further information. Provide positive feedback. Encourage progress by praise and general positive reinforcement (that's good, well done, you're doing well). Avoid the negative. If a trainee is not getting much out of the session, try to analyse where the problem is or who is at fault.

## Assessing and recording learner performance

If you have clear definitions of your competency goals (e.g. NVQ targets) then you have a structure with which to work, both in terms of checking competence (can they do it to the right standard in the required time?) as well as a system of recording achievement.

There are a variety of systems for keeping records. Most use a tick box system based on observing practical skills plus oral and written assessment. This is a good starting point although you may wish to adapt it to the salon's requirement. The important point is that the system of recording progress is quick, clear and can be modified if required in the future. When a recording system is established it provides a structure for reviewing the training requirements with a trainee.

A **review session** should be carried out on a one-to-one basis and in a situation where disturbance and interruptions are minimal. Both the trainee and the supervisor should prepare for the review session. If you have a clear set of criteria for competence in an area, the trainee can independently assess their own level of competence and then compare it with the supervisor. This encourages the trainee to feel they have some role in the process and to take it seriously. In addition, it concentrates time on the areas of mismatch, where the supervisor and the trainee have different opinions. If both assessments agree then the review can move straight on to producing a plan to achieve the missing or underdeveloped skills.

## Evaluating the training

Evaluation is judging the worth of something (its value) and any evaluation of training hinges on whether it has been worthwhile and has achieved its objectives. Even if it has, could it be improved? Perhaps it could be more efficient (using less time and resources) or more effective (with better learning opportunities).

Spend as much time on the evaluation as you spent on the planning. There is a tendency to finish and run; that is, to finish the programme and let that be the end of the supervisor's involvement. This is particularly true if the training has been successful. Post-mortems should not be reserved for the bad ones.

A careful, step-by-step review of all parts of the programme using **feedback** from the trainees, management and the supervisor's own feelings and perceptions can save time in the future and improve even the most successful programmes. This feedback will arise:

- **During the sessions** – verbal and non-verbal communication of the level of involvement, enjoyment and learning.
- **During the review** – with trainees before and after the programme.
- **During discussion** – meet with the salon management to discuss the content and outcomes of the training.

You can also use questionnaires to obtain anonymous feedback from participants, session by session if required. However, if questionnaires are used they should be short, tick box questionnaires with some space for a written comment.

Following the evaluation, ensure any notes on improvement, etc., are kept for reference in the future. It is surprising how even the best memories lose details of the evaluation after six busy months. Writing short notes will ensure that lessons learnt are taken into consideration and do not have to be relearnt at a later date.

## Influences on training and development activities

The influences are factors which produce a need for training and may well form part of the content of the activity. There are a large number of influences (Fig. 3.11.4).

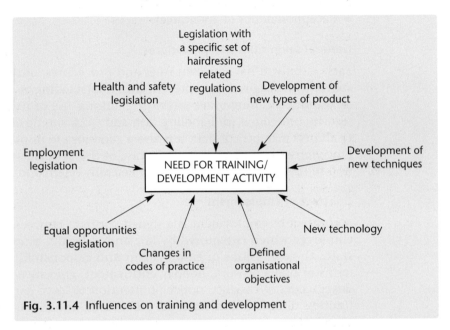

**Fig. 3.11.4** Influences on training and development

## Key areas for training

### Inducting new staff

Inducting means giving a new employee all the information they will need and settling them into their new environment as quickly and painlessly as possible. Starting somewhere new can be a bewildering process and a lack of induction can leave the employee feeling confused, anxious and frustrated.

Very often a large amount of information needs to be taken in at once, so an induction programme spread over a period of time is a useful way to ease the learning process. Some salons have a probationary period of about three months when the salon and the new staff member can decide whether they are compatible with one another. Any induction programme should be well planned with sessions built in to assess how the new employee is coping with their new environment and whether there are any problems. Solving any initial difficulties prevents problems becoming insurmountable and helps to create a bond between the employee and the organisation.

The induction programme should include the following items:

- General salon rules and procedures.
- Contract of employment.
- Protective clothing and use of equipment.
- Roles and responsibilities of the staff.
- Training, monitoring and appraisal systems.
- Reception duties (if applicable).

### General salon rules and procedures

Each salon will have its own rules and procedures, and they should be clearly stated at the beginning to prevent misunderstanding at a later date. Issues such as laundry, cleaning rotas, safety precautions, use of hazardous substances and security procedures for handling cash and stock should all be carefully explained to all new members of staff. It is also a good idea to display notices on important procedures (such as what to do in case of fire or accident) in a prominent position in the staffroom, then they can be easily referred to at any time.

### Contract of employment

A contract of employment is a signed contract between the employer and the employee which is required by law and is legally binding by both parties. It states the conditions of employment and responsibilities of the employee in terms of hours of work, holiday entitlement, grievance procedures, health and safety, codes of conduct, notice of intention to leave employment, equal opportunities, discipline and dismissal procedures, and it usually includes a restraint on working in another salon via a radius clause. Thus, it is in the interests of both the employer and employee to ensure that the contract and its contents are fully understood and agreed upon before it is signed.

### Protective clothing and use of equipment

Some salons provide overalls or uniforms for the staff, others make employees buy their own or allow them to wear whatever they wish. However, remember that the salon must project a professional image and its staff should be dressed accordingly. A salon uniform helps to maintain this professional image and also protect clothing from the effects of strong chemicals such as bleaching and tinting agents. New staff should be shown the safe use and maintenance of all salon equipment to minimise the risk of any accidents. All staff should be encouraged to report any faulty equipment so it can be rectified immediately.

### Roles and responsibilities of the staff

All new staff members must be encouraged to acquire a thorough knowledge of the work of the team, the policies of the organisation and how they themselves fit into the organisation's structure. They must also know what responsibilities they have towards their peers, seniors, clients and the salon. A job description is useful to enable the employee to know their duties exactly and to establish who is responsible for what. If staff do not know what they are supposed to do, it is difficult for them to do it well.

Take time introducing new staff to the other team members and use everyone's names as often as possible. It can be embarrassing at first to try to remember names, particularly in large organisations. Asking a more experienced member of staff to act as a mentor to the new member can sometimes help them to settle in more easily and quickly. This system helps a new person to become part of the team more quickly and to ask questions which they may be reluctant to ask an employer or senior member of staff. A new team member can be a little disturbing to established relationships, so it is important to give existing staff time to adjust.

### Training, monitoring and appraisal systems

Training has been described as the transfer of knowledge and skills from one person to another. It plays an important role in any organisation as it is the mechanism which enables each individual to be effective and produce work of a high standard. A new member of staff must be made aware of the salon's training programme and how it is to be implemented.

Staff must also be aware of the salon's system of monitoring and assessing their progress and performance to enable them to measure their success and increase their motivation. Appraisal systems are a useful way of monitoring staff performance. Their aim is to identify strengths and weaknesses and provide a means of setting goals and improving performance standards.

### Reception duties (if applicable)

Larger organisations employ a receptionist who takes over these duties in their entirety. However, in smaller salons the reception duties may be carried out by all members of staff, so guidance must be given on the salon's policies and procedures regarding the use of the telephone, booking and cancelling appointments, behaviour towards clients, taking messages and handling cash. Most salons have strict rules regarding these areas and each system should be carefully explained to avoid future mistakes.

## Activity

Write an outline handbook for new staff either as an individual or as part of a team. In a team give different sections to different team members. If your salon already has a handbook, evaluate its contents and suggest any improvements.

## Product knowledge

There is a constant flow of new products onto the market. Updating on these can be obtained from:

- Trade journals.
- Manufacturers' marketing materials and representatives.
- Seminars.

Product knowledge is essential in order to:

- Meet client requirements.
- Sell the product.
- Protect the client against possible hazards.

The key areas of product knowledge are:

- Applicability.
- Cost-effectiveness.
- Health and safety implications (if applicable).

These are best discussed with the supplier or the company directly. All of these factors are important in providing the best standard of client care.

# Activity

Choose a product you would like to know more about. Plan how you would get this product knowledge.

## Developing training plans for individual learners

Training plans are really action plans based on outcomes of review activities. They often come down to the same three questions:

- **Where are we now?** What skills, expertise and knowledge do we have? What is our *current competence*?
- **Where do we want to get to?** What do we need to develop? What is our *potential competence*?
- **How do we get there?** What is our *training* or *development* plan?

The specific objectives of this plan, however they are arrived at, need to be clearly stated. There is a natural tendency to rush into planning actions often before it is entirely clear what the plan is supposed to do. It is well worth spending significant time on carefully stating exactly what the objectives of the plan are and this will be a tremendous help in deciding how best to get there. Make sure that the plan is:

S   Specific

M   Measurable in its outcomes (how will you judge if the objectives have been met?)

A   Achievable ⎫ with the potential of the individuals involved and the
R   Realistic  ⎭ resources available

T   Time limited (carried out within a particular length of time)

Where are we now? Finding the starting point is a key part of managerial and supervisory activity. Assessment of potential performance and learning ability is very important in making sure that the plan is achievable and realistic. The best method is to encourage staff through listening, support and review meetings, in order to identify training and development needs. This will ensure a commitment to the process and encourage staff motivation. In addition, any planned outcomes need to be worked out by the individual or team concerned so that they feel an ownership of the process. The NVQ training base can be very useful in helping people identify what they can or cannot do. Competency statements mean staff can tick off those areas where they consider themselves to be competent and thus identify areas for development.

There will be times when there are tensions, or even conflicts, between some of the specific objectives used to develop training and development plans. Long-term objectives may not fit well with short-term objectives; individual needs may not rest within those identified for the team; and so on. There will also be constraints on resources, such as time, materials and money, which will need to be considered. The strategy here is to prioritise – decide which are the most important and put them top of the list. This should be discussed openly and fairly among the whole team. Staff morale can be severely damaged if decisions are perceived as being made behind closed doors. Besides that, teams are a good way of sorting out complex issues.

## Updating and improving training plans

It is good practice to review planned activities at regular intervals. The more clearly the specific objectives, activities and outcomes have been planned, the easier this review will be. The review process is a chance to evaluate effectiveness, sort out problem areas and move on. It fits into the **management cycle** shown in Fig. 3.11.5.

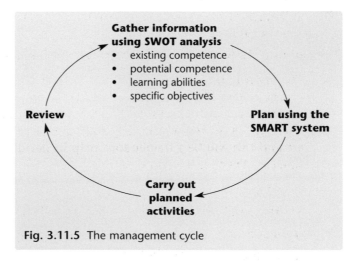

Fig. 3.11.5 The management cycle

## Things to do

1. You have been asked to help organise the training of a trainee in fashion colouring techniques. What method (or methods) of training would you use? Explain your choice. How would feedback on the person's performance be provided?

2. (a) List areas of the salon's activities which are fully under your control.
   (b) List areas decided jointly by yourself and salon management.
   (c) List areas decided by management.

## What do you know?

- What is meant by the induction of new staff?

- List **six** areas that an induction programme may cover.

- List the most important rules or guidelines which exist in your salon.

- What is a training plan?

- What is usually included in a training plan?

- Give your ideas of how staff within your organisation could be made more aware of health and safety within the salon.

- State the staff members of your organisation and list their specific responsibilities.

- What is the main aim of any review system?

- What are the key areas of product knowledge?

# 12

In this unit you will learn about:

- Fair, valid, reliable and efficient assessment.
- NVQ and the philosophy of a competence-based system.
- Types of assessment.
- Assessment planning.
- Judging candidate performance.
- Testing knowledge and understanding.
- Giving feedback and keeping records.

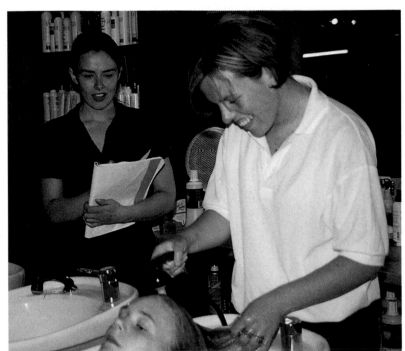

Plassey Hair Studio, Wrexham

# Assessing performance

## Assessing candidate performance

Part of the role of the manager or supervisor within an organisation is to monitor the progress, efficiency and effectiveness of their working team. This is carried out by **assessing** performance, which is something that we do all the time – not only in the work situation. For example, when someone is seen for the first time, judgements are made about that person through the clothes that they wear, the way that they talk and their manner, etc. These judgements are usually very subjective – in other words, they are only a personal opinion and may be totally incorrect. The old saying 'never judge a book by its cover' shows that snap judgements are not very desirable and in some cases can be damaging. Indeed, subjective judgements of staff could have far-reaching implications in terms of their future training and career prospects.

Assessments involve making judgements about someone's ability to carry out specific tasks or work roles to a specified standard. The **criteria** for making judgements as to whether a person is competent as a hairdresser have been devised by the Hairdressing and Beauty Industry Authority (HABIA), which is the industry lead body for hairdressing and beauty therapy, and the strategies used for testing these criteria have been designed by the awarding body, which is also responsible for application and verification of all assessments. The standards required by industry are built into the criteria and they are called **National Standards**.

Assessment, if carried out correctly, is a means of ensuring quality control within the organisation and will also help to determine future training needs of the staff. However, to be effective the assessment process has to be fair, valid, efficient and reliable.

### Fair assessment

The assessment can only be fair if it is carried out by a person qualified to National Standards. In other words, the assessor should have adequate experience in the industry and should have had training in assessment procedures and methods to be able to make convincing judgements. In addition, the person being assessed should have access to the criteria by which they are being judged so that they know in advance what is expected of them. It is unrealistic and unfair to expect anyone to succeed if they do not know what it is they are supposed to be doing and what exactly the assessor is looking for.

### Valid assessment

A valid assessment is sound and it tests what it is supposed to test. For example, if a trainee were questioned on how to brew tea this would not be valid as it does not test their practical hairdressing skills. For certification purposes, staff should be assessed to the criteria specified in the National Standards, and only to these criteria, to make sure that the assessment is carried out objectively. Assessing to the National Standards makes the assessments valid because it tests what the hairdressing industry has decided are the skills necessary for their trained workforce. In addition, having a National Standard means that everyone's competence or skill is measured to the same standard. Thus, it is the same throughout the country and should not matter whether the assessment is carried out in salons, colleges or training centres as the outcome should be identical.

## Reliable assessment

To be reliable, the assessment should have the same outcome (result) no matter who does the assessment, where the assessment is carried out, the time of day or month of the year. By using only the criteria stated in the National Standards and by having trained assessors, the assessment becomes as reliable as possible.

## Efficient assessment

Efficient assessment is cost-effective and tests the relevant skills in a productive manner. Carrying out the assessment with the minimum disruption to normal routines and incorporating the assessment into the normal working week, at the salon and/or at the college or training centre, will encourage the assessment to become an integral part of the training process and ongoing staff development.

But before anyone can begin to make assessments, it is necessary to have some underpinning knowledge of the systems and structure of the standards to be achieved. Without an overall understanding of the system it is very difficult to carry out the assessments in the correct manner. Thus, it is perhaps useful now to take an overview of the National Vocational Qualification system and its historical perspective.

## Overview of National Vocational Qualifications

In 1985 the government proposed a review of all vocational education and training. This led to the setting up of the **National Council for Vocational Qualifications (NCVQ)** which in turn led to the reform and rationalisation of existing vocational qualifications. A new framework of qualifications was introduced called **National Vocational Qualifications (NVQs)** and **Scottish National Vocational Qualifications (SNVQs)**. These qualifications are based on standards of competency, which indicate whether someone is skilled in their work role. These standards are defined by industry through their industry lead body (ILB), and in the case of hairdressing this was the Hairdressing Training Board (now the Hairdressing and Beauty Industry Authority).

The framework has five levels which create a system allowing for progression upwards, or across to other work areas, e.g. from hairdressing to beauty therapy or retailing, etc. It also provides a national and clear indication of the level of attainment achieved by those completing their award.

## The five levels

### Level 1

Competence in the performance of a range of varied work activities, most of which are routine and predictable. This first level is particularly useful for staff who carry out an assisting role and are not expected to make decisions, e.g. Saturday staff.

### Level 2

Competence in a significant range of varied work activities performed in a variety of contexts; some of them are complex and non-routine, involving some individual responsibility. In other words, this level is concerned with the knowledge of how to carry out basic hairdressing skills without supervision.

### Level 3

Competence in a broad range of varied work activities performed in a wide variety of contexts, most of which are complex and non-routine. There is considerable responsibility, and control and guidance of others is often required. Level 3 begins to look at the managerial role, the training and assessing of others, and the more intricate and specialised practical hairdressing skills.

### Level 4

Competence in a broad range of technical or professional work activities performed in a wide variety of contexts and with a substantial degree of personal autonomy and responsibility. Responsibility for the work of others and the allocation of resources is also important. This level is management-orientated and is therefore particularly relevant to those who are aspiring to be, or already are, salon owners.

### Level 5

Competence which involves the application of a significant range of fundamental principles and complex techniques across a wide variety of contexts, substantial personal autonomy, responsibility and accountability. This is the highest standard attainable and is equated with the academic standard of postgraduate studies.

## NVQs should be

- Based on national standards required for performance in employment – standards written by industry for industry.
- Based on an assessment of the outcome of learning – what the trainee can do regardless of when and how it was learnt.
- Awarded on the basis of sufficient, valid and reliable assessment of current competence.
- Without fixed periods of study – candidates work at their own pace.
- Open to all – no age barriers, no specific entry requirements, no specific ways of studying.
- By credit accumulation – candidates can be accredited for the units they wish to achieve then build on them as and when they wish.
- Assessed when the candidate is ready, in the workplace or in a realistic, simulation.

## The NVQ framework

The NVQ framework has many implications for the hairdressing industry. Firstly, trainees can learn their skills wherever they wish and the length of time it takes them to become competent becomes their own responsibility. Therefore, how quickly they attain the desired level of competence depends on their commitment and level of skill.

It is also the responsibility of the trainee to decide when *they* think they are competent enough to be assessed, and this assessment can take place in the workplace (on the job) or in a simulated environment such as a college or training centre (off the job). This split may mean that trainees will be assessed by different people in different locations, hence the need for trained assessors both on and off the job who understand the underlying principles and who know what, when, and how they are to make assessments.

## The structure of NVQs

There is a formal structure for all NVQ schemes outlining what stages a candidate has to go through to gain their award. Each NVQ is given a title which will identify the job role it relates to and the level within the NVQ framework, e.g. NVQ Level 3 in Hairdressing.

The NVQ is then subdivided into units (Fig. 3.12.1). A unit is like a mini qualification because each unit can have separate accreditation; therefore it is possible for an individual to build up separate units in their own time at their own pace until they have been accredited enough units to make up a qualification. Thus, the unit structure of NVQs allows individual choice and enables the candidate to select relevant units to suit their individual requirements. The final certificate will show each successful unit obtained.

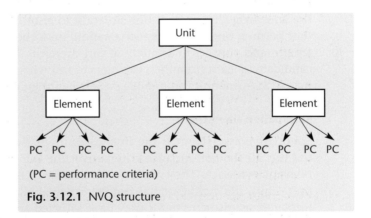

(PC = performance criteria)

**Fig. 3.12.1** NVQ structure

Each unit is broken down into National Standards. These standards are used to describe what performance is expected of the candidate in the working environment. In other words, what a competent person would be expected to be able to do in the salon and what is considered to be an acceptable level of performance by the hairdressing industry. Each standard has three components:

- **Element titles** – for example, Level 3, Unit 312.4, Giving feedback and keeping records.
- **Set of performance criteria** – each performance criterion (PC) describes one characteristic of satisfactory performance for the element. All the performance

criteria of the element have to be met in order to claim competence and all of the elements have to be completed to pass the unit. Each performance is judged on a 'can do/cannot do yet' basis, and there are no grades or marks.

- **Range statement** – each element is accompanied by a range statement which describes the various circumstances in which the competence must be applied. It may refer to differences in physical location, employment contexts, equipment used, etc.

## Assessing the competence of a candidate

Competence is concerned with what people can do and if the assessment is carried out correctly it becomes not only a means of judging that person's skill, but also a very valuable learning tool. Most of the time, in everyday life, we learn through our mistakes – a small child learns by this method constantly – so if the assessment is carried out in a supportive and non-threatening manner with mistakes treated as a means of improving future performance, the assessment process becomes a valuable experience instead of a fearsome ordeal.

### Formative and summative

#### Formative assessment

Formative assessment is ongoing and means that the candidate has not yet fulfilled all the performance criteria over the full range. Anyone in training will need to prove that they can do the task or skill in a variety of situations and can transfer the knowledge learnt from one situation to another. For example, to be a competent permer, one would expect a candidate to be able to perm hair of different lengths and porosity in a variety of curl strengths. Formative assessment allows the candidate to learn from their experience, and when used in conjunction with summative assessment it can provide evidence of their competence over the full range.

#### Summative assessment

Summative assessment is the final assessment (summing up) when a candidate has met all the performance criteria over the full range and has produced all the relevant evidence. They are therefore ready to be accredited in that particular unit. Thus, if a candidate has not yet satisfied all the performance criteria it is a formative assessment, but if they have satisfied all the performance criteria it is a summative assessment.

## What makes an effective assessor?

To be effective, an assessor must be fully aware of the performance criteria, range statements, and what evidence is required from the candidate to prove their competence. The candidate will also need to be asked oral and/or written questions to test their underpinning knowledge; in general terms, do they know and understand what they are doing? This is not always the case.

The candidate must also have a clear understanding of why they are being assessed, by what criteria, when and by whom. This means they should have an opportunity to discuss these issues and be given the relevant guidance and documentation to help them understand how the assessment will operate. It is far easier to arrive if you know where you are supposed to be going and are given a route to go by.

Letting people know where they have gone wrong and how they can remedy any faults is not easy but it is an essential, and perhaps the most important, aspect of the assessment process. Always comment on the task, not the person, and use only the performance criteria, not your own personal preferences (again, this tends to be difficult when first assessing). Limit any comments to praise of where the candidate has been successful and constructive suggestions of how they can improve where they have not. Make specific references to the performance criteria, as it reinforces that this is the standard the candidate should be working towards and it also takes some of the blame away from you personally if they have been unsuccessful.

The feedback given on any performance should be a two-way process to allow the candidate the opportunity to question any assessment decisions. Encouraging them to identify how they think they have performed in relation to the criteria and allowing them to suggest ways in which they could improve will help them to make their own decisions and be more responsible for their own actions in the future.

Interpersonal skills are extremely important when assessing. A good assessor is firm and fair but also supportive and approachable. Remember that effective assessment should also be used as an aid to learning and, as such, it should leave the candidate feeling they are able to move forward in a positive way.

## Assessment procedure

Bear in mind that assessment is not a competition and is certainly not a method of catching people out. It should be a well-planned operation that enables people to be accredited for their achievements and encouraged to improve. There are four broad areas of activity (Fig. 3.12.2) to ensure the assessment is carried out fairly and effectively: preparation, observation, testing, feedback.

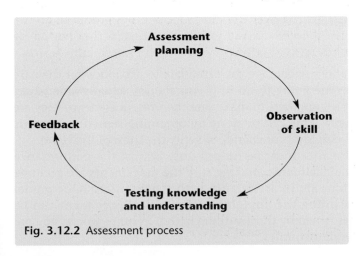

Fig. 3.12.2 Assessment process

### Preparing for the assessment

Preparing is planning the actual assessment with the candidate. It is very important that the candidate is fully involved in this stage of the procedure as it is their responsibility to decide when they are competent. To make sure everyone knows what they are expected to do, draw up an **assessment plan** which is negotiated between the assessor and the candidate.

When the plan has been finalised it should be agreed by both parties and anyone else who may be affected; this ensures it causes the minimum disruption to normal working duties and makes the best use of situations which occur naturally, e.g. assessing shampooing competence when a candidate is carrying out a shampoo on a regular client. Make sure the assessment is carried out in a suitable place and at a suitable time.

If the assessor is unsure when a candidate offers alternative forms of evidence (perhaps a roller set on a practice block) then expert advice should be sought. Should there be any difficulties, the notes supplied by the awarding body, the internal verifier, the external verifier and the awarding body itself are all sources of expert advice.

### Drawing up the assessment plan

The following information should be included in the plan: **when** the assessment is to take place; **where** (workplace, college or training centre); **who** will be carrying out the assessment; **what** evidence the candidate can provide to support their claim of competence. To make sure the assessment procedure is fully understood and documented, it is also necessary to answer these questions:

- Who is the candidate being assessed?
- What National Standard is the candidate being assessed against?
- What elements of competence are being assessed?
- What are the assessment requirements of the elements?
- What opportunities will be used for the assessment?
- What assessment methods will be used to assess the candidate?

## Observing the evidence

Watching people work, judging their capabilities and asking them questions are things we do all the time, particularly if we are watching someone perform a skill. For example, anyone baking a cake in the home could be asked questions such as: What type of cake is it? What's in it? Will it have cream on top? etc. These questions check what the cake will be like and whether the person knows what they are doing; they also provide a yardstick by which to judge the final result and see whether it has turned out as predicted. Exactly the same process is used when assessing a candidate's performance but because it is about their work role, it is done in a more specialised way.

### Judging performance

At the start of the observation, encourage the candidate to explain what they are going to do and how they are going to do it. If you are not actually able to see them carry out the task, it is important to make sure the work or evidence they are submitting is actually theirs. This can be done by obtaining signed statements from people involved, e.g. employers or clients, to verify the truth of the claim.

The evidence or performance must be judged only against the performance criteria within the National Standards, making sure the judgements are accurate and any tests or simulations are in accordance with the awarding body guidelines (all information regarding the implementation of the assessment can be found in the scheme notes issued by the awarding body). In other words, you are not allowed to make up your own rules.

The assessor should not overpower the candidate. Standing next to them and watching their every move will make them extremely nervous and prevent them from giving a natural performance. It is therefore important to be as unobtrusive as possible, although there will obviously be times that require a close look at what the candidate is doing. If any difficulties or misunderstandings do occur, it is always better to ask an appropriate authority; ultimately, a final decision will always rest with the awarding body after weighing up all the evidence.

## Testing knowledge and understanding

Anyone can be taught to demonstrate a skill – animals are frequently used to carry out specific roles or tasks either to entertain or to help the human race. However, this does not automatically mean they also understand what they are doing or why. By watching someone do something, we often presume or infer that they are competent, but how do we know whether they truly are? A hairdressing candidate could prove a positive danger to the client without an awareness of how salon chemicals affect people and objects, or without a full understanding of what they are doing in addition to their practical skills. Therefore, to prove that they really are competent, candidates also have to demonstrate their knowledge. This can be done using written evidence and oral evidence.

### Written evidence

Written evidence of underpinning knowledge can be supplied in many different forms, through projects, assignments, case studies, reports, testimonials, diaries and appointment books, job appraisals and specifications, letters, minutes and agendas, action plans, assessor-devised written questions, etc. In some instances the awarding body supply their own written questions which must be completed before competence can be claimed by the candidate.

Written questions are usually carried out after the observation of the candidate's practical skill but within a certain time limit so that the theory of the task is easily related to what they are doing – it should never be thought of as a separate entity. Specific guidelines on how to administer these written tests are always stipulated by the awarding body and must be strictly adhered to at all times. Traditional examinations were always administered and marked by the awarding body but this is inappropriate for candidates on a competence-based scheme where they work at their own pace. Consequently, the responsibility now rests with the assessor, together with the incumbent ethical and moral issues.

The candidate must sit the written test in a quiet place, away from any distractions, and they must be invigilated or supervised by the assessor to ensure the work is theirs. Books or other aids are not allowed and the assessor should not help with the questions. The test should be completed within the stipulated timescale, then the answers collected and marked as soon as possible. Marked papers must be kept in a locked, secure place and filed as evidence that the external verifier may wish to see on their verification visit.

### Oral evidence

Oral evidence takes place either during or just after the observational assessment. Questions should be phrased so the candidate understands exactly what is being asked, but if there is any misunderstanding of the question, it should be worded differently. It would be very unfair for the candidate if they were penalised because of this. Alternatively, the questions should not lead the candidate; in other words, they should not tell them the answer in a roundabout way otherwise there would be no point to the questioning.

Do not harass the candidate while they are trying to demonstrate their competence. If the questioning seems to be affecting their performance either by making them nervous or distracting them, then the questions should be asked when they have finished, again in a quiet, private area without distractions. The assessor is not supposed to be an inquisitor.

As with written questions, oral questions should also be relevant to the task or skill and should not be personal opinions but based on the performance criteria of the national standards.

It is possible for the assessor to devise their own written and oral questions which can be used as forms of evidence, but if this is the case then they must make sure the questions are unambiguously worded and are testing what they are supposed to test according to the specifications contained within the performance criteria. It is not permissible to test people on your personal preferences. When devising the questions it is always useful to look at the range that has to be covered by the candidate and to use questions that test their understanding in these areas.

### Recorded evidence

A very cost-effective method of gathering evidence is by use of audio tape or videotape. These are very useful as they provide a wealth of valid evidence easily collected and unlike written methods do not act as a barrier to those who have difficulty writing things out. They are also very good for internal and external verification of assessment decisions as the verifier can see or hear what is being assessed and judge the assessment decision with some precision.

## Giving feedback and keeping records

### Giving feedback

Giving feedback is a very, very important part of the assessment process for it is at this stage that the candidate will gain the most learning from their experience. Think of your own past experiences. How did you feel when you were praised? How did you feel when you were criticised? How did you feel when no one would tell you if you had done something wrong? You need to bear these feelings in mind when you are giving feedback. It is important to all of us to know what we do well and what we need to improve on, because if we never know these things then we will never be able to give a better performance.

Feedback should always be given as soon as possible following an assessment otherwise both the assessor and the candidate will have forgotten a good proportion of what happened and also the momentum will be lost. Again, the session should not be an ordeal for the candidate and the aim should be to give encouragement and advice where needed.

**POINTS TO REMEMBER**

- Encourage the candidate to carry out a self-evaluation of their performance at the beginning of the session.
- Always begin the feedback with a positive statement of the candidate's performance.
- Comment only on the task not the person.
- Go through the performance criteria identifying weak and strong areas. This process should also lead to discussion regarding further training, practice and progression.
- Encourage the candidate to ask questions and identify ways in which they can improve.
- Keep a record of the discussion for future reference and review sessions.

### Keeping records

Record keeping is extremely important because the awarding body will require evidence that the assessor is carrying out duties correctly and in accordance with awarding body specifications. Records also enable the assessor to keep track of how the candidate is progressing and where they need additional training, as well as providing a basis for future discussions.

Records are private documents and as such must not be used for general viewing. The candidate should have the right of access to them whenever they wish, except for the awarding body written answer sheets, which should be stored in accordance with the body's specifications. However, if the assessments have been carried out correctly there should be no secrecy regarding what the candidate has attained.

All records must be clear, legible and accurate, particularly dates. They must be completed in accordance with verification requirements otherwise they could be considered invalid by the awarding body and the candidate will fail to gain their certificate. When completed, records are usually passed on to the person in overall charge of the assessments, usually the internal verifier; and to ensure that their records are up to date it is necessary to pass on the results of a successful assessment as soon as possible.

# 13

In this unit you will learn about:

- Different types of evidence to prove competence.
- How to assess a candidate lacking in confidence.
- What is meant by special assessment requirements.
- The main points when compiling a portfolio of evidence.

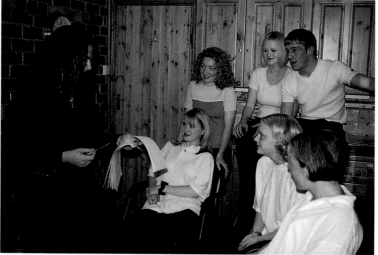

Plassey Hair Studio, Wrexham

# Assessing performance and other evidence

## Assessing candidates using different sources of evidence

There are many ways of assessing a trainee; earlier units have covered observation of a natural performance and assessments by oral and written questioning. However, there are other sources of evidence which can be shown to the assessor to prove that a trainee can carry out the requirements of their work role competently and to the required standard. Here are some of them.

### Simulations

To gain an NVQ qualification, a trainee must show they are able to competently meet all the performance criteria over the stated range. However, in certain circumstances it may not be possible to have access to the necessary specialised equipment or situation to enable the trainee to do this, e.g. a fire alarm – carrying out a fire drill. If this is the case it will be necessary to devise a suitable simulation of the real situation. Any simulation must be carefully planned to enable the trainee to practise the required skills beforehand so they are ready to be assessed when the simulation is carried out.

### Projects and assignments

Projects and assignments are means of encouraging trainees to actively find out relevant information and gain the underpinning knowledge needed to understand more fully what they are doing and why. However, trainees will not automatically know where and how to gather the information they require, and it is the responsibility of the person delivering the training to give adequate support and guidance on the necessary study skills. Study skills could include how to:

- Use a library.
- Extract information from textbooks, magazines or journals.
- Use a computer (CD-ROM, Internet).
- Summarise information.
- Write for information from manufacturers and other sources.
- Present any findings.
- Work fairly and effectively as a member of a group.

Themes for assignments may be negotiated with the trainees or devised by the tutor, trainer or supervisor, or they may be supplied by the awarding body. However the assignment theme is arrived at, it is very important that sufficient information is given to the trainee to ensure they fully understand exactly what the expected outcomes are and how they should achieve them. The assignment criteria should be very specific to aid objectivity when assessing, and they should also be in writing so the trainee can refer to them as and when necessary.

## Case studies

Case studies are a useful means of enabling the trainee to examine and solve difficult situations and potential problems. They also allow practice in working things out for themselves, encouraging autonomy and less reliance on senior staff members. Case studies enable trainees to practise dealing with problems in a safe environment without the additional stress and responsibility of a real situation. In this way, should an accident or problem actually occur, it is less traumatic for the trainee and they will be more confident and competent to deal with it. Providing evidence via case studies helps to illustrate the trainee's depth of understanding and knowledge, particularly if used in conjunction with oral questioning.

## Trainee reports

Trainee reports are explanations of the process or processes that have been carried out and why certain techniques were used. They are often submitted as evidence with photographic proof of competence. A photograph by itself may not prove that the trainee actually carried out the work or that it was what the client wanted. Thus, a written statement or report is a means of helping to ensure sufficiency of evidence to enable the assessor to make an informed judgement through the additional evidence.

## Witness testimonies

Witness testimonies can be used by the employer to state that they believe the trainee is competent if the employer, manager or supervisor is not a qualified assessor. They can also be used by clients to show that they are satisfied with the service they have received and they can also be done by the trainee's colleagues. Allowing trainees and other working colleagues to assess each other's performance is a good learning tool, in that it again increases autonomy, and also responsibility, on behalf of all the staff members. Remember that trainees need to be able to make objective judgements about themselves and others if they are to develop and improve.

Any witness testimony must be relevant to the NVQ criteria and should include the name of the trainee, the date of the assessment, what was carried out, the name and status of the witness, and any other relevant information. Special pro formas can be easily filled in and they are often supplied by the awarding body for greater coherence and ease.

## Videos

If a trainee cannot be directly observed, a video of them carrying out the skill or process can be a very effective form of evidence. Very often a lot of evidence can be generated if the salon carries out a promotional hair show which is videoed. However, to be valid, the video needs to show the trainee actually carrying out the task and this may require close-ups. It is therefore useful to bear this in mind when organising what type of photographic shots are needed prior to the event.

## Prior learning (APL)

APL is a means of accrediting people for what they have already achieved or what they can do. Sometimes this is quite easily done by matching any previous certification to the current performance criteria of the qualification they wish to gain. However, it can be very time-consuming as it is usually carried out on a one-to-one basis and the trainee usually requires a great deal of help and guidance in deciding what past experience is relevant and what is not. It is also important that all the evidence is current as well as relevant.

After an initial consultation, the trainee usually tries to match any evidence they may have against the performance criteria and range statements. An individual training plan is then negotiated to provide training and/or assessment of any shortfall or areas where the performance criteria and range cannot be met by past experience. The main points to consider are whether the evidence is:

- Current enough.
- Sufficient.
- Authentic.
- Valid.

## Trainees who lack confidence

A trainee who is nervous will not perform to the best of their ability, particularly if the assessor increases their nervousness through an unsympathetic, abrupt manner. The trainee should never feel intimidated by the assessor either before or during the assessment process, and the feedback given should emphasise strengths and provide guidance on ways of eliminating any weaknesses. Nothing succeeds like success and it is possible to increase trainee confidence by providing a supportive and positive environment.

## Trainees with special requirements

All trainees are special and all require individual support and guidance. However, some trainees have obvious disadvantages and an example of this would be deafness or dyslexia. These trainees should never be penalised or patronised because of their disability and ways must be sought to enable them to succeed in spite of their difficulties. Any queries regarding problems with trainees should initially be referred to the internal verifier, and if they remain unresolved then consult the external verifier.

## Summary

The process for assessing trainees using different sources of evidence (T&D D33) is slightly different to assessing the trainee merely by observation and questioning (T&D D32). The process is summarised in Fig. 3.13.1. Here are the main questions to ask when dealing with different sources of evidence:

- Does the evidence belong to the trainee?
- Is there enough evidence to be able to make a truthful decision?

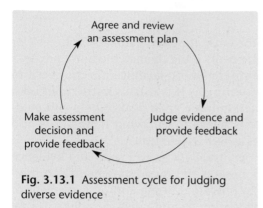

**Fig. 3.13.1** Assessment cycle for judging diverse evidence

- Is it valid evidence? Does it show what it is supposed to show?
- Is it reliable evidence? Would other assessors, including the internal and external verifiers, agree with your decision?

If in doubt always seek advice from other assessors and ask to see additional evidence as proof of competence until you are satisfied. But remember that the trainee must always be assessed to the national standards for their qualification and not yours.

## Compiling a portfolio of evidence

The amount of evidence produced for any portfolio depends on the individual. However, the evidence should be:

- **Valid** – relating only to the elements and performance criteria used.
- **Sufficient** – covering what is outlined in the performance criteria and range statements for each element.
- **Authentic** – belonging to the person who presents it.

Before starting the portfolio, read through the performance criteria and range statements of each element thoroughly to be familiar with what is required. It is then useful to prepare a file to collate the evidence. Divide the file into the required elements before beginning to collect the evidence; this will enable it to be systematically filed in the correct place as it is collected. Each piece of evidence should be labelled to correspond with the relevant element and performance criteria and filed accordingly. In the final portfolio there should be a contents list and an indexing system to enable all the evidence to be easily found.

When all the evidence has been collected, it is usually necessary to describe how the evidence matches the performance criteria. This provides written evidence of understanding the performance criteria and is often known as an **achievement record**. Here is an example of what an achievement record may look like:

**Level 3 Unit 312.1 Agree and review a plan for assessing performance**
The evidence I am submitting for 312.1 can be found in Appendix 1 of the attached file.

Sample 1 shows the assessment plans drawn up by me and vocational candidate Karen Barrell on [date]. These plans are submitted as evidence for performance criteria a, b, c and d.

Sample 2 shows observation notes made by my assessor on [date] when she observed me drawing up an assessment plan with vocational candidate Karen Barrell. They show how discussion between myself and the candidate was used to identify assessment opportunities and they are submitted as evidence for performance criteria a, b, d, e and f.

## Things to do

This task has been devised to give you practice in formulating oral and written questions which can then be given to a trainee to test their understanding and knowledge of a topic area.

1. Choose a topic area within the hairdressing NVQ, e.g. shampooing. Read the performance criteria for the topic area thoroughly and carefully devise:
   (a) ten questions that you could ask the trainee orally
   (b) ten questions that would require a written response by the trainee

2. Write down or print out the questions then try them out on a trainee in the workplace.

3. Evaluate whether the questions were suitable by discussing the outcome of the test with the trainee. Were the questions valid and reliable?

### Useful guidelines

- Make sure the questions relate to the performance criteria, i.e. make sure they test what they are supposed to.

- Make the questions clear.

- Do not use language that the trainee finds difficult to understand; check that they understand the terms you have used.

- Do not make the questions too long or complicated.

## What do you know?

- Explain the difference between a subjective judgement and an objective judgement.

- What **four** things are necessary to ensure the assessment process is effective?

- What is the meaning of a valid assessment?

- Give the definition of a Level 3 NVQ.

- What is the current name of the industry lead body for hairdressing and beauty therapy?

- What is a range statement?

- Explain the difference between a formative assessment and a summative assessment.

- What makes an effective assessor?

- List the **four** areas of activity for the assessment procedure.

- List **six** points to consider when giving feedback.

# Unit

# 14

In this unit you will learn about:

- Identifying development needs.
- How to create a development plan.
- Contributing to development activities.
- Appraisal methods and assessing progress.

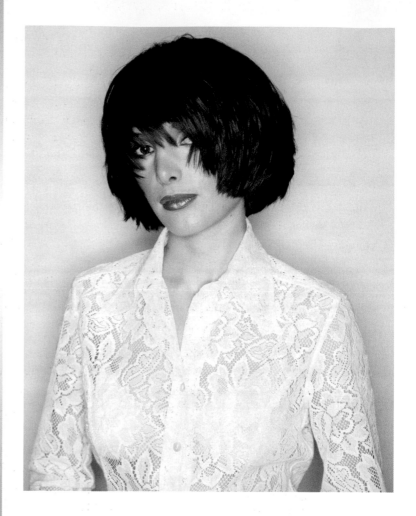

# Developing teams and individuals

## How teams are created

Teams do not just happen. Indeed, to encourage a group of people to work efficiently and creatively together as a team requires planning, organisation and sheer hard work on behalf of the supervisor or manager. One aspect of being a supervisor or manager is to act as a role model for the team. This includes setting a good example to other staff members by acting professionally at all times and maintaining standards by supporting the salon's procedures and activities. Teams consist of individuals and the contribution of each member is important for the team's success.

**POINTS TO REMEMBER**

Two important terms are training and development. This unit concentrates on development.

- **Training** – any kind of action to impart or improve the knowledge and skills, attitudes and sensitivity of an employee.
- **Development** – systematic planning and application of training and other activities to thoroughly provide a person with the whole range of knowledge, skills and experience needed for effective performance in current and future roles.

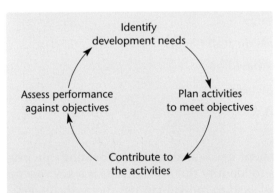

**Fig. 3.14.1** Development of training needs cycle

This unit covers the component parts of the **development cycle**, sometimes called the training needs cycle ( Fig. 3.14.1). The role of management is to:

- Match the plan against organisational values, i.e. what is important to the organisation.
- Link it to team objectives; the management will have agreed their definition earlier on.
- Agree to support training that meets the development objectives identified in the action plan.

## Writing an action plan

Having discussed the development needs with the individual concerned, some aims and objectives will begin to emerge:

- **Aims** – general statements, often vague.
- **Objectives** – specific, measurable things to achieve.
- **SMART system** – a way to write down objectives in an action plan.

| Specific | the more specific the better |
| Measurable | essential to assess and appraise progress |
| Achievable | reasonable step on from current competence |
| Realistic | can the organisation afford the training? |
| Time limited | achieved after a certain length of time |

**POINTS TO REMEMBER**

## Why write objectives?

Objectives are precise statements that help define the changes the training has to achieve. They provide a summary of any course intended to meet development needs. They require knowledge of the subject (in terms of pre- and post-training expectations) to enable the trainer to:

- Limit ambiguity of interpretation.
- Measure the training's effectiveness.
- Decide on the best learning strategy.

# Identifying needs

## Two key questions

### What training and development needs do staff have?

The answer to this question is usually based on:

- Improving technical skills and knowledge.
- Broadening experience (education).
- Changing attitudes.

Involving team members in development needs analysis and providing opportunities and supporting team members to identify their own needs is a key role for a team leader. Delegating the needs analysis to individuals has three advantages:

- It gives freedom and authority to handle matters.
- It encourages initiative.
- It builds confidence.

All are team-building, positive activities. Appraisal systems are good at facilitating this process. There are various systems but the key points are summarised in Fig. 3.14.2. The time to complete the cycle is often one year with an interim review after six months.

### What can be done to met these needs?

This depends on appraisal in the formal context of a regular review and as the ongoing observation or interaction between supervisor and staff. Both of these contribute to the needs analysis which produces the development objectives.

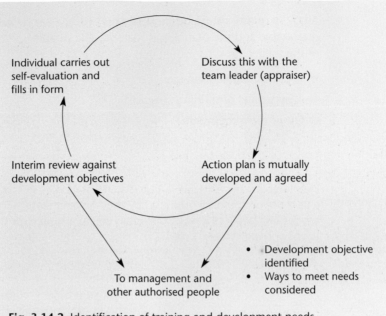

**Fig. 3.14.2** Identification of training and development needs

## Development needs analysis

A good starting point is to consider two factors:

- What are the objectives of the development? This will be based on the team objectives and the individual's aspirations for their own development.
- What is the current position? This baseline is defined in terms of attitude, skills and understanding in the individual and/or team.

The gaps between future objectives and the baseline form the basis of the **development plan**. These gaps may need to be prioritised as a needs analysis will usually generate a large number of them. Management have a role deciding the priority areas. That is, deciding which needs are most strategically important to the business.

## Activity

Using the MCI competencies listed on page 510 carry out a needs analysis on yourself. Ask yourself these questions and make a note of your thoughts:

- Where am I up to in terms of the competencies I need in order to fulfil this role effectively?
- In what areas do I need training and development?
- What are the best development activities to meet these identified needs?

All three questions are best investigated with other people to ensure the analysis is reasonable and the planning is realistic. The people involved could be one or more of the following. Who would you involve and why?

- Your immediate manager.
- A personnel or training specialist.
- Other team members.

## POINTS TO REMEMBER

Developing teams and individuals requires competence in a wide range of skills. Here is a very useful summary produced by the Management Charter Initiative. These competencies also apply to many other areas where a supervisor has a role, including leading teams and individuals (Unit 3.15).

**Acting assertively**
- State your own position and views clearly in a conflict situation.
- Maintain your beliefs, commitment and effort in spite of setbacks or opposition.

**Building teams**
- Make time available to support others.
- Encourage and stimulate others to make the best use of their abilities.
- Evaluate and enhance people's capability to do their jobs.
- Provide feedback designed to improve people's future performance.
- Use power and authority in a fair and equitable manner.
- Keep others informed about plans and progress.
- Invite others to contribute to planning and organising work.
- Set objectives which are both achievable and challenging.

**Communicating**
- Listen actively, ask questions, clarify points and rephrase others' statements to check mutual understanding.
- Identify the information needs of listeners.
- Adopt communication styles appropriate to listeners and situations, including selecting an appropriate time and place.
- Use a variety of media and communication aids to reinforce points and maintain interest.
- Present difficult ideas and problems in ways that promote understanding.
- Confirm listeners' understanding through questioning and interpretation of non-verbal signals.
- Encourage listeners to ask questions or rephrase statements to clarify their understanding.
- Modify communication in response to feedback from listeners.

It can be very useful to use already existing lists of criteria. These criteria are available from a number of sources, including:

- NVQ criteria for hairdressing and for other areas such as team leadership, management, accountancy procedures, etc. All NVQ programmes are organised as **competence statements** and they provide a useful checklist to use as a basis for a skills or competences audit.
- Personal identification of the compentencies needed for the job rule.
- Detailed job description, outlining the work role and team requirements.
- Appraisal or review criteria used in the organisation, which may include additional performance criteria.
- Informal comments by people whose opinion you would particularly value.

Once specific competence-based objectives have been identified, the next step is to discuss and decide proposals for the training and learning strategies to meet the identified development objectives. Here are some of them:

- Work activities will develop skills.
- Training courses and seminars.
- Open learning activities are flexible and can be accomplished at an individual's own speed.
- Assignments and projects can be part of external programmes or developed by individuals or teams in the salon.
- Job rotation on a planned basis helps to fill any gaps in work experience.
- Mentoring and coaching activities develop compentencies in supervisory and management skills.
- Job shadowing develops an appreciation of the qualities, skills and competencies required for a particular role. Conversely, an individual can agree to be shadowed so that their performance can be evaluated as a means of identifying points for personal development.

## Role and qualities of a manager

The manager's role is to seek to achieve the objectives of an organisation by controlling and organising its resources, including human resources, in the most efficient way possible. The manager acts as a link between the employer and the workforce, so they must be a good communicator and well aware of current legislation in addition to the salon's rules, procedures and policies and how they affect the workforce.

Managers are not always expected to carry out manual work as their role is to delegate tasks to other people, leaving themselves free to oversee the running of the salon, solve problems and make decisions as and when necessary. In order to delegate effectively, the manager must be fully aware of the abilities of each staff member, including their strengths and their weaknesses. Knowing their strengths enables them to select the most suitable person for each task; knowing their weaknesses allows extra training to be given where it is needed (often called staff development).

A manager must also have good administration skills and be able to write reports, keep or check records of staff attendance and try to ensure that all the salon paperwork is in order. In addition, it is usually the manager's responsibility to listen to the views and problems of staff and clients, often relayed through the supervisor. A good manager should identify and solve each problem as it arises, before it has a chance to affect the efficiency and goodwill of the salon.

## Role and qualities of a supervisor

A supervisor is a 'person responsible for others but also having operative duties with limited formal authority and with responsibility to management'. The supervisor is expected to keep the manager informed of what is happening within the salon and to contribute ideas for improvement. However, he or she must be very much a people person with a key role in ensuring that the salon runs efficiently with a well-motivated team producing work of a high standard. The main duties and qualities of a supervisor include:

- Set a good example to the other salon staff and know where the limits of their authority lie.
- Know when to operate on their own and when to involve management.
- Work with the rotas and schedules as the other staff are expected to.
- Provide a lead in working to organisational standards.
- Show a high awareness of health and safety.
- Prioritise work efficiently and carry it out effectively and within a recognised time limit.
- Encourage cooperation between staff and set a good example of this through liaising constructively with the salon management.
- Participate in an appraisal system which identifies problem areas and seek help and advice on these areas from salon management.
- Be prepared for unforeseen events and emergencies where changes to the planned work schedule become necessary.
- Show a lead in client care, taking client requirements into account in their operations.

## Training and development

### Resourcing the plan

There are three main benefits to developing teams and individuals:

- It secures the future of the business.
- It improves team cohesion.
- It prioritises and identifies where to put resources.

The last of these items is considered here. Management needs to be sure that scarce resources are used to the best effect, and information which helps them decide is based on a **cost-benefit analysis**. As the name suggests, this system allows a balancing of the cost to the business with the benefit in terms of increased performance or progress towards team objectives. These benefits may be direct or indirect. Any proposals for development should be put in this form.

## Activity

Outline two main arguments you would put to management to justify training investment in your team.

### Delivering the training

Having identified the training and development needs and the planning to meet these needs, the next step is to carry out the planned activities. Here are some possibilities.

#### Training in the workplace

- **Delegation** – giving subordinates the freedom and authority to handle certain matters on their own initiative, confident they can do the job successfully.
- **Coaching** – development at work turning problems into learning situations in a planned way under guidance.
- **Action learning** – provide conditions for a manager to recognise any attitude problems, unfreeze and change attitudes.

#### Group-based training

- Updated courses.
- Teambuilding activities.
- Group or team discussions.

### Private study

Private study means using magazines, journals, books, videos, TV, CD-ROMs (and other computerised systems) and discussions (formal and informal).

### Summary

Supervisors can play a key role in encouraging all three types of training and can be directly involved in training and advice in all these areas. Unit 3.11 gives details on organising effective training and assessment programmes, but here is a summary:

- Clearly identify objectives.
- Carefully plan activities.
- Carry them out.
- Review and evaluate using feedback from participants.
- Keep notes.

## Team and individual needs

### Team needs

It cannot be stressed too often that to create the right atmosphere within the salon and to work efficiently and effectively, the staff must work as an integrated team. Building a team requires special skills of the supervisor as it is never easy to bring together a group of people with different personalities and backgrounds to work together in harmony. However, the following points can be helpful to satisfy the needs of the team and aid cohesion:

- Make use of individual talents.
- Speak up for the team and put their views to management.
- Consult the team and involve them in the organisation and decision-making process.
- Establish standards and maintain them with the help of the team.
- Encourage group identity and help the team to give other members mutual support.
- Book a regular meeting slot and keep the team fully informed of what is happening.

### Individual needs

Various studies have shown that work plays an important role in most people's lives. People do not always work for financial rewards alone although they are obviously an important incentive. Often people work for other reasons such as personal satisfaction, challenge and status. People do not work well if there are bad working conditions, fear of redundancy or change, personal worries, lack of incentives or information, lack of importance, boredom or poor relationships with colleagues. The supervisor must therefore take into consideration the needs of the individual and try to provide the right atmosphere and opportunity for personal growth and satisfaction. This can be done in the following ways:

- Ensure the working environment is as pleasant as possible.
- Understand the organisation's policies and keep staff fully informed of any decisions and changes by holding regular meetings.
- Be approachable so that staff feel they can discuss any problems freely and with confidentiality.
- Ensure there is a structured training programme with a system for progression within the organisation.
- Encourage staff to use and broaden their individual talents and skills.
- Delegate responsibility and encourage staff to take pride in their work and the salon.
- Offer incentives to increase productivity and standards.

## Giving information and advice

An important role of the supervisor is to help staff with any queries or problems, offering help and guidance as and when necessary. Good interpersonal skills are essential to be able to communicate with other staff members at a variety of levels.

Communication is defined as the transfer of information from one person to others. It sounds easy but poor communication is the cause of more interpersonal problems than almost anything else in the salon. Communication goes wrong due to a combination of the speaker not being clear about their message and/or the listener picking out (perceiving) things in the message that are not there or taking the wrong emphasis.

The important thing is to be clear on the key points of the message and to relay them carefully to the listener. Good communicators do not have to speak loudly, fast or often. They put the message clearly and simply and they make sure the listener understands it. A similar approach also works for written communication.

### Meetings

Meetings are an excellent means of passing on information and receiving staff opinions, ideas and suggestions – if they are conducted properly. They should be held on a regular basis at a regular time slot to ensure that all staff are available. If possible, they should be well planned in advance and staff should be informed of the topics that are to be discussed. To be successful, the meeting should be kept strictly to time and within the limits of the agreed topics on the agenda. If other issues are raised, they should be included at the end under 'any other business' or retained for a future meeting. Make sure that any decisions made are implemented as soon as possible and any tasks allocated to staff are followed up soon after the meeting to ensure they have been done or are in hand.

### One-to-one discussion

During a busy working day one-to-one discussion is not always as simple as it seems. However, finding time to talk to staff very often pays dividends as problems are more easily solved and good ideas can be implemented. Being available to staff also enables the supervisor to be aware of the opinions and feelings of their team and therefore puts them in a better position to put their point of view across to higher management when required.

### Telephone conversation

A business telephone is not for social chatting and any conversation or instructions need to be kept clear and short. It is important to identify the essential information and concentrate on this. Question the listener to ensure they have taken in the message and that it has no ambiguity.

### Written communication

Written communication can be in the form of a business letter or a report. In giving a report or set of instructions to salon personnel (at a staff meeting for example), write down and try out (rehearse) what you want to say. A memo is the most usual form of written communication used in the salon. It is a condensed message and the key points to remember are to keep it clear and short, as with a telephone conversation. Use note form and include lists as often as possible.

## Record keeping

Good record keeping is essential to the smooth operation of the salon and enables senior management to acquire any relevant information which it may require as quickly as possible. The supervisor usually has responsibility for keeping the following records accessible and up to date:

- Recording of work done by each stylist and other staff members to enable any training needs to be quickly identified.
- Staff attendance and sickness.
- Staff appraisal, training and assessment so that the progress of each member of staff is monitored.
- Any disputes, grievances and discipline procedures.
- Updating of personnel records of employees to ensure that any change in address, circumstances, staff development, etc., is duly recorded for future reference.
- Results of any marketing exercises.
- Resource allocation including stock control and maintenance of equipment.

## Supervision and support

How much help and support a person needs involves a delicate balance between too much and not enough. When the requirements of work activities have been identified and written down, it facilitates the mutual process of deciding how much support an individual feels they need and in which areas. It is well worth keeping a record for each individual and the task carried out.

Involving both the individual and the supervisor means that:

- Problem areas can be precisely and objectively defined.
- Agreement is reached on what action to take, the nature of the action and the time span. This action may involve other members of staff who can help the

individual develop their competence. There needs to be agreement on when and how this assistance is to be provided and the person involved informed.

- Feedback to individuals is objective and positive. The objectivity is provided if a person's performance is rated against specific criteria rather than just on a subjective 'it seems to me' basis. Objectivity keeps feelings out of the process as far as possible.

## Working with management

Establishing a good working relationship between supervisor and manager is very important for, although the manager has overall responsibility, the supervisor is between other staff and the manager, a supervisor could feel too insecure to offer suggestions or, alternatively, the manager may dismiss good ideas out of hand, without considering them fully, because of personal animosity.

When putting forward any proposals, always make sure they have been thought through thoroughly. It is a good idea to write down any ideas on paper, then try to imagine any difficulties and how they can be overcome. By preparing in advance, proposals are more likely to be considered and accepted.

## Assessment of progress

Clearly identified objectives with specific review dates lead to efficient and effective progress which can be easily assessed. Without the clarity and timescale, assessment becomes very difficult and very subjective. A good performance appraisal system incorporates features which help ensure:

- Individuals being involved in their own needs analysis, target setting and assessment of progress towards targets.
- The system is objective and fair.
- Feedback on the effectiveness of the training and development is provided.
- Identification of further training and development needs by review.
- Information is in a useful format and is produced by a specific time.
- Confidentiality of information to just those who are authorised, e.g. appraisee, appraiser and managers.
- Recognition and reinforcement of the development of knowledge, understanding and improved performance.

Other methods of assessment are:

- Testing knowledge, understanding and skills levels.
- Observation of ongoing day-to-day activities and informal discussions of this.

## A typical appraisal system

The system is a cycle (Fig. 3.14.3). The appraisal report form can also set out:

- Timescale to review and assessment of progress to meet agreed targets.
- To whom and by when the report form needs to be distributed.

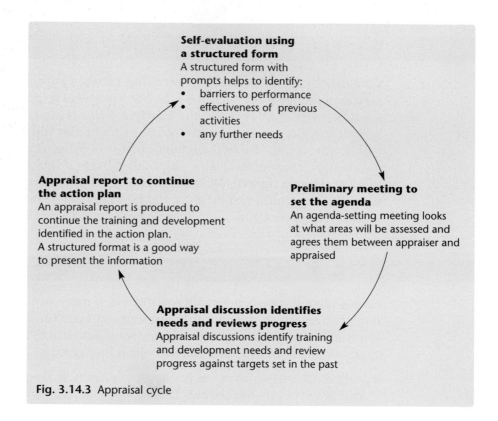

**Self-evaluation using a structured form**
A structured form with prompts helps to identify:
- barriers to performance
- effectiveness of previous activities
- any further needs

**Preliminary meeting to set the agenda**
An agenda-setting meeting looks at what areas will be assessed and agrees them between appraiser and appraised

**Appraisal discussion identifies needs and reviews progress**
Appraisal discussions identify training and development needs and review progress against targets set in the past

**Appraisal report to continue the action plan**
An appraisal report is produced to continue the training and development identified in the action plan. A structured format is a good way to present the information

**Fig. 3.14.3** Appraisal cycle

### Things to do

Analysis of training needs is a fundamental starting point for a systemic process of identifying and the meeting training and development needs. List **five** skills that a trainer should possess to be competent to carry out a training needs analysis. Rate yourself (e.g. marks out of 10) against each one. If you feel a lack of confidence in any of the five areas, what action would you take to remedy these difficulties?

## What do you know?

- What is the difference between development and training?
- Outline the development cycle.
- Identify a good starting point for development needs analysis.
- What are the **two** key questions to ask when identifying development needs?
- Give **three** reasons why it is good practice to involve individual staff members in analysis of their own development needs.
- Describe the SMART system of planning that can be used to help produce a development and training plan.

- List **four** ways a supervisor can provide information and give advice to teams and individuals.
- Outline what is meant by cost-benefit analysis of a training and development plan.
- Give examples of the types of delivery for training and development programmes.
- Explain why it is good practice for a supervisor to be involved in the delivery of training.
- Explain the necessity for good open communication between a supervisor and their manager.
- What are the main stages of a performance appraisal cycle?

# 15

In this unit you will learn about:

- The PERL system of leadership.
- Planning work for teams and individuals.
- Assessing the work of the team and individuals.
- Supervising and supporting individuals.
- Providing feedback to the team.

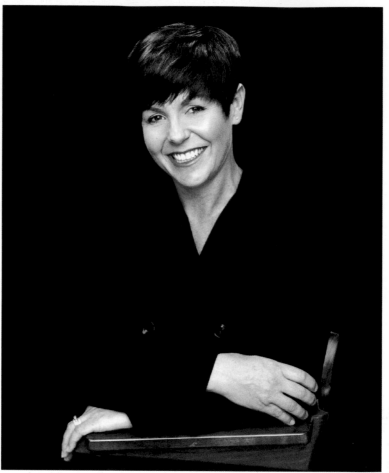

L'Oreal

# Leading teams

## The PERL system

The PERL system of leadership is summarised in Fig. 3.15.1. The first element of this unit concentrates on planning, the second on assessment involving large amounts of review. The third and last element looks at feedback, which is essential for learning to take place.

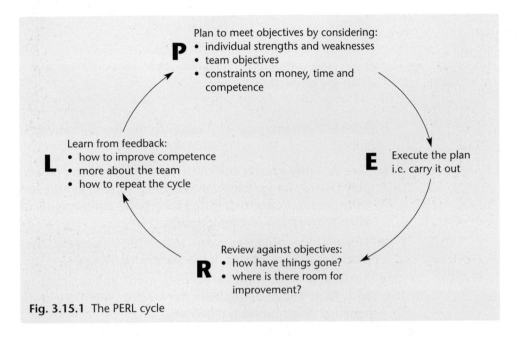

**P** Plan to meet objectives by considering:
- individual strengths and weaknesses
- team objectives
- constraints on money, time and competence

**E** Execute the plan i.e. carry it out

**R** Review against objectives:
- how have things gone?
- where is there room for improvement?

**L** Learn from feedback:
- how to improve competence
- more about the team
- how to repeat the cycle

**Fig. 3.15.1** The PERL cycle

## Planning work

Planning is about a careful and effective approach to the work of the salon team. There is always a need for **reactive planning**, often called fire-fighting; quickly made plans may be needed to deal with unexpected problems. The problem is that reactive planning can become far too common, and although it is not possible to plan for every contingency, the expected and anticipated events and activities do provide a good opportunity to plan effectively.

Planning is best carried out as a **team activity**; this has three advantages:

- Promoting team cohesion.
- Pooling experience.
- Opportunities for initiative.

Salon teams often contain a variety of backgrounds, work histories, approaches and perspectives. Pooling experience can contribute to effective planning. Individuals need opportunities to show initiative and enthusiasm, and to identify training and development needs. For example, if the objective is to increase the range of salon services, this will focus on present competences and training needs of the team.

# Activity

List the main activities in the salon. Against this list put the members of your team and code them with these letters:

M = the person who usually does it
C = a person competent to stand in
T = training required to carry out activity
V = no one can do it – a vacancy exists

You will have competed a **versatility chart** for your team and outlined potential training and development needs.

The SMART system (page 450) can help to plan the activities of the team and its members:

- **S**pecific – the greater the clarity and detail of the objectives, the better the plan. There is a very human tendency to rush at this; resist it. Take time to write specific objectives from the general aims (vague and ambiguous) that often provoke the planning session.

- **M**easurable – once again the better the objectives, the easier this is. This process is the assessment of the planned activities.

- **A**chievable – given the relative strengths and weaknesses of the team members, their personal qualities, how effectively they work together, and the organisational and team objectives.

- **R**ealistic – within the constraints of time, competence and money which often limit and restrict planning.

- **T**ime constraints – a time element to be introduced; the final element of the action planning sequence: what, how, who, when?

## The role of communication

Good communication is at the heart of effective teams. People feel listened to and valued. Team and individual objectives are clearly stated. Plans are discussed clearly, openly and in a supportive and trusting atmosphere. This encourages and reinforces the team members to support plans and their realisation.

Good communication involves:

- Active listening.
- Summarising.
- Moving on the discussion.
- Being clear and concise.

Finally, good communication is needed to ensure management are kept informed, understand the team's planned activities, and are helped to run through a **cost-benefit** analysis which produces a positive outcome.

## Handling conflict

Conflict can arise for any number of reasons – a difference of opinion, a personality clash, someone breaking the rules or behaving inappropriately, sexist or racist issues, or it could merely be caused by a misunderstanding. How the conflict is handled depends on the gravity of the situation and the issues involved. The important thing to note is that any potential disagreement is identified as soon as possible and dealt with in an appropriate manner immediately to prevent the situation getting out of control. If small problems are not resolved quickly, they can snowball with the next small problem until eventually the supervisor has a crisis on their hands.

The supervisor must be aware of the legal rights of the staff as ignorance of the law is no excuse for wrong decisions and, certainly, issues involving equal opportunities, racism, sexism and working conditions are all covered by legislation in addition to any salon policy. However, trying to resolve disputes informally through good communication skills is usually preferable to more formal disciplinary action or eventual legal proceedings.

Because of their liaising role, the supervisor will have to learn to deal not only with different forms of conflict but also contention between staff on the one hand and management on the other.

## Dealing with staff conflict

Misunderstandings can be minimised if all staff know the standards they are expected to adhere to. This includes not only their practical skills but their behaviour towards the clients and each other. If they are disruptive or behaving inappropriately, the supervisor will need to find out the reason why. There must therefore be opportunities available for staff members to talk over their problems or difficulties in a quiet place away from interruptions. It is advisable to keep confidential records of both informal and formal interactions; it is also advisable to ensure management is aware of any difficulties and how they are being resolved.

The main point here is listening to problems, as opposed to solving them. There is always a natural inclination to look for solutions to other people's problems but this is not what the listening role is about. If the solutions offered are unsuccessful then the situation will be made far worse as the blame will automatically be transferred to the person giving the advice. You need to be a sympathetic ear and, if necessary, a shoulder to cry on. Any solutions need to come from within the person, not from outside.

It is important to bear in mind the confidential nature of the conversations. The staff should feel they can talk to you and be absolutely sure you will not divulge any of what they tell you. Even if you feel the manager ought to know about the conversation, you must first obtain the permission of the staff member.

Although this rarely happens, it is possible that someone who has told you of various troubles will then use your knowledge of this to attempt to manipulate you over such matters as pace and standard of work. If you feel this is the case, tell the individual concerned that this is not really fair and that at the end of the day, however sympathetic you are, there is a limit to the amount of consideration a person can have in a salon operating as a business in a competitive environment.

It is essential to be very careful in any form of counselling role and refer the person to professional counselling help if appropriate.

## Conflict with management

Any disagreements with the line manager should be sorted out as amicably as possible – at the end of the day, both parties usually have to remain working together. It is also demotivating to the staff and detrimental to the organisation if senior staff members are continually at loggerheads with each other.

It is often difficult to give criticism and even harder to accept, particularly if you feel it is unjustified or too personal. Conflict is almost always disturbing to deal with and it is therefore important to keep calm, stick to the facts and act in an adult fashion. Do not revert to child mode and have a tantrum if things do not go exactly as you would wish.

Very often people only listen selectively to what they hear and therefore misinterpret what is being said, particularly if one or both of the two parties lack interpersonal skills. The golden rule is to listen to the comments, weigh up what is being said and then make a reasoned judgement before deciding on the course of action.

## Assessing the team's work

The purpose of the assessment has been clearly identified by the Management Chapter Initiative (Element C12.2):

- Assurance of achieving the objective.
- Assurance of quality and meeting customer requirements.
- Appraisal of team or individual performance.
- Recognition of competent performance and achievement.

These assessments may be general or specific:

- **Specific** – one person, one activity, etc.
- **General** – whole team performance, etc.

Any kind of assessment needs to be based on information in order to measure performance of the plan against the plan's objectives. This information can be from a variety of sources (Fig. 3.15.2). Much of this is built into an effective **performance appraisal system** to ensure that assessment is fair and objective.

## Activity

Read the section on performance appraisal systems. Outline the main sequence of events. How does the system help ensure clear, fair and objective assessments?

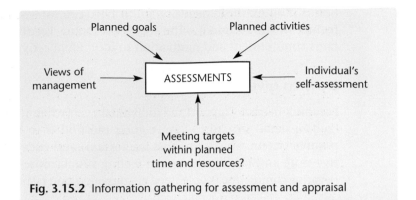

Fig. 3.15.2 Information gathering for assessment and appraisal

## Supervision and support of individuals

How much help and support to give a person is a delicate balance between too much and not enough. When the requirements of work activities have been identified and written down, it facilitates the mutual process of deciding how much support an individual feels they need and in which areas. It is well worth keeping a record for each individual and the task carried out. Involving the individual and the supervisor means that:

- Problem areas can be precisely and objectively defined.
- Agreement is reached on what action to take.
- Feedback to individuals is objective and positive.

It is important to agree the nature of the action and the time span. The action may involve other members of staff who can help the individual develop their competence. There needs to be agreement on when and how this assistance is to be provided and the person involved should be informed. Objectivity is provided if a person's performance is rated against specific criteria rather than on a subjective 'it seems to me' basis. Objectivity keeps feelings out of the process as far as possible.

## Providing feedback to the team

Feedback on performance is the information you give to team members on how well they are performing against the objectives which have been agreed. Research shows that humans do not learn in a vacuum, they need feedback on how they are doing. This can be intrinsic feedback or extrinsic feedback:

- **Intrinsic** – internal feedback, self-evaluation and feelings of pleasure and contentment at having achieved.
- **Extrinsic** – external feedback, such as the opinions of others and incentives, e.g. money, status.

Intrinsic feedback is more powerful than extrinsic feedback; and in order to be effective, extrinsic quantities have to be internalised. For example, a performance bonus is an extrinsic quantity and it becomes internalised if it produces a good feeling in the recipient – the feel-good factor. Feedback encourages and maintains commitment and motivation to individual activities and teamwork.

## How to give feedback

Feedback needs to support the individual even when it is negative (this is also covered in detail in Unit 3.12). A good method is to use the positive–negative–positive system. This starts (first impression) and ends (last impression) on a positive note and leaves the person feeling much more motivated than undiluted negative comments. People need encouraging and respond best to feedback that is:

- Clear, objective and constructive.
- Shows they are valued.
- Encourages them to suggest how they could improve.
- Confidential to those directly involved and to management.

Feedback provides the opportunity to positively reinforce individuals and teams. So often the only news is bad news. Mistakes, omissions, etc., are quickly reacted to but the mass of good work is seemingly ignored and taken for granted by the management. Acknowledging this good work and competence as part of the **culture** of the salon is extremely powerful in motivating staff (assuming it is genuine, not overdone and devalued).
Feedback can be given:

- As part of ongoing general activities.
- As a motivator.
- As part of the appraisal system.
- During formal and informal discussions and meetings.

Formal contexts, such as performance appraisal and team meetings, often put feedback in writing, whereas other contexts tend to use verbal feedback. Whether written or verbal, good feedback relies on good communication skills.

## Things to do

1. What written comments could be put into the supervision record (Fig. 3.15.3) for
   (a) an excellent performance?
   (b) a poor performance?
   (c) a reasonable level of competence?

2. Contingency plans are needed to cover abnormal staffing situations. Devise plans to cope with the following contingencies:
   (a) staff absence through sickness – an extreme example would be all the staff away through illness
   (b) unexpected increase in clients – a nearby salon closing could cause this.

3. Explain how you would manage each of the following:
   (a) Persistent lateness or excessive time off work.
   (b) Attitude problems shown by being offhand or rude to colleagues and clients.
   (c) Slovenly or low standards of practical skills.

| | Time and date | Place | Services performed and by whom | Comments | Signed |
|---|---|---|---|---|---|
| A | | | | | |
| B | | | | | |
| C | | | | | |

SUPERVISION RECORD

**Fig. 3.15.3** Sample supervision record card

## What do you know?

- List the **three** main elements of leading teams or individuals.
- Give **three** advantages of planned activities.
- What does SMART stand for in planning?
- What are the **four** components of effective communication?.
- Outline the effective management of conflict (a) between staff and (b) with managers.
- List **four** purposes of assessment.
- Define **five** types of information that can feed into the assessment process.

- Outline the features of a supportive approach to individuals as they carry out tasks.
- What is meant by feedback?
- Distinguish between intrinsic and extrinsic feedback.
- Outline an effective method of giving negative feedback without profoundly reducing motivation.
- List **five** qualities of the type of feedback that people generally respond to in a positive way.
- Outline the times when feedback can be given. What is positive reinforcement? Why is it important?

# Glossary

**acid** Any substance which when dissolved in water gives off hydrogen ions. It produces a solution with a pH value below 7.

**acid conditioners** Conditioners which help to restore the hair to an acid state.

**acid mantle** Idea that natural oil (sebum) and sweat produce a slightly acid condition on the skin.

**acid perms** Perms which operate at an acid pH. Cause less damage to hair than traditional alkaline perms.

**action learning** Learning by doing; a very effective way of learning new skills.

**action plan** A detailed plan of what is to be done, how it is to be carried out, by whom and by what date.

**activators** *see* **boosters**

**added hair** Extra pieces of hair wound or plaited into the client's style.

**aerosol** Fine droplets of a liquid in the air, produced by sprays.

**aesculap scissors** Scissors which have one (or both) blades serrated.

**afro comb** A comb with thick, large prongs usually made from vulcanite that can be used to create volume without frizz on African Caribbean or extremely curly hair.

**afro hair** African Caribbean hair which is usually extremely curly and brittle.

**AIDS** Stands for Acquired Immune Deficiency Syndrome. This very dangerous disease could possibly be transmitted from one person to another in the salon by blood contamination. For example, when someone is cut by a razor and the razor is not cleaned, and then it is used again and cuts another person. There is some risk but there have been no recorded cases of transmission in this way in the hairdressing salon.

**alkali** *see* **base**

**alkaline bleach** A type of simple bleach using an alkali to speed up the bleaching action.

**allergic dermatitis** *see* **dermatitis**

**allergy test** *see* **skin test**

**alopecia** The general name for hair loss or balding. There are a number of different types including:

  **alopecia areata** Hair loss in patches, cause not known.

  **circatrical alopecia** On scars and scar tissue.

  **alopecia diffusa** General thinning of hair, can be due to a number of causes, e.g. some drugs.

  **traction alopecia** Hair is pulled out by tension applied to the hair, e.g. some hairstyles.

**alpha keratin** Hair protein in an 'unstrectched' form.

**alternative tools, equipment and techniques** The improvised use of tools, equipment and techniques to enable an effect to be achieved which cannot be achieved using conventional means.

**amino acids** Building blocks of protein. They make up polypeptide chains.

**ammonium sulphite** Used in some hair straighteners (relaxers).

**ammonium thioglycollate** Active ingredient in traditional alkaline (pH 9.5) perm lotions. Acid perms contain glycerol thioglycollate.

**appraisal** An assessment of staff performance, potential and action planning to encourage development.

**assertive action** Firm, clearly defined, non-aggressive activities done to acheive a goal.

**assessment (of client)** Judging a client's requirements in terms of their face, shape, lifestyle, hair types and condition before a treatment.

**assessment (of staff)** Often called 'appraisal'. This should be done against specific criteria and is a positive process of finding out what staff can or cannot do well.

**back brushing** Pushing the hair back on itself using a brush to create volume to the hairstyle when dressing hair.

**back combing** Pushing the hair back on itself at the roots to produce a padded effect which gives volume to the hairstyle. Backcombing on top of the hair mesh to blend the hair is termed 'teasing'.

**bacteria** Type of micro-organism which can be neutral or useful or harmful (pathogenic) and cause disease.

**balance** Term used in hairdressing to refer to the shape of the final hairstyle in relation to the client's face, head, neck and body. The silhouette of a hairstyle helps to show up any defects in its balance.

**balding/baldness** *see* **alopecia**

**barber's itch (sycosis barbae)** Caused by staphylococci bacteria which cause inflammation of the beard hair follicles.

**barrier cream** A cream used to protect the client's skin when carrying out processes which could cause skin irritation or staining, e.g. when perming, tinting or bleaching.

**base** Any substance which can react with an acid to form a substance called a salt and water. Soluble bases are called alkalis and have pH values above 7.

**bevel cutting** Club cutting the hair on a curve. The hair is held between the fingers and then bent up and in towards the scalp; when this hair is then cut straight across, graduation is created on the ends of the hair.

**bleach** Chemicals used to lighten or decolorise the colouring pigment of the hair. Types include simple, oil, powder (or paste) and emulsion bleaches.

**blepharitis** *see* **styes**

**block colouring** A fashion colouring technique usually used to emphasise the shape of a short hairstyle by graduating various colours in 'blocks' through the hair from the nape through to the front of the head.

**blowdrying** A method of drying the hair with the aid of brushes, combs and/or hands to create a natural, soft effect which can be either curly or smooth depending upon the desired result.

**blow waving** A method of waving the hair with the aid of a comb or brush and the heated air from a hand drier.

**boil (furuncle)** Caused by staphylococci bacteria. Symptoms are red, round area which is very sensitive with a central core containing pus.

**boosters (activators)** Oxidising agents which add to the action of the main oxidiser (often hydrogen peroxide).

**brighteners (brightening shampoos)** Mild bleaches which lift the hair base colour shade slightly.

**by-laws** Local regulations.

**canities** Technical name for hair growing without pigment. Produces 'white' hair.

**chipping in** Haircutting technique used to remove bulk or weight from the ends of the hair and for softening the outline shape of the haircut.

**chlorofluorocarbons** The materials once widely used in aerosol spray cans to propel the liquid out. Their use has now been phased out since they were shown to cause damage to ozone layer in the Earth's atmosphere.

**chopsticks** A perming rod which produces a considerable volume with uniform angular curl.

**circuit breakers (earth leakage devices)** Automatic switches which switch the electrical supply off in the event of overloading or a fault.

**citric acid** Technical term for lemon juice.

**client care** All the aspects of making a client feel valued, satisfied with the service received and protecting them from hazards in the salon.

**client image** That which is projected through personality, appearance and lifestyle.

**club cutting** Cutting the hair straight across to remove length but not bulk.

**cohesive set (wet setting)** Hair that is wet then moulded and dried in the moulded position, e.g. setting, blowdrying.

**cold sores (herpes)** Caused by a virus. The symptoms are cracking and oozing of skin around the mouth.

**colleagues** People who form the staff in the salon.

**colour flashes** Fashion tinting technique of lightening a band of hair around the front hairline.

**colour reducer** Used to remove unwanted artificial colour pigments from the hair.

**communication** The key process of passing information from one person to another. Sounds easy but is not.

**compound henna** An inorganic dye which is a mixture of vegetable henna and a metallic dye. It reacts with hydrogen peroxide and is therefore not used in salons any more as the chemical processes available to the client are severely restricted if the hair has been treated with metallic salts.

**concave cutting** *see* **inversion**

**condition** An overall summary of the client's hair type, damage (if any) to the hair and amount of oil present, etc.

**conditioner** A product designed to leave the hair in good condition. types include: oil-based (emollients), substantive and mild acid rehabilitating rinses.

**conjunctivitis** Eye infection which causes a general inflammation and weeping of the front of the eye.

**consultation** A detailed discussion and assessment of the client and the client's requirements.

**contact dermatitis** *see* **dermatitis**

**contagious** Spread by direct or indirect contact, e.g. touch.

**contingency plans** Plans ready for likely but unpredictable events. staff off ill is a good example.

**contra-indications** Things to look for which would prevent hairdressing operations.

**conventional tools, equipment and techniques** Those which are commonly used in a traditional way by the hairdressing profession.

**cornified layer** Dead, protective outermost layer of the skin.

**cortex** *see* **hair cortex**

**COSHH** Short for Control of Substances Hazardous to Health Act.

**covering dyes** Dyes which tint hair darker or a similar shade (tone) to the natural, base colour shade of the hair.

**cow's lick** Hair tending to stick up around the crown. caused by hair growth pattern.

**creativity/creative techniques** Methods using original combinations of existing techniques to produce attention grabbing looks.

**critical influencing factors** Anything that could affect a given service.

**croquignole** A term used for winding the hair from the hair points down towards the roots.

**cross-checking** A procedure to check that a hairdressing treatment, e.g. cutting, tinting, bleaching, has been thoroughly and correctly carried out.

**cross-linkages (cross-links)** Hold the polypeptide chains in place in the hair cortex.

**curl test** Used to monitor reagent action during perming or relaxing/straightening hair.

**cuticle** *see* **hair cuticle**

**cutting comb** A pliable comb that is smaller and thinner than most other combs to enable the hair to be cut nearer to the scalp when using the 'scissor over comb' method of cutting hair.

**damaged cuticle** Caused by chemicals or physical damage. Causes hair tangle.

**dandruff** *see* **pityriasis**

**data protection** The Data Protection Act requires the strict confidentiality of personal information kept in computerised systems, and (with some exceptions) also gives people the right to see what information is being held.

**decolorising** Removal of colour from a pigment by either oxidation, e.g. bleaching or reduction.

**delivery note** A document that is usually received with an order. The contents of each should be checked not only against one another but also against the original order to ensure that the correct stock has been delivered in good condition.

**depilatory** A product used to remove hair. Generally works by breaking down the hair structure so that the hair disintegrates.

**demonstrations** Are very effective if properly planned. They can be used to show staff techniques and to promote/publicise the salon.

**density** *see* **abundance**

**dermal papilla** A bundle of blood vessels and fat cells in the centre of the hair bulb. It provides the chemicals for hair growth.

**dermatitis** Inflammation, swelling and cracking of the skin: contact dermatitis is a response to a substance (called the primary irritant) which may need previous exposure until body 'over-reacts' to it, i.e. a period of sensitisation.

**dermis** Inner layer of the skin which gives it its elasticity.

**development (developing)** Producing the final colour of hair tints and bleaches or the transition from straight to curled hair during the softening and moulding stages of perming.

**development plans** *see* **training plans**

**diagnostics** Means looking at the client's hair and scalp. Recognising skin and scalp condition and knowing what to do about them. Particularly important is knowing which conditions prevent hairdressing operations and which do not.

**disciplinary procedures** A statement of the steps involved in taking such action against someone.

**double crown** Two crowns, caused by hair growth patterns.

**dressing comb** A comb (usually made of vulcanite) with a fine end and a rake end that is used for disentangling and dressing the hair.

**dressing hair** The final stage of the hairdressing process when the hair is arranged into the finished style using a variety of techniques (brushing, combing, teasing, etc.), tools (brushes, combs, fingers), and dressing aids (dressing creams, sprays, etc.).

**earthing** A part on an electrical system that provides an 'easy' route for electricity into the ground. It helps to prevent electric shock.

**eczema** Similar to dermatitis, words are often used interchangeably. The general distinction is weeping of the skin and eczema is caused by internal factors.

**effleurage** Hand massage involving slow, stroking movements. Used at the beginning and end of every massage treatment.

**elasticity test** Test of hair conditioning by stretching it and allowing the hair to return to its unstretched length.

**emollients** *see* **conditioners**

**emulsions** Droplets of one liquid suspended in another. Emulsifying agents help this process.

**epidermis** The upper layer of the skin which has an outer horny layer of dead, flattened cells that are constantly flaking off to be replaced by cells that have been produced in the basal, the lowest layer of the epidermis.

**evaluation** A judgement (or series of judgements) about somebody or something based on specific criteria.

**exothermic perm** A perming technique which uses heat.

**feedback** Obtaining information about performance. How well something has gone.

**finger waving** Setting the hair using 'S' shaped movements formed with the fingers and a comb.

**first aid** Measures designed to help an injured person until help arrives.

**fish-hook ends** Hair points which are bent back on themselves. Creates a 'frizzed' look on the ends of the hair which can be removed by wetting when caused during setting but can only be removed by cutting if the hair has been permed in this position.

**flea (pulex irritans)** A blood sucking parasite on the body, in clothing, bedding etc. Moves by jumping.

**flying colours** *see* **painted lights**

**foam perm** A perming technique where the perm lotion is applied as a mousse.

**follicle** *see* **hair follicle**

**folliculitis** Swelling and reddening of the hair follicle often with pus formation.

**formative assessment** Judgements made about a process while it is happening.

**fragilitis crinum (split ends)** Where the points of the hair fray and split. No 'cure': they must be cut off.

**freehand** The cutting of hair without holding it in place not to be confused with texturising).

**fresh air** Air which is usually cool, dry and free from contamination.

**fungi (tinea)** Are plants made up of tiny threads called hyphae, some of which are parasites on humans, e.g. ringworm.

**furuncle** *see* **boil**

**gel** A thickened liquid (technically, a liquid with high viscosity).

**germinative layer** Growing layer of the skin epidermis.

**glimmering (polishing)** Adding colour to the hair using tin foil painted with tint in a polishing motion.

**graduation** A hair cutting term used to describe the effect created when the top layers of the hair lie above the underneath layers. A steeply graduated haircut is referred to as high layering, while very little graduation in a haircut is referred to as low layering.

**grievance procedure** A statement of the steps to be taken if someone has a grievance against something or somebody.

**hair bulb** Bulge on lower part of the hair root. The area from which hair grows.

**hair colour restorer** Metallic dye containing lead acetate and sodium thiosulphate.

**hair cortex** Inner bulk of hair made up of fibres.

**hair cuticle** The outer layer of the hair, made of overlapping scales.

**hair cuttings** Cuttings of hair taken from various parts of the head to enable certain tests to be carried out, e.g. incompatibility, porosity, elasticity, etc.

**hair extensions/hair pieces** Additional pieces of hair woven in the client's hair as part of the hairstyle design.

**hair fixing sprays** Developed from plastic polymers dissolved in alcohol which coat the hair with a plastic film.

**hair fly** When hair tends to lift away from the scalp due to static electricity.

**hair follicle** Tiny pit in the skin from which hair grows.

**hair growth cycle** Consists of three phases (stages): anagen – active growth; telogen – resting; catagen – hair replaced by new one.

**hair growth pattern** The growth direction of the hair due to the angle of the follicle in the scalp.

**hair medulla** Possible third, central area of hair.

**hair mesh** A section of hair gathered together in some way for a hairdressing operation.

**hair root** The part of the hair which is buried in the skin.

**hair root sheath** Lining of hair follicle which holds the hair in the skin.

**hair shaft** The part of the hair which is visible beyond the skin surface.

**hard pressing** A hair straightening technique where more heat is used, which consequently removes more of the hair curl.

**hazards** Potential or actual risks to people's health and safety. They may be biological, chemical, or physical.

**head louse** *see* **lice**

**hepatitis** A very dangerous disease which can be transmitted in the salon.

**herpes simplex** *see* **cold sores**

**highlighting** Technique of lightening fine strands of hair using bleach and/or tint.

**hirsutism** Literally means 'very hairy'. What happens in practice is that the areas which usually have the fine vellus hair grow darker, thicker secondary hair.

**hone** To sharpen, e.g. a razor, before shaving.

**horny layer** *see* **cornified layer**

**hydrogen peroxide** An effective oxidising agent which decomposes to produce water and oxygen. Used for oxidising permanent waves, para dyes and bleaches.

**hydrometer** Used for measuring the density of liquids. One type, a peroxometer can be used for direct measurement of the strength (concentration) of hydrogen peroxide solutions.

**hygiene** Practices likely to reduce the chances of infection or infestation.

**hygrometer** Device for measuring the amount of water vapour (humidity) in the air.

**hygroscopic** Ability of some materials (including hair) to absorb water vapour (moisture) from the air.

**hypertrichosis** The growing in specific place of thick pigmented hair in areas where usually only fine vellus hair grow.

**images** *Fantasy* – that which is extreme, imaginative and often theme-based. *Avant garde* – that which is a fore-runner of fashion. *Commercial* – that which is popular with the mass market.

**impetigo** Caused by staphylococci bacteria. Characteristics include blisters and weeping, formation of yellow crusts. Common as a secondary infection.

**incentive** Anything which is used to encourage or reward people for taking certain actions.

**incompatibility test** A test to determine whether the hair has been previously treated with an incompatible chemical (e.g. metallic dye); if positive, hairdressing treatments should be avoided.

**induction** The process where a person new to a salon is informed on the policies, procedures, work patterns, etc.

**infection** Invasion of the body by pathogens (germs).

**infectious** Of a disease spread by air or water.

**infestation** Animal parasites living on the body. Sometimes used to refer to premises, e.g. a house 'infested' with mice.

**inversion (concave)** Refers to a rounded inwards shape that is cut into the hair.

**invoice** A document which lists and gives the price of the various products contained in an order. It should be checked against the delivery note to ensure that the order is correct before paying for the goods.

**itchmite (sarcoptes scabiei)** Causes scabies (or the itch). Very small parasites which are almost invisible to the unaided eye. The females burrow into the skin and lay eggs which causes intense itching (usually at night). Scratching often leads to secondary infections, e.g. impetigo.

**job role/job description** A detailed description of a person's role and responsibilities in the salon.

**karaya gum** An Indian gum used in some setting agents. Requires a preservative to prevent it going mouldy.

**keratin** Hard, fibrous protein found in hair, skin and nails.

**keratinisation** Process by which skin, hair, and nail cells become filled with keratin.

**lanolin** A wax which is obtained from sheep's wool, and is often used in traditional conditioning agents, shampoos and hand creams.

**lanugo hair** The first hair produced by babies, often while in the womb.

**layering** A form of graduation. High layering has steep graduation. Low layering has very little graduation.

**legislation** Laws affecting the conduct of business, the premises or working environment, persons employed and systems of work.

**leuco-compounds** Breakdown products produced by decolorising (removing colour) from a developed para tint.

**liaison** Communicating with someone, working with them.

**lice** Parasitic insects (all have six legs, none can fly). Headlouse (pediculus capitis) produces an infestation called pediculosis. The adults are small and lay pearl-coloured eggs (nits) which are cemented to the hair shafts particularly in the nape and behind the ears. Other types of lice include the body louse (pediculus corporis) and pubic louse (phthirus pubis).

**lightening dyes** Para dyes which tint the hair lighter than the hair's natural colour.

**limits of own authority** Individual's extent of responsibility as determined by own job description and organisational policy.

**line and balance** The relationship between the finished hairstyle and the shape of the client's face, facial features and body size.

**local by-laws** Special rules, issued normally by a local authority, affecting certain parts of the business and often relating to health and safety.

**looks** *Classic* – that which is recognised by clients and the profession as having timeless appeal. *Fashion* – that which is recognised by clients and the profession as being currently in vogue. *Avant garde* – that which is a fore-runner of fashion.

**lowlights** Adding small strands of colour to the hair either throughout the head or where necessary to emphasise and enhance the finished hairstyle.

**male pattern baldness** An inherited condition that affects approximately 40% of males by the age of 40.

**management** All the processes and methods used to ensure a salon operates effectively, efficiently and economically.

**massage** The general name for rubbing and kneading actions. It generally increases blood flow to the massaged area.

**medulla** A third central layer sometimes present in hair.

**melanin** Black/brown natural pigment in the hair and skin.

**melanocytes** Cells which produce and lay down natural pigments in the hair and skin.

**mesh (or section)** *see* **hair mesh**

**monilethrix** A rare condition where there are bead-like swellings along the hair shaft.

**mousses** Foams produced by a propellent gas blowing through a liquid.

**nape whorls** Patterns of hair growth.

**nascent oxygen** Single atoms of oxygen (unlike oxygen gas which has two atoms, $O_2$). Highly reactive and responsible for developing tints, bleaches and oxidising ('neutralising') perms.

**National Vocational Qualifications** A national system of vocational qualifications.

**neutralisation** The oxidation stage of perming/straightening where the hair is fixed in the new style.

**nits** Eggs of the parasitic louse (*see* **lice**).

**non-verbal communication** The very powerful transfer of information by body movements, eye contact, facial expression and tone of voice.

**normalisation** A term sometimes used in perming to mean 'neutraliser'.

**NVQ** *see* **National Vocational Qualifications**

**oil bleach** A bleach contained in an oil emulsion.

**operational requirements** A statement of what is needed and/or what needs to be done for a particular salon operation.

**oral communication** Spoken words, often less important than **non-verbal communication**.

**organisational requirements** Procedures and arrangements issued by a given salon management, affecting the conduct of its business.

**overbooking** Booking too many appointments into the salon; often salon services and staff will be unable to cope.

**oxidation** The addition of oxygen or the removal of hydrogen from a substance. Chemicals that can do this are called oxidising agents or oxidisers.

**painted lights (flying colours)** The technique of tinting fine strands of hair using a 'vent' brush, wide-toothed comb or fine artist's brush to emphasise the shape of a hairstyle.

**para dye (aniline dye)** Permanent, semi-permanent, synthetic, organic dye. Must be mixed with hydrogen peroxide to be effective.

**parasite** A living thing that lives on or in another living thing (called the parasite's host).

**patch test** *see* **skin test**

**pathogenic** Disease causing. Pathogenic micro-organisms (pathogens) are germs.

**pediculus capitis** Infestation of the scalp by head lice (*see* **lice**).

**percentage strength (%)** A way of expressing strength (concentration) of hydrogen peroxide solutions (see volume strength). Based on parts per hundred (%) of 'pure' peroxide in a solution.

**performance criteria** The specific method and standard to which something is to be done.

**perimeter lines** Important in cutting in the outside profile or shape of the haircut.

**peroxometer** *see* **hydrometer**

**petrissage** Massage movements involving kneading actions.

**pH balance** A product designed to leave the hair/skin slightly acid.

**pH scale** A scale of acidity or alkalinity. Has 14 points; 7 is neutral (neither acid nor alkaline), below 7 is acid and above 7 is alkaline.

**pheomelanin** Red/yellow natural pigment in the hair and skin.

**pin curls** Type of setting where the hair is wound flat. Types are: clockspring, barrel spring, stem and sculptured curls.

**pityriasis (pityriasis simplex)** The technical name for dandruff (scurf) due to the flaking of the scalp skin.

**plaiting** Various techniques where the hair is weaved together.

**pointing** *see* **chipping in**

**policy** A statement (written or oral) issued by a given salon management, setting out its considered approach to the conduct of its business. It may be required by legislation, e.g. a Health and Safety policy.

**polypeptide chains** The smallest chains in the hair cortex made up of amino acids.

**polyvinyl accetate/polyvinyl pyrollidone (PVA/PVP)** Adhesives used in hair-holding products, such as a setting lotion.

**porosity test** A test to assess the state of the hair cuticle. The more open or damaged it is the more porous is the hair.

**portfolio** A set of evidence of competence in a particular area. Can be used as a basis for assessment.

**post-damping** Applying perm reagent to the curlers after they have been wound.

**postiche** Collective name for wigs and hair pieces.

**posture** The way in which someone stands.

**powder bleach** Where the liquid bleach is made into a paste with a powder.

**predisposition test** *see* **skin test**

**pre-perm test** A test cutting perm carried out before perming the whole head.

**prepigmentation** Tinting bleached hair to its original colour.

**pre-saturation** Applying perm reagent to the hair mesh as it is wound.

**pressing combs** Used for straightening hair.

**primary colours** The three colours, yellow, red and blue, from which all others can be made.

**primary irritant** *see* **dermatitis**

**professional image of the salon** That which the salon wishes to portray to achieve a targeted position within the commercial market.

**promotion** A variety of techniques designed to market the salon and its services.

**psoriasis** A non-infectious skin condition. Often seen as silvery scales with red skin underneath; the silvery scales flake off when rubbed.

**pulex irritans** Human flea. It has long back legs which allow it to jump from one person to another.

**pull-burn** A burn on the skin caused by winding the hair too tightly when perming.

**reduction** The opposite of oxidation. It involves removal of oxygen from or addition of hydrogen to a substance. Chemicals that do this are reducing agents.

**reduction dye** A metallic dye which uses pyrogallol as a reducing agent.

**regrowth** The hair nearest the scalp which has grown since the last hairdressing treatment, therefore has natural colour and wave.

**rehabilitating rinse** *see* **conditioners**

**relaxer cream** Reagent for straightening hair.

**relaxing hair** *see* **straightening**

**repetitive strain injury** Painful reaction to using the same muscles and joints with a high frequency over a long period.

**resources** Whatever is needed to carry out an activity: products, tools, equipment, people, time, electricity, etc.

**restructurant** Type of conditioner which is substantive, 'adds to' the hair shaft. Makes hair less porous.

**re-style** A change of look which is significantly different from that which existed before cutting commenced.

**retouch** Applying a chemical treatment to a regrowth.

**reverse graduation** A haircutting term used to describe the effect created when the top layers of the hair lie below the underneath layers.

**ringworm (tinea)** Caused by a parasitic fungus. When present on the scalp it produces reddened, round patches with a stubble of hair. Tinea capitis – fungal infection of the scalp.

**risk assessment** The process of looking at the hazards and chances of accidents in the salon.

**roller setting** A wide variety of setting techniques using rollers (rods).

**root** *see* **hair root**

**root sheath** *see* **hair root sheath**

**rota** A list of the duties of salon staff at different times.

**salon requirements** Procedures and arrangements issued by a given salon management, which must include the minimum health, safety and hygiene requirements of the service being provided.

**saponification** Technical name for soap making process.

**sarcoptes scabiei** *see* **itchmite**

**scabies** An infection of the skin caused by the itchmite. Causes intense itching.

**schedule** *see* **rota**

**scrunching** When used in relation to fashion colouring it is a method of lightening the ends of the hair using either tint, bleach or a combination of both.

**scurf** *see* **pityriasis**

**sebaceous cyst (wen)** A raised lump on the skin caused by a blockage of the sebaceous gland.

**sebaceous gland** Produces natural oil sebum which coats the hair and the skin. A blocked gland can lead to a build up of sebum in a wen (sebaceous cyst).

**seborrhoea** Is an overproduction of sebum. Causes oily hair and skin, it can be triggered by hormone changes at puberty. It may also cause swelling, itching and reddening on the scalp, called seborrhoeic dermatitis.

**sebum** Natural oil made by sebaceous gland in hair follicles. It waterproofs and conditions the hair and skin.

**secondary hair** Sometimes called terminal hair. It is the thick, usually darker hair on the scalp and body.

**secondary infection** It occurs where an earlier infection produces conditions which encourage a second type of pathogen to invade the body, e.g. impetigo is a common secondary infection of scabies caused when the skin is broken through scratching.

**self-development** The process of increasing knowledge, understanding and skill level.

**selenium sulphide** A substance used in shampoo to combat dandruff. It reduces the activities of the germinative layer of the skin thus reducing flaking

**sensitisation** *see* **dermatitis**

**sensitivity test** *see* **skin test**

**setting** Various methods both wet and dry, used to give hair a temporary style. Setting aids help to produce and prolong the set.

**shampoo** A solution for cleaning hair. Usually a soapless base containing a mixture of ingredients to remove dirt and oil from the hair.

**shimmer lights** A tinting technique that produces a similar effect to painted lights. The hair is combed into position with a gel, then the raised part of the ridges has tint applied to it with a fine brush.

**shingle** A graduated hair cut where the nape hair is cut extremely short, usually with the clippers or scissors over comb.

**simple bleach** A bleach made with hydrogen peroxide as a liquid.

**skin epidermis** The outer part of the skin, made up of layers. The bottom layer (germinative) grows and moves towards the surface, eventually producing the dead outer layer of the skin (cornified).

**skin test** A test taken to see if a person has an allergy to a substance. The material to be tested is placed on the skin and checked to see if a 'rash' develops. If such a reaction takes place the person is probably allergic to that substance.

**slicing (tramming)** A method of tinting whereby slices of colour are placed in the hair where required.

**slither cutting** *see* **tapering**

**sodium lauryl sulphate** Common base ingredient in cleaning products, such as shampoos.

**soft pressing** A relaxing technique where heat is used to produce some hair straightening.

**specified procedures** Those requirements which relate to the conducting of tests carried out on hair, skin and scalp and are in accordance with manufacturer's instructions.

**spot tinting/bleaching** Tinting or bleaching the hair where required to correct uneven colour faults.

**sterilisation** A process which kills all micro-organisms.

**stock control** Procedures designed to ensure that stock is available when needed and is rotated to ensure it is used before deterioration.

**straightening (relaxing) hair** Methods used to remove curl/wave from the hair.

**strand test** A test used to monitor the development of the hair colour during tinting.

**streptococci** Bacteria which cause infections, e.g. sore throat. Divide to form chains.

**strop** A leather strap used to sharpen open, cut-throat razors.

**styes (blepharitis)** Caused by bacteria invading the hair follicle of eye lashes (commonly of the lower eyelid) causing reddening and swelling.

**substantive** Something which joins with or enters the hair shaft (*see* **conditioners**).

**sulphide dye** An inorganic metallic dye.

**sulphur bonds** Cross linkages that hold the polypeptide chains, sometimes referred to as 'S' bonds', di-sulphide bonds, cystine linkages or sulphur bridges.

**summative assessment** The final stage in an assessment of performance. Based on the whole process and overall performance.

**supervisor** A person with a degree of responsibility. Generally concerned with carrying out policies rather than determining them.

**sycosis barbae** *see* **barber's itch**

**tail comb** A comb used for sectioning, lifting or weaving the hair. It has a fine end and a tail end. A variation of the tail comb is the pin-tail comb which has a thin, metal, stiletto tail end.

**tapering (slither cutting)** A method of cutting hair using a 'slithering' movement which removes bulk and length.

**technical services** The group name for the large range of services a salon may offer.

**telogen** The stage in the hair growth cycle where hair growth stops; a resting stage.

**terminal hair** *see* **secondary hair**

**test curl** A wind on a small sample of the client's hair to check if the intended process will work satisfactorily.

**test cutting** Taken before a hairdressing process to ensure the best choice, and to determine the effects of the products to be used on the hair.

**texture** The texture of the hair refers to its diameter. Fine hair is narrow in diameter while thick hair has a much larger diameter.

**texturising** Cutting into the hair to increase movement, volume and create a non-uniform effect.

**thinning** A haircutting method that removes weight and bulk from the hair.

**tinea** *see* **ringworm; fungi**

**tints** Dyes used to colour the hair. They can be lightening or covering, temporary, semi-permanent or permanent.

**toners** Tints used to 'mask' unwanted colour tones.

**tortoiseshell highlights** Woven strands of hair which are then tinted with three or four different colours throughout the head or where required.

**traction alopecia** *see* **alopecia**

**tragacanth gum** White powder obtained from the bark of a shrub grown in Turkey, which can be used in setting agents.

**training plan** A statement showing the steps to meeting a person or staff team's identified training needs.

**tramming** *see* **slicing**

**translucent** Allows light to pass through, and scatters (diffuses) it.

**trichorrhexis nodosa** Condition where hair splits and frays at swellings along the length.

**ultra-violet radiation** Part of electromagnetic spectrum not visible to the eye, which is used in UV sterilisers and triggers melanocytes in the skin, producing a sun-tan.

**uni perm** A perming technique using heated rollers.

**vegetable dye** A dye obtained from plants, e.g. camomile.

**vellus hair** The fine, often unpigmented (or slightly pigmented) downy hair, e.g. present on the female face.

**verrucae** *see* **warts**

**vibro machine** A mechanical form of massage. The machine has various attachments, the most common of which are the spiked applicator, the sponge applicator and the bell-shaped applicator. It is used in conjunction with hair/scalp treatments to stimulate blood flow, and promote healthy hair.

**virus** The smallest type of micro-organism; it cannot survive long outside the body. It causes colds, 'flu, 'cold sores' (herpes) and some types of wart.

**volume strength (vol. strength; 'vols')** A way of expressing strength (concentration) of hydrogen peroxide solutions. It means the number of volumes of oxygen gas given off by one volume of peroxide. For example, when completely broken down 1 cm$^3$ 20 vol. hydrogen peroxide would give off 20 cm$^3$ of oxygen gas.

**warts (verrucae)** Some warts are caused by a virus (papova virus) which makes the skin produce raised lumps. On the feet, the pressure of the body weight can cause the wart to grow inwards creating a verruca (plantar wart).

**wen** *see* **sebaceous cyst**

**wet setting** *see* **cohesive set**

**widow's peak** A natural wave in the fringe area caused by hair growth direction.

**winding** Term for insertion and rolling up of rollers, curlers, etc., in the hair.

**zinc pyrithione** Substance found in medicated or anti-dandruff shampoos.

# Index